PROVIDER MANUAL
SIXTH EDITION

ENPC®

EMERGENCY NURSING PEDIATRIC COURSE

An ENA® Course

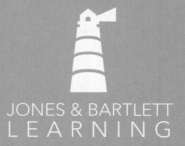

JONES & BARTLETT
LEARNING

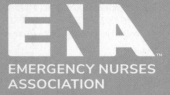

ENA
EMERGENCY NURSES
ASSOCIATION

World Headquarters
Jones & Bartlett Learning
25 Mall Road
Burlington, MA 01803
978-443-5000
info@jblearning.com
www.jblearning.com

ENA
EMERGENCY NURSES ASSOCIATION

Emergency Nurses Association
930 E. Woodfield Road
Schaumburg, IL 60173
847-460-4000
education@ena.org
www.ena.org

Jones & Bartlett Learning books and products are available through most bookstores and online booksellers. To contact Jones & Bartlett Learning directly, call 800-832-0034, fax 978-443-8000, or visit our website, www.jblearning.com.

Substantial discounts on bulk quantities of Jones & Bartlett Learning publications are available to corporations, professional associations, and other qualified organizations. For details and specific discount information, contact the special sales department at Jones & Bartlett Learning via the above contact information or send an email to specialsales@jblearning.com.

Production Credits
Vice President, Product Management: Marisa R. Urbano
Vice President, Content Strategy and Implementation: Christine Emerton
Director, Product Management: Matthew Kane
Product Manager: Tina Chen
Director, Content Management: Donna Gridley
Manager, Content Strategy: Carolyn Pershouse
Content Strategist: Christina Freitas
Content Coordinator: Samantha Gillespie
Director, Project Management and Content Services: Karen Scott
Manager, Project Management: Jackie Reynen
Project Manager: Kelly Mahoney
Senior Digital Project Specialist: Angela Dooley
Content Services Manager: Colleen Lamy
Vice President, Manufacturing and Inventory Control: Therese Connell
Product Fulfillment Manager: Wendy Kilborn
Composition: S4Carlisle Publishing Services
Cover and Text Design: Michael O'Donnell
Senior Media Development Editor: Troy Liston
Rights & Permissions Manager: John Rusk
Rights Specialist: Maria Leon Maimone
Cover Image (Title Page, Chapter Opener): © antishock/iStockphoto.
Printing and Binding: LSC Communications

Library of Congress Cataloging-in-Publication Data
Names: Emergency Nurses Association, issuing body.
Title: Emergency nursing pediatric course : provider manual / Emergency
    Nurses Association.
Description: Sixth edition. | Burlington, MA : Jones & Bartlett Learning,
    [2023] | Includes bibliographical references and index. | Summary: "ENPC
    is designed for the graduate, professional nurse looking to gain
    certification in the pediatric emergency course administered by ENA"--
    Provided by publisher.
Identifiers: LCCN 2022026672 | ISBN 9781284272628 (paperback)
Subjects: MESH: Pediatric Nursing | Emergency Nursing | Pediatric Emergency
    Medicine--methods | Outline
Classification: LCC RJ370 | NLM WY 18.2 | DDC
    618.92/0025--dc23/eng/20220727
LC record available at https://lccn.loc.gov/2022026672

6048

Printed in the United States of America
26 25 24 23 22   10 9 8 7 6 5 4 3 2 1

Contents

The Pedagogy

These features of the provider manual support your learning.

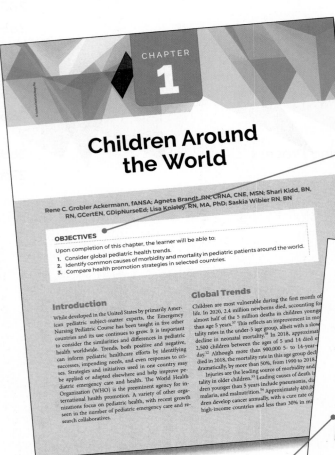

Objectives Each chapter begins with a list of the chapter learning objectives.

Figures Full-color illustrations, diagrams, and photographs aid your learning.

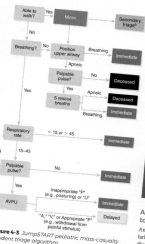

Clinical Pearls Each Clinical Pearl emphasizes an important point of clinical practice.

Notes The Note element provides brief but important bits of information that do not fit neatly into the flow of the text.

Boxes The Box element is another type of sidebar or aside for exploring additional points or concepts requiring longer, more expansive explanations.

Red Flags The Red Flag element flags anything that could become a serious threat to health.

Neonates are known to be viable at as early as 22 weeks' gestation, but survivability is based on the social and medical conditions in which the neonate was born and the access to and capability of the neonatal care in that region.[46]

Neonatal Resuscitation

A neonate may be born having experienced an interruption in the normal transition to extrauterine life. Interruptions in this transition can stem from birthing difficulties such as placental abruption, nuchal cord (when the umbilical cord is wrapped around the baby's neck), and congenital abnormalities.[37] In such a case, the neonate's organs will not receive an adequate amount of oxygen and the neonate may decompensate. Assessment findings of an abnormal, or interrupted, transition include the following:

- Absent, rapid, or irregular breathing
- Tachycardia or bradycardia
- Decrease in muscle tone
- Pale or blue skin of lips, head, or trunk (central cyanosis)
- Low oxygen saturation
- Low blood pressure

If any of these findings are present, neonatal resuscitation interventions are performed.[52(Ch3)]

> ### NOTE
> **Central Cyanosis Versus Acrocyanosis: Is Cyanosis Normal in a Neonate?**
>
> Acrocyanosis is a normal finding in a neonate. Acrocyanosis includes paleness or blueness of the hands, feet, and the skin around the lips. This finding can be present during the neonatal phase when the infant becomes cold, such as after a bath. Warming methods will resolve the cyanosis.
>
> Central cyanosis refers to paleness or blueness of the more central parts of the body, including the lips, the head, and the trunk. It is an abnormal finding in a neonate and indicates a lack of oxygen in the blood. Consider abnormalities of the heart, lungs, or blood. A neonate born presenting with central cyanosis requires resuscitation interventions.[12]

Preparing for Resuscitation

When anticipating a birth in the emergency department (ED), collect the necessary equipment for possible neonatal resuscitation. Ask the following pre-birth questions[52(Ch2)]:

- What is the expected gestational age?
- Is the amniotic fluid clear?
- Are there any additional risk factors?
- What is our umbilical cord management plan?

Steps in Neonatal Resuscitation

Once the neonate is born, an immediate assessment is performed. Three questions are addressed during this assessment:

- Does the baby appear to be term?
- Does the baby have good muscle tone?
- Is the baby breathing or crying?

If the neonate appears to be term, has good muscle tone, and is crying vigorously, the neonate is placed with the mother. If the neonate does not appear to be term, does not have good muscle tone, or is not breathing regularly, then immediate resuscitation is required.

The interventions for neonatal resuscitation are as follows:

- Warm, dry, and stimulate the neonate. Provide warmth by placing the neonate under a radiant warmer. Use a towel or blanket to dry the neonate. Stimulate the neonate while drying or rub the neonate's back, trunk, or extremities.
- Position the neonate's head and neck to open the airway. Use a suction bulb syringe to clear the mouth and then the nose.
- If the neonate is not breathing or is gasping, or if the neonate is breathing but the heart rate is less than 100 beats per minute, initiate positive-pressure ventilation (PPV) at 21% oxygen and 40 to 60 breaths per minute. After the first 15 seconds of PPV, assess the neonate's heart rate and chest rise.
- If the heart rate is not increasing or the chest is not rising with breaths, use the MRSOPA acronym for corrective interventions[52(Ch4)]:
  - Mask adjustment
  - Reposition head and neck
  - Suction the mouth and nose
  - Open the mouth
  - Pressure increase using PPV
  - Alternative airway
- If there is no improvement after the pressure increase, insert an endotracheal tube or place a laryngeal mask in the neonate and provide 30 seconds of PPV.[52(Ch5)]

---

when presenting to the ED. Communication regarding baseline behavior and the differences that prompted the current visit is essential to understanding why the caregivers are bringing the child in for evaluation. Caregivers are typically well versed in the patient's history and medical needs, making them expert historians. CSHCN can all be quite different at baseline, but the caregiver's information can ensure the exceptions are identified and included in the plan of care. Partnering with the caregivers in the plan of care will ensure collaboration and a cohesive relationship aimed at ensuring quality care for the child. This, in turn, establishes a trusting relationship that will aid future healthcare visits as well.

Glossary of Conditions with Nursing Considerations

The conditions discussed in this section are more commonly seen in children visiting the ED, but are not meant to be an exhaustive list of all possibilities. A knowledge base regarding those conditions seen more frequently gives the nurse more opportunity to provide safer and better-quality care.

> ### RED FLAG ⚠
> Fever is an emergent condition in many CSHCN. Immunocompromise can be caused by the disease itself or by medical management of the disease, such as chemotherapy for cancer, immunosuppressant drugs given post transplant, and immunologic therapies for autoimmune conditions and asthma.

Cancer

After traumatic injury, pediatric cancer is the second leading cause of death in children.[35] Occasionally, pediatric patients will receive a new cancer diagnosis in the ED (**Box 18-1**). More commonly, children with cancer will seek care for treatment-related complications or side effects. These visits are increasing as more effective cancer treatments and home therapies have evolved (Stephanos & Picard, 2018).[35]

Presentations During Treatment

The cancer itself may cause bleeding, anemia, and cardiorespiratory compromise. Chemotherapy, immunotherapy, radiation, and surgical resection are just a few cancer therapies with complications that may necessitate an ED visit.

> ### BOX 18-1 New Cancer Diagnosis
>
> Childhood cancer can be difficult to detect early. Parents may have multiple interactions with medical providers in which symptoms are overlooked or attributed to more common conditions. The following signs and symptoms are associated with a new diagnosis of cancer[35,36]:
>
> - Abdominal pain
> - Blood count abnormalities
> - Bruising
> - Fatigue
> - Headache
> - Limping
> - Long bone pain
> - Lump or swelling
> - Pallor
> - Persistent fever, nausea, or vomiting
> - Vision changes
> - Weight loss
>
> Sometimes, imaging or blood work will suggest or confirm a cancer diagnosis. At other times, follow-up with a pediatric oncologist is required for definitive diagnosis. Partner with the physician or advanced practice provider to have a private discussion with the parents. Work with the parents to determine the best age-appropriate manner (with consideration of how, who, and when) to inform the child. Delayed information sharing fosters anxiety and distrust; effective communication is key to creating a trusting relationship. Be prepared for the family and child to be overwhelmed. Provide supportive information, balancing uncertainty with hope.[17,35]
>
> Data from Stephanos, K., & Picard, L. (2018). Pediatric oncologic emergencies. Emergency Medicine Clinics of North America, 36(3), 527-535. https://doi.org/10.1016/j.emc.2018.04.007; Steuber, C. P. (2021). Overview of common presenting signs and symptoms of childhood cancer. UpToDate. Retrieved March 9, 2022, from https://www.uptodate.com/contents/overview-of-common-presenting-signs-and-symptoms-of-childhood-cancer; Dobrozsi, S., Trowbridge, A., Mack, J. W., & Rosenberg, A. R. (2019). Effective communication for newly diagnosed pediatric patient with cancer: Considerations for the patients, family members, providers, and multidisciplinary team. American Society of Clinical Oncology Educational Book, 39, 573-581. https://doi.org/10.1200/EDBK_238181

Chemotherapy and radiation target rapidly growing cancer cells, but also damage healthy cells such as those found in gastric mucosa and blood. Mouth sores, nausea,

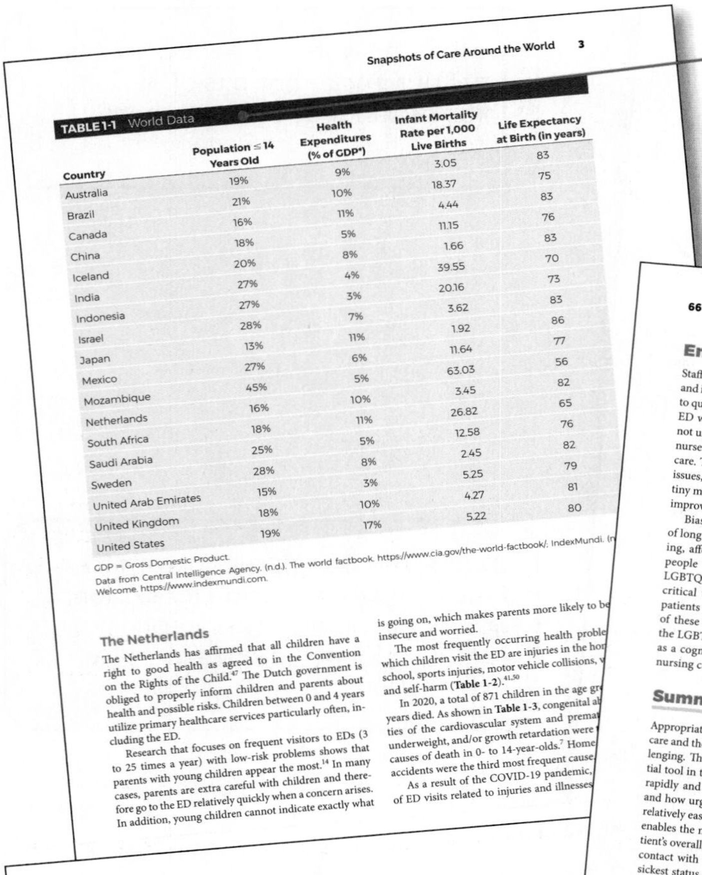
Snapshots of Care Around the World 3

TABLE 1-1 World Data

Country	Population ≤ 14 Years Old	Health Expenditures (% of GDP*)	Infant Mortality Rate per 1,000 Live Births	Life Expectancy at Birth (in years)
Australia	19%	9%	3.05	83
Brazil	21%	10%	18.37	75
Canada	16%	11%	4.44	83
China	18%	5%	11.15	76
Iceland	20%	8%	1.66	83
India	27%	4%	39.55	70
Indonesia	27%	3%	20.16	73
Israel	28%	7%	3.62	83
Japan	13%	11%	1.92	86
Mexico	27%	6%	11.64	77
Mozambique	45%	5%	63.03	56
Netherlands	16%	10%	3.45	82
South Africa	18%	11%	26.82	65
Saudi Arabia	25%	5%	12.58	76
Sweden	28%	8%	2.45	82
United Arab Emirates	15%	3%	5.25	79
United Kingdom	18%	10%	4.27	81
United States	19%	17%	5.22	80

GDP = Gross Domestic Product.
Data from Central Intelligence Agency. (n.d.). The world factbook. https://www.cia.gov/the-world-factbook/. IndexMundi. (n... Welcome. https://www.indexmundi.com.

The Netherlands

The Netherlands has affirmed that all children have a right to good health as agreed to in the Convention on the Rights of the Child.[47] The Dutch government is obliged to properly inform children and parents about health and possible risks. Children between 0 and 4 years utilize primary healthcare services particularly often, including the ED.

Research that focuses on frequent visitors to EDs (3 to 25 times a year) with low-risk problems shows that parents with young children appear the most.[14] In many cases, parents are extra careful with children and therefore go to the ED relatively quickly when a concern arises. In addition, young children cannot indicate exactly what is going on, which makes parents more likely to be... insecure and worried.

The most frequently occurring health proble... which children visit the ED are injuries in the hor... school, sports injuries, motor vehicle collisions, ... and self-harm (**Table 1-2**).[41,50]

In 2020, a total of 871 children in the age gr... years died. As shown in **Table 1-3**, congenital ab... ties of the cardiovascular system and prema... underweight, and/or growth retardation were ... causes of death in 0- to 14-year-olds.[7] Home... accidents were the third most frequent cause...

As a result of the COVID-19 pandemic, ... of ED visits related to injuries and illnesses...

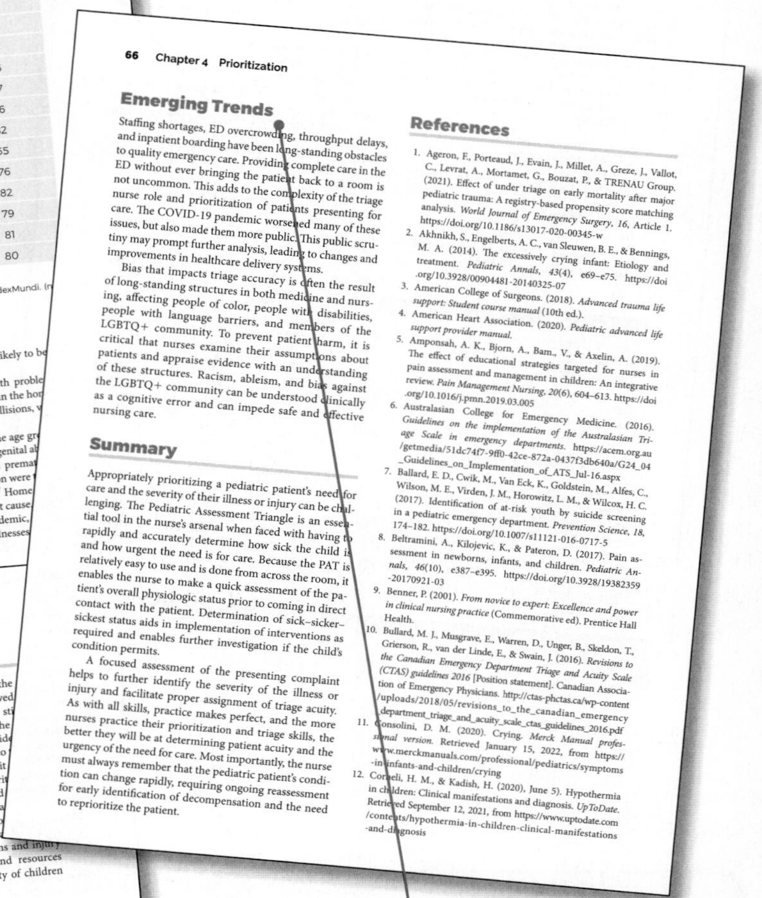
66 Chapter 4 Prioritization

Emerging Trends

Staffing shortages, ED overcrowding, throughput delays, and inpatient boarding have been long-standing obstacles to quality emergency care. Providing complete care in the ED without ever bringing the patient back to a room is not uncommon. This adds to the complexity of the triage nurse role and prioritization of patients presenting for care. The COVID-19 pandemic worsened many of these issues, but also made them more public. This public scrutiny may prompt further analysis, leading to changes and improvements in healthcare delivery systems.

Bias that impacts triage accuracy is often the result of long-standing structures in both medicine and nursing, affecting people of color, people with disabilities, people with language barriers, and members of the LGBTQ+ community. To prevent patient harm, it is critical that nurses examine their assumptions about patients and appraise evidence with an understanding of these structures. Racism, ableism, and bias against the LGBTQ+ community can be understood clinically as a cognitive error and can impede safe and effective nursing care.

Summary

Appropriately prioritizing a pediatric patient's need for care and the severity of their illness or injury can be challenging. The Pediatric Assessment Triangle is an essential tool in the nurse's arsenal when faced with having to rapidly and accurately determine how sick the child is and how urgent the need is for care. Because the PAT is relatively easy to use and is done from across the room, it enables the nurse to make a quick assessment of the patient's overall physiologic status prior to coming in direct contact with the patient. Determination of sick–sicker–sickest status aids in implementation of interventions as required and enables further investigation if the child's condition permits.

A focused assessment of the presenting complaint helps to further identify the severity of the illness or injury and facilitate proper assignment of triage acuity. As with all skills, practice makes perfect, and the more nurses practice their prioritization and triage skills, the better they will be at determining patient acuity and the urgency of the need for care. Most importantly, the nurse must always remember that the pediatric patient's condition can change rapidly, requiring ongoing reassessment for early identification of decompensation and the need to reprioritize the patient.

References

1. Ageron, F., Porteaud, J., Evain, J., Millet, A., Greze, J., Vallot, C., Levrat, A., Mortamet, G., Bouzat, P., & TRENAU Group. (2021). Effect of under triage on early mortality after major pediatric trauma: A registry-based propensity score matching analysis. *World Journal of Emergency Surgery, 16*, Article 1. https://doi.org/10.1186/s13017-020-00345-w
2. Akhnikh, S., Engelberts, A. C., van Sleuwen, B. E., & Bennings, M. A. (2014). The excessively crying infant: Etiology and treatment. *Pediatric Annals, 43*(4), e69–e75. https://doi.org/10.3928/00904481-20140325-07
3. American College of Surgeons. (2018). *Advanced trauma life support: Student course manual* (10th ed.).
4. American Heart Association. (2020). *Pediatric advanced life support provider manual.*
5. Amponsah, A. K., Bjorn, A., Bam., V., & Axelin, A. (2019). The effect of educational strategies targeted for nurses in pain assessment and management in children: An integrative review. *Pain Management Nursing, 20*(6), 604–613. https://doi.org/10.1016/j.pmn.2019.03.005
6. Australasian College for Emergency Medicine. (2016). *Guidelines on the implementation of the Australasian Triage Scale in emergency departments.* https://acem.org.au/getmedia/51dc74f7-9ff0-42ce-872a-0437f3db640a/G24_04_Guidelines_on_Implementation_of_ATS_Jul-16.aspx
7. Ballard, E. D., Cwik, M., Van Eck, K., Goldstein, M., Alfes, C., Wilson, M. E., Virden, J. M., Horowitz, L. M., & Wilcox, H. C. (2017). Identification of at-risk youth by suicide screening in a pediatric emergency department. *Prevention Science, 18*, 174–182. https://doi.org/10.1007/s11121-016-0717-5
8. Beltramini, A., Kilojevic, K., & Pateron, D. (2017). Pain assessment in newborns, infants, and children. *Pediatric Annals, 46*(10), e387–e395. https://doi.org/10.3928/19382359-20170921-03
9. Benner, P. (2001). *From novice to expert: Excellence and power in clinical nursing practice* (Commemorative ed). Prentice Hall Health.
10. Bullard, M. J., Musgrave, E., Warren, D., Unger, B., Skeldon, T., Grierson, R., van der Linde, E., & Swain, J. (2016). *Revisions to the Canadian Emergency Department Triage and Acuity Scale (CTAS) guidelines 2016* [Position statement]. Canadian Association of Emergency Physicians. http://ctas-phctas.ca/wp-content/uploads/2018/05/revisions_to_the_canadian_emergency_department_triage_and_acuity_scale_ctas_guidelines_2016.pdf
11. Consolini, D. M. (2020). Crying. *Merck Manual professional version.* Retrieved January 15, 2022, from https://www.merckmanuals.com/professional/pediatrics/symptoms-in-infants-and-children/crying
12. Corneli, H. M., & Kadish, H. (2020, June 5). Hypothermia in children: Clinical manifestations and diagnosis. *UpToDate.* Retrieved September 12, 2021, from https://www.uptodate.com/contents/hypothermia-in-children-clinical-manifestations-and-diagnosis

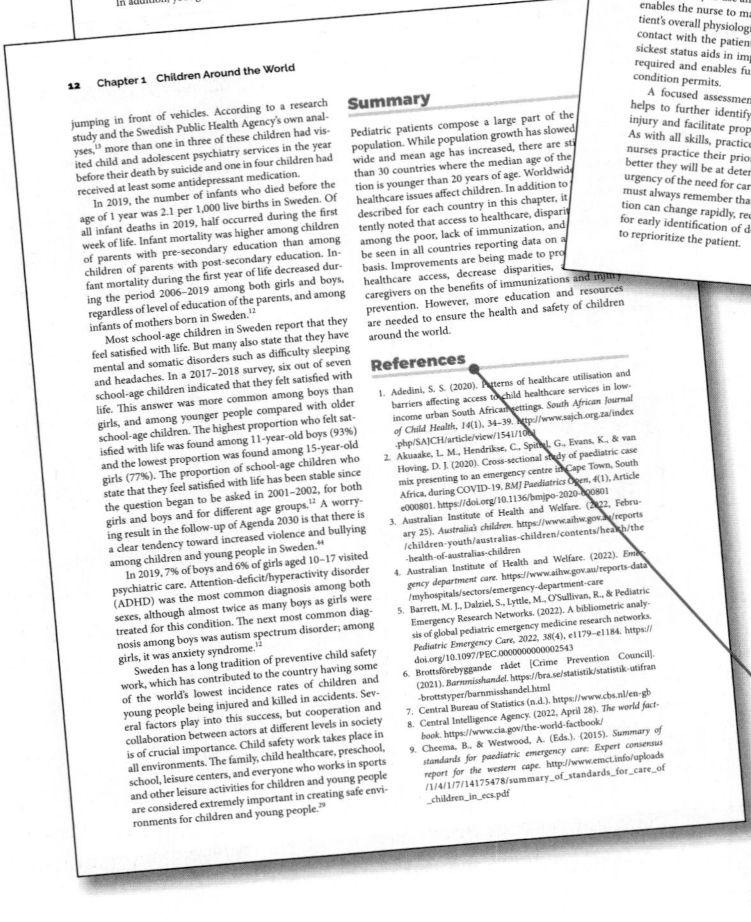
12 Chapter 1 Children Around the World

jumping in front of vehicles. According to a research study and the Swedish Public Health Agency's own analyses,[13] more than one in three of these children had visited child and adolescent psychiatry services in the year before their death by suicide and one in four children had received at least some antidepressant medication.

In 2019, the number of infants who died before the age of 1 year was 2.1 per 1,000 live births in Sweden. Of all infant deaths in 2019, half occurred during the first week of life. Infant mortality was higher among children of parents with pre-secondary education than among children of parents with post-secondary education. Infant mortality during the first year of life decreased during the period 2006–2019 among both girls and boys, regardless of level of education of the parents, and among infants of mothers born in Sweden.[12]

Most school-age children in Sweden report that they feel satisfied with life. But many also state that they have mental and somatic disorders such as difficulty sleeping and headaches. In a 2017–2018 survey, six out of seven school-age children indicated that they felt satisfied with life. This answer was more common among boys than girls, and among younger people compared with older school-age children. The highest proportion who felt satisfied with life was found among 11-year-old boys (93%) and the lowest proportion was found among 15-year-old girls (77%). The proportion of school-age children who state that they feel satisfied with life has been stable since the question began to be asked in 2001–2002, for both girls and boys and for different age groups.[12] A worrying result in the follow-up of Agenda 2030 is that there is a clear tendency toward increased violence and bullying among children and young people in Sweden.[44]

In 2019, 7% of boys and 6% of girls aged 10–17 visited psychiatric care. Attention-deficit/hyperactivity disorder (ADHD) was the most common diagnosis among both sexes, although almost twice as many boys as girls were treated for this condition. The next most common diagnosis among boys was autism spectrum disorder; among girls, it was anxiety syndrome.[12]

Sweden has a long tradition of preventive child safety work, which has contributed to the country having some of the world's lowest incidence rates of children and young people being injured and killed in accidents. Several factors play into this success, but cooperation and collaboration between actors at different levels in society is of crucial importance. Child safety work takes place in all environments. The family, child healthcare, preschool, school, leisure centers, and everyone who works in sports and other leisure activities for children and young people are considered extremely important in creating safe environments for children and young people.[29]

Summary

Pediatric patients compose a large part of the ... population. While population growth has slowed ... wide and mean age has increased, there are sti... than 30 countries where the median age of the ... tion is younger than 20 years of age. Worldwide ... healthcare issues affect children. In addition to ... described for each country in this chapter, it ... tently noted that access to healthcare, disparit... among the poor, lack of immunization, and ... be seen in all countries reporting data on a... basis. Improvements are being made to pro... healthcare access, decrease disparities, ... caregivers on the benefits of immunizations and injury prevention. However, more education and resources are needed to ensure the health and safety of children around the world.

References

1. Adedini, S. S. (2020). Patterns of healthcare utilisation and barriers affecting access to child healthcare services in low-income urban South African settings. *South African Journal of Child Health, 14*(1), 34–39. http://www.sajch.org.za/index.php/SAJCH/article/view/1541/1061
2. Akuaake, L. M., Hendrikse, C., Spittal, G., Evans, K., & van Hoving, D. J. (2020). Cross-sectional study of paediatric case mix presenting to an emergency centre in Cape Town, South Africa, during COVID-19. *BMJ Paediatrics Open, 4*(1), Article e000801. https://doi.org/10.1136/bmjpo-2020-000801
3. Australian Institute of Health and Welfare. (2022, February 25). *Australia's children.* https://www.aihw.gov.au/reports/children-youth/australias-children/contents/health/the-health-of-australias-children
4. Australian Institute of Health and Welfare. (2022). *Emergency department care.* https://www.aihw.gov.au/reports-data/myhospitals/sectors/emergency-department-care
5. Barrett, M. J., Dalziel, S., Lyttle, M., O'Sullivan, R., & Pediatric Emergency Research Networks. (2022). A bibliometric analysis of global pediatric emergency medicine research networks. *Pediatric Emergency Care, 2022, 38*(4), e1179–e1184. https://doi.org/10.1097/PEC.0000000000002543
6. Brottsförebyggande rådet [Crime Prevention Council]. (2021). *Barnmisshandel.* https://bra.se/statistik/statistik-utifran-brottstyper/barnmisshandel.html
7. Central Bureau of Statistics (n.d.). https://www.cbs.nl/en-gb
8. Central Intelligence Agency. (2022, April 28). *The world factbook.* https://www.cia.gov/the-world-factbook/
9. Cheema, B., & Westwood, A. (Eds.). (2015). *Summary of standards for paediatric emergency care: Expert consensus report for the western cape.* http://www.emct.info/uploads/1/4/1/7/14175478/summary_of_standards_for_care_of_children_in_ecs.pdf

Tables Tables summarize multidimensional information in clear, succinct fashion.

Emerging Trends The Emerging Trends section features new evidence or procedures that may eventually make their way into everyday practice.

References The information in the chapters is evidence-based and extensively documented through citations and the corresponding references.

Preface

Student, you do not study to pass the test. You study to prepare for the day when you are the only thing between a patient and the grave.

—Mark B. Reid, MD, @medicalaxioms

Medical centers with comprehensive pediatric specialty resources and pediatric emergency departments are not immediately accessible to many children in need of emergency care. Most children are seen in emergency departments that do not specialize in pediatric care. The Emergency Nursing Pediatric Course (ENPC) was introduced in 1993 to address the educational needs of nurses faced with pediatric emergencies in a variety of healthcare settings. It was developed and continues to evolve thanks to the work of Emergency Nurses Association (ENA) volunteers committed to improving pediatric emergency care.

ENPC frames pediatric emergency care within the context of family, healthcare team, and regional resources. A systematic assessment process founded on pediatric anatomy, growth and development, and pathophysiology is used to guide care and promote optimal outcomes. Children and their families come to the emergency department for an event, situation, or symptom of concern. Patient presentation, however, is not always easily correlated to the underlying pathophysiology. The systematic assessment process is useful for all children but is particularly vital to identify signs of pediatric compensation for illness or injury and conditions that can be reversed with early intervention.

This provider manual is not meant to be a comprehensive tome detailing every pediatric condition that might possibly be seen in the emergency department. Rather, it is the basis for a course designed to help nurses systematically assess a child and recognize abnormal findings requiring immediate intervention or further investigation. Emphasis is placed on early identification of pediatric patients experiencing life- or limb-threatening illness or injury and providing appropriate interventions. Some children will present with needs that exceed the department's or facility's capabilities. Early recognition of these patients, timely consultation with experts, and transfer to definitive care will improve pediatric outcomes.

A multitude of clinical resources with continuously updated medication information (indications, dosing guidelines, and precautions), assessment tools and calculators, diagnostic criteria, medical management, and standards of care are available to the emergency department nurse. Use of peer-reviewed, reputable, and reliable electronic resources is highly encouraged. In all cases, patient care should be delivered in accordance with facility policy, regional statutes, and device manufacturer recommendations.

What's New and Different?

The sixth edition of ENPC has been reorganized according to patient presentation. Previous editions have included much more comprehensive information about a variety of infrequently seen pediatric conditions. That content, while valuable, detracts from the core knowledge necessary to provide safe pediatric care. The critical functions of nursing are the focus of this course. Nurses recognize abnormal findings, anticipate potential interventions, and assess for the effectiveness of interventions within the nursing scope of practice and according to the best-available evidence. A team approach includes communication with healthcare providers, regional resources, the patient, and the family to maximize the nurse's ability to advocate for the patient.

The intention behind the ENPC course is to prevent the need for pediatric resuscitation by teaching early recognition of and intervention for critical illness or injury. Sometimes, however, the child may present too late for interventions to be effective in preventing decompensation and/or cardiac arrest. The 2020 American Heart Association guidelines are incorporated into Chapter 7, "The Child in Need of Stabilization."

ENA recognizes that health outcomes for children are directly impacted by systemic racism, bias, and stigmatizing language. In turn, ENA is committed to promoting diversity, equity, and inclusivity with a focus on achieving health equity. Throughout the ENPC course, efforts have been made to change language and content to better represent and respect all patients. For example, describing skin as "pink, warm, and dry" does not encourage nurses to consider what pallor looks like in patients with darker skin tones. There are subtle but important differences in introductions starting with "What do you like to be called?" as opposed to "What are your chosen or preferred pronouns?" The word "chosen" or "preferred" is much less accepting of the individual we are accompanying in care, while "What do you like to be called?" promotes openness and the opportunity to engage in respectful communication. ENA welcomes feedback on how we can continue to improve the content we teach and the language we use in ENA educational materials.

Acknowledgments

ENPC, Sixth Edition Work Team

Shellie Bumgarner, MSN, RN, CEN, CPEN, TCRN
Clinical Educator
Spectrum Education & Consulting, LLC
Hickory, North Carolina

Margot Daugherty, MSN, MEd, RN, CEN
Education Specialist II, Trauma Service
Cincinnati Children's Hospital
Maineville, Ohio

Margaret M. Dymond, BSN, RN, ENC(C), DCS
Clinical Nurse Educator
University of Alberta Hospital
Alberta, Canada

Krista Easley, MSN, RN, TCRN
BSW-McLane Children's Medical Center
Killeen, Texas

Tracey Gates, RN, CEN, CPEN
TNCC & ENPC Coordinator
Mission Hospitals
Asheville, North Carolina

Diana Giordano, DNP, RN, FNP-BC
Critical Care Educator
Franciscan St. Margaret Health
Hammond, Indiana

Robin Goodman, MSN, RN, CPEN
Emergency Medical Services for Children
    Innovation and Improvement Center
The Lundquist Institute
Torrance, California

Lisa Jamerson, DNP, RN, NRP
Assistant Professor of Nursing
University of Lynchburg
Evington, Virginia

Tina Johnson, MSN, RN, SCRN, CPEN, CFRN, CEN, CMTE
PI/Stroke Coordinator
Northeast Georgia Health System
Hoschton, Georgia

Josephina (Josie) Kik, BSN, RN, CPEN
Emergency Services Educator
Spectrum Health/Helen Devos Children's
    Hospital
Grand Rapids, Michigan

Patricia (Dusty) Lynn, RN, MSc, TCRN, EMT-P
RN Administrative Coordinator
University of Virginia
Earlysville, Virginia

Kimberly MacKeil-White, MSN, BN, RN, CPEN, BC-NPD
Nursing Education Specialist
Vanderbilt Children's Hospital
Franklin, Tennessee

Roberta Miller, DNP, RN, CPN, CPEN, TCRN
Education Coordinator
Cook Children's Medical Center
Fort Worth, Texas

Shannon Miller, MSN, TNS, SANE-P, CPNP, DNP
Pediatric Nurse Practitioner
St. Louis Children's Hospital
Saint Louis, Missouri

Robin S. Powers-Jarvis, PhD, RNC, CEN, CCRN, TCRN, CPEN
St. Mary's Medical Center
West Palm Beach, Florida

Lisa Smotrich, BSN, RN, CPEN, NPD-BC, CCRN-K
RN Education Specialist
Johns Hopkins All Children's Hospital
St. Petersburg, Florida

Geraldine Siebenga St. Jean, RN, BScN, ENC(C)
Clinical Nurse Educator
University of Alberta Hospital
Alberta, Canada

Jane Stuart-Minaret, RN, BScN, MN, RN
Staff Nurse
Sick Kids Toronto
Ontario, Canada

Anne-Marie Sweeney, DNP, RN(EC), CNCC(C), CNN(C)
Nurse Practitioner
Cambridge Memorial Hospital
Ontario, Canada

Jennifer (Gigi) K. Taylor, MSN, RN, EMT, CEN, TCRN
Coordinator, Trauma Services
University of Tennessee Medical Center
Knoxville, Tennessee

Kelly Williams, MSN, RN, CEN, CPN, CPEN, NPD-BC, CNE
Children's National Hospital
Annapolis, Maryland

Mindy B. Yorke, MSN, APRN, CEN, CPEN, FNP-BC
Staff Nurse
Wuesthoff Memorial Hospital
Melbourne, Florida

Reviewers

René Ackermann, RN, fANSA
Group Trauma, Emergency and Transplant Manager
Lenmed Hospital Group
Alberton, South Africa

Amy Boren, MS, BSN, RN, CEN, CPEN, TCRN
RN Professional Development
UC Health
Greeley, Colorado

Agneta Brandt, RN, CRNA, CNE, MSN
President
Swedish Association of Nurses in Trauma
Åkersberga, Sweden

Cam Brandt, MSN, RN, CEN, CPEN
Educator, Emergency Services
Cook Children's Medical Center
Keller, Texas

Elizabeth (Dixie) Bryant, MSN, RN, CEN
ED Nursing Manager
University of Kentucky
Berea, Kentucky

Joop Breuer, FNA, FAEN
Staff Nurse
Leiden University Medical Center
Rijnsburg, The Netherlands

Janet Jenista, MSN, RN, Grad Cert Tertiary Education
Faculty Manager
Edvoke Education
Kingston Foreshore, ACT, Australia

Sharolyn Kidd, BN, RN, GCertEN, GDipNurseEd
Nurse Educator, Statewide Trauma
Western Australia Trauma Training and Education Unit
Government of Western Australia, Department of Health
Clinical Nurse, Emergency Department
Sir Charles Gairdner Hospital
Perth, Western Australia

Lisa Knisley, RN, MA
Executive Director, Translating Emergency Knowledge for Kids (TREKK)
The Children's Hospital Research Institute of Manitoba
Manitoba, Canada

Justin Milici, MSN, RN, CEN, FAEN
Clinical Editor
Elsevier Clinical Solutions
Dallas, Texas

Julie Miller, BSN, RN, CEN
Nurse Manager
Stormont Vail Health
Manhattan, Kansas

Dawn Peta, BSN, RN, ENC(C)
Clinical Instructor
Alberta Health Services
Alberta, Canada

Claudia Phillips, MSN-ED, RN, CEN, CPEN
Registered Nurse
Sandoval Regional Medical Center
Rio Rancho, New Mexico

Kristine Powell, MSN, RN, CEN, FAEN
NTX Division Director, Emergency Services
Baylor Scott & White Health–North Texas
Grandview, Texas

Judy Stevenson, DNP, RN, CEN
Emergency APRN
St. John Medical Center
Tulsa, Oklahoma

Julie Tseh-Willcockson, RN
Registered Nurse
Colorado Springs, Colorado

Anna Valdez, PhD, MSN, RN, CEN, CFRN,
CNE, FAEN
Department Chair
Sonoma State University
Windsor, California

Rebecca VanStanton, MSN, RN, CEN,
CPEN, TCRN
Pediatric Trauma Clinical Reviewer
Baylor Scott & White Medical Center
West Bloomfield, Michigan

Steve Weinman, MSc, RN, CEN, TCRN,
NHDP-BC, EMT, TR-C
Division of Trauma, Acute Care Surgery &
Surgical Critical Care
St. Joseph's University Medical Center
Paterson, New Jersey

Saskia Wibier, RN, BN
Nurse ED Medicine
Slingeland Hospital Doetinchem
Aerdt, The Netherlands

ENA Staff

Katrina Ceci, MSN, RN, TCRN, CPEN,
NPD-BC, CEN
Director of Educational Content

Sharon Graunke, APRN, MSN-CNS, CEN
Exam Development Specialist

Yolanda Mackey, BA, PMP
Education Project Manager

Chris Zahn, PhD
Developmental Editor

Children Around the World

Rene C. Grobler Ackermann, fANSA; Agneta Brandt, RN, CRNA, CNE, MSN; Shari Kidd, BN, RN, GCertEN, GDipNurseEd; Lisa Knisley, RN, MA, PhD; Saskia Wibier, RN, BN

OBJECTIVES

Upon completion of this chapter, the learner will be able to:

1. Consider global pediatric health trends.
2. Identify common causes of morbidity and mortality in pediatric patients around the world.
3. Compare health promotion strategies in selected countries.

Introduction

While developed in the United States by primarily American pediatric subject-matter experts, the Emergency Nursing Pediatric Course has been taught in five other countries and its use continues to grow. It is important to consider the similarities and differences in pediatric health worldwide. Trends, both positive and negative, can inform pediatric healthcare efforts by identifying successes, impending needs, and even responses to crises. Strategies and initiatives used in one country may be applied or adapted elsewhere and help improve pediatric emergency care and health. The World Health Organization (WHO) is the preeminent agency for international health promotion. A variety of other organizations focus on pediatric health, with recent growth seen in the number of pediatric emergency care and research collaboratives.

Global Trends

Children are most vulnerable during the first month of life. In 2020, 2.4 million newborns died, accounting for almost half of the 5 million deaths in children younger than age 5 years.[57] This reflects an improvement in mortality rates in the under-5 age group, albeit with a slower decline in neonatal mortality.[58] In 2018, approximately 2,500 children between the ages of 5 and 14 died each day.[12] Although more than 900,000 5- to 14-year-olds died in 2018, the mortality rate in this age group declined dramatically, by more than 50%, from 1990 to 2018.[53]

Injuries are the leading source of morbidity and mortality in older children.[53] Leading causes of death in children younger than 5 years include pneumonia, diarrhea, malaria, and malnutrition.[54] Approximately 400,000 children develop cancer annually, with a cure rate of 80% in high-income countries and less than 30% in middle- to low-income countries.[56] The significantly lower cure rates are attributed to obstacles to accessing care, including delayed diagnosis and medications that are readily available in higher-income countries.[56] Emerging pediatric health threats include air pollution, obesity, marketing of addictive or unhealthy goods, and violence.[58]

Great strides have been made in reducing global pediatric morbidity and mortality through implementation of preventive health measures such as increased access to immunizations, safe food and water, and healthcare, but there remains much room for improvement.[54]

International Pediatric Research

The year 1994 marked the first publication by a pediatric emergency medicine (PEM) research network, the PEM Collaborative Research Committee of the American Academy of Pediatrics.[5] In the intervening years, 493 articles have been published by nine PEM research networks.[5] The Pediatric Emergency Research Network (PERN) includes representatives from PEM research networks in Europe, the Middle East, the Americas, and Australasia (**Box 1-1**).[31]

Comparison Data

The global population has tripled since 1950,[60] with continued, but slower, growth expected through the 21st century.[48] In 2019, the estimated global population was 7.7 billion people; the world population is expected to total 8.5 billion people in 2030, 9.7 billion people in 2050, and 10.9 billion people in 2100.[48] Monitoring trends in pediatric population distribution enables pediatric health champions to anticipate and fill gaps in health services. Are there areas with an increasing pediatric population but limited access to primary care? Is increased funding needed, and what is the best use of existing funds to improve pediatric health? Where does it make the most sense to concentrate scarce pediatric specialty services? Globally, 25% of the population is less than 14 years old,[51] with a life expectancy of 73 years.[52] The global infant mortality rate is 30.8 per 1,000 live births.[18] See **Table 1-1** for some global statistics that inform pediatric health initiatives.[8]

Snapshots of Care Around the World

It is enlightening to consider what pediatric healthcare looks like in different geographic regions and countries. Challenges to accessing care in sparsely populated, mountainous, or other remote locations require creative solutions that can be implemented with minimal

---

BOX 1-1   Pediatric Emergency Research Network

Member organizations: https://pern-global.com

- Paediatric Emergency Research in the UK and Ireland (PERUKI): https://www.peruki.org/
- Paediatric Research in Emergency Departments International Collaborative (PREDICT): https://www.predict.org.au
- Pediatric Emergency Care Applied Research Network: https://pecarn.org
- Pediatric Emergency Medicine Collaborative Research Committee (PEM CRC): https://www.pemcollaborativeresearchcommitteepemcrc.org
- Pediatric Emergency Research Canada: https://perc-canada.ca
- Research in European Paediatric Emergency Medicine (REPEM): https://eusem.org/sections-and-committees/sections/paediatric-section/research-in-european-pediatric-emergecny-medicine
- Red de Investigación de la Sociedad Española de Ugerncias de Pediatría (RISeuP)/ Spanish Pediatric Emergency Research Group (SPERG): https://sperg.es/en/borrador-automatico/
- Red de Investigación y Desarrollo de la Emergencia Pediátrica Latino-America (RIDEPLA): Website pending

---

resources. People living in densely populated areas may have adequate access to care but deal with problems such as pollution, overcrowding, and violence. This section provides a glimpse of our global colleagues' practice environment and solutions.

Australia

Australia is the seventh largest country in the world and the only country that spans a whole continent. Its population of more than 26 million people makes Australia the 54th largest country in the world.[8] About 4.7 million of these people, or 19% of the population, are 14 years of age or younger.[8] In 2020 and 2021, patients younger than 4 accounted for 10% of emergency department (ED) presentations, despite representing only 7% of the population.[3,4]

The Netherlands

The Netherlands has affirmed that all children have a right to good health as agreed to in the Convention on the Rights

	TABLE 1-1 World Data			
Country	**Population ≤ 14 Years Old**	**Health Expenditures (% of GDP*)**	**Infant Mortality Rate per 1,000 Live Births**	**Life Expectancy at Birth (in years)**
Australia	19%	9%	3.05	83
Brazil	21%	10%	18.37	75
Canada	16%	11%	4.44	83
China	18%	5%	11.15	76
Iceland	20%	8%	1.66	83
India	27%	4%	39.55	70
Indonesia	27%	3%	20.16	73
Israel	28%	7%	3.62	83
Japan	13%	11%	1.92	86
Mexico	27%	6%	11.64	77
Mozambique	45%	5%	63.03	56
Netherlands	16%	10%	3.45	82
South Africa	18%	11%	26.82	65
Saudi Arabia	25%	5%	12.58	76
Sweden	28%	8%	2.45	82
United Arab Emirates	15%	3%	5.25	79
United Kingdom	18%	10%	4.27	81
United States	19%	17%	5.22	80

GDP = Gross Domestic Product.

Data from Central Intelligence Agency. (n.d.). *The world factbook.* https://www.cia.gov/the-world-factbook/; IndexMundi. (n.d.). *Welcome.* https://www.indexmundi.com

of the Child.[47] The Dutch government is obliged to properly inform children and parents about health and possible risks. Children between 0 and 4 years utilize primary healthcare services particularly often, including the ED.

Research that focuses on frequent visitors to EDs (3 to 25 times a year) with low-risk problems shows that parents with young children appear the most.[14] In many cases, parents are extra careful with children and therefore go to the ED relatively quickly when a concern arises. In addition, young children cannot indicate exactly what is going on, which makes parents more likely to become insecure and worried.

The most frequently occurring health problems for which children visit the ED are injuries in the home or at school, sports injuries, motor vehicle collisions, violence, and self-harm (**Table 1-2**).[41,50]

In 2020, a total of 871 children in the age group 0–14 years died. As shown in **Table 1-3**, congenital abnormalities of the cardiovascular system and premature birth, underweight, and/or growth retardation were the leading causes of death in 0- to 14-year-olds.[7] Home and sports accidents were the third most frequent cause.[7]

As a result of the COVID-19 pandemic, the number of ED visits related to injuries and illnesses in 2020 was fewer than in previous years. Measures aimed at preventing the spread of the virus, such as mandatory working from home and the (temporary) closure of schools and sports facilities, changed the activity patterns of the inhabitants of the Netherlands. In addition, people were less likely to go to the hospital, so as not to burden the care system even more and/or from fear of contracting a COVID-19 infection in the hospital.

TABLE 1-2	Health Issues Bringing Children to the Emergency Department by Age and Sex		
Age	**Male**	**Female**	**Total**
Private Accidents (Home or School) per 100,000 Inhabitants			
0–4	14,800	12,200	27,100
5–9	12,800	11,100	23,900
10–14	10,700	8,800	19,600
15–19	7,600	5,600	13,100
Sports Injuries per 100,000 Sports Hours			
0–4	300	200	500
5–9	3,300	3,500	6,800
10–14	12,000	8,800	20,800
15–19	10,300	5,200	15,400
Traffic Accidents per 10 Million Kilometers			
0–5	2,600	1,900	4,500
6–11	3,000	2,300	5,200
12–17	7,000	3,900	11,000
18–24	7,700	4,800	12,400
Violence per 100,000			
0–9	< 100	100	200
10–14	400	200	600
15–19	1,400	600	2,000
Self-Harm per 100,000			
0–9	< 100	< 100	< 100
10–14	< 100	200	300
15–19	300	2,000	2,400

Data from Stam, C., & Blatter, B. (2021). Letsels 2020: Kerncijfers LIS. VeiligheidNL; VZinfo.nl. (n.d.). Letsel informatie system.

As mentioned previously, the government is obliged to properly inform children and parents about health and possible risks. It does so with the help of social media with sites such as www.Rijksoverheid.nl, www.veiligheid.nl and www.nji.nl (Netherlands Youth Institute), and www.RIVM.nl. Meanwhile, health and injury information is mainly provided at the municipal level. This is typically done through the local Municipal Health Service (gemeentelijke gezondheidsdienst or GGD), one of the Netherlands' decentralized health organizations.

TABLE 1-3	Top Eight Causes of Death of Children 0–14 Years of Age in 2020	
Rank	**Cause of Death**	**Number of Deaths in Dutch Population per 100,000**
1	Congenital abnormalities of the cardiovascular system	44
2	Premature birth, underweight, and/or growth retardation	41
3	Private, occupational, and sports accidents	24
4	Transportation accidents	21
5	Injuries resulting from violence	11
6	Brain cancer	10
6	Epilepsy	10
6	Intellectual disability	10

Data from Central Bureau of Statistics. (n.d.). *Manufacturing output almost 14 percent up in April.* https://www.cbs.nl/en-gb

South Africa

South Africa is a diverse country and is often referred to as the rainbow nation. The colors of the rainbow represent South Africa's diverse races, tribes, creeds, languages, and landscapes and are reflected in the six colors of the national flag (**Figure 1-1**).

The South African Constitution guarantees everyone "access to health care services" and states that "no one may be refused emergency medical treatment." Hence, all South African residents, including refugees and asylum seekers, are entitled to access to healthcare services.[39] Access to healthcare varies, as levels of care span from services provided at the rural clinic level, to care at tertiary hospitals (public healthcare), to First World private healthcare facilities. Delayed and limited access are often factors that compromise care of pediatric patients, especially in the emergency setting. Overcrowding of facilities and lack of training in the management of this special population group place an additional burden on both the care of the pediatric patient and the healthcare and trauma/emergency system.

Population Distribution by Age

South Africa has a total population of 56.9 million people.[20] In 2015, 28.34% of South Africa's population was 14 years old or younger,[42] with that percentage decreasing to 27.94% in 2020 (**Figure 1-2**)[19] and then increasing to 28.8% in 2021. This large young population has a direct effect on the nation's key socioeconomic issues, placing demands on the education and healthcare systems, particularly opportunities for preventive health measures (e.g., immunizations).

The distribution of children across the provinces (regions/states) in South Africa is slightly different from that of adults, with a larger share of children living in provinces with large rural populations (**Figure 1-3**).[43] Collectively, KwaZulu-Natal, the Eastern Cape, and

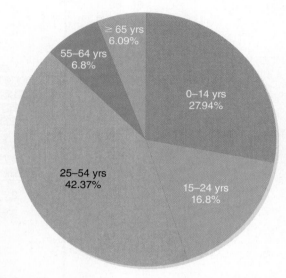

Figure 1-2 *Age structure as a percentage of the South African population, 2020.*

Data from IndexMundi. (2021). *South Africa age structure.* Retrieved May 12, 2022, from https://www.indexmundi.com/south_africa/age_structure.html

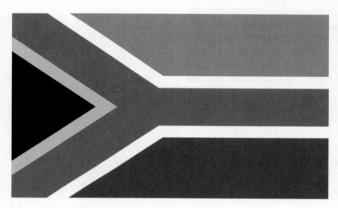

Figure 1-1 *The South African flag.*

© flowgraph/iStock/Getty Images Plus/Getty Images.

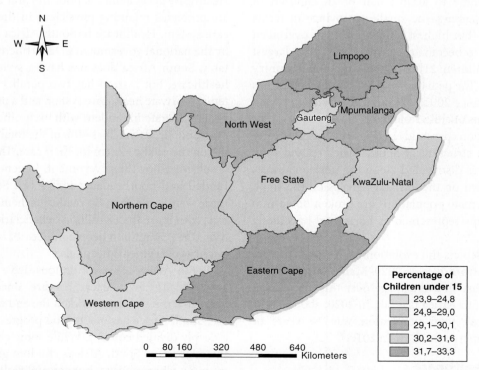

Figure 1-3 *Percentage of South African population younger than 15 years of age per province.*

Reproduced from Statistics South Africa. (2020). *Mid-year population estimates: 2019.* Republic of South Africa. https://www.statssa.gov.za/publications/P0302/P03022019.pdf

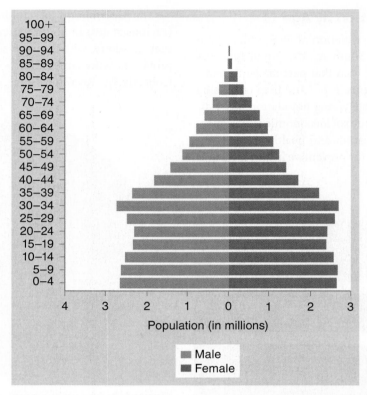

Figure 1-4 *Population pyramid in South Africa, 2020.*

Modified from Central Intelligence Agency. (n.d.). *The world factbook.* https://www.cia.gov/the-world-factbook/countries/south-africa/images/cG9zdDoxODYzNTE=

Limpopo are home to almost half of all children in South Africa. Gauteng, the smallest province in terms of physical size (but highest population), has overtaken KwaZulu-Natal to become the province with the largest population of children: 21% of all children in the country live in Gauteng. The pediatric population of Gauteng has grown by 42% since 2002, making it the fastest-growing province in terms of child residents.[16]

The population pyramid in **Figure 1-4** illustrates the age and sex structure of South Africa's population. The population is distributed along the horizontal axis, with males shown on the left and females on the right. The male and female populations are broken down into 5-year age groups represented as horizontal bars along the vertical axis.[19]

Figure 1-5 depicts the evolution of the age structure in South Africa from 2010 to 2020. Many countries have shown an increase in average age over this period, but this trend in South Africa is weak. In 2020, about 28.8% of South Africa's total population was 14 years or younger, as compared to 29.7% in 2010.[30]

Access to Healthcare

The 2020 Global Healthcare Index reported that South Africa's healthcare system ranked 49th out of 89 countries.

Healthcare accessibility is poor in rural areas, and there are problems retaining physicians in the public healthcare system. Healthcare in South Africa is administered by the national government's Department of Health. Notably, South Africa does not have a system of universal healthcare, but instead has two parallel healthcare systems. A private healthcare system and a public healthcare system operate in tandem with each other. The majority of the public, as much as 80% of the total population, relies on the public system for their care. The public system is subsidized by the government. In general, it is underfunded and poorly managed.[22] As of September 2020, there were more than 80 medical schemes in South Africa, with more than 8 million beneficiaries, compared to more than 51 million people in need of care provided by public (government) hospitals.[40]

South Africa has a continuous drive to enhance access to healthcare at all levels of care. Since 1994, when its first universal elections marked the end of the Apartheid era, South Africa has made good progress, yet it remains a deeply divided country. While some children flourish, the majority of South Africa's children grow up in communities where poverty, hunger, and violence continue to compromise their health, development, education, and future employment prospects.[34]

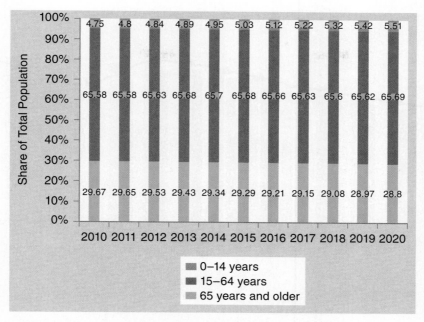

Figure 1-5 *Evolution of the age structure in South Africa, 2010–2020.*

Data from O'Neill, A. (2022, February 2). *South Africa: Age structure from 2010 to 2020.* Statista.

The government hospitalization system is graded from community-based small hospitals, to regionalized facilities with specialist capabilities in the larger centers, to super-specialized academic teaching hospitals. Pediatric specialized care is available at regional centers of the country, although this is often limited to the private health system.

Article 27(3) of the South African Constitution addresses the right to emergency care as a basic right.[9] The government's policy decision to prioritize primary health was reinforced by two other health rights in the Constitution: every child's immediate and unqualified right of access to "basic health care services" and the right of everyone to an environment "not harmful to health or wellbeing."[24]

Adedini et al. reported in 2020 that 81.9% of South African parents (public sector—no medical insurance) prefer clinics (public healthcare) as their first choice when seeking care for their children, and 84.2% prefer hospitals (public healthcare) as their second option. About 5% of caregivers prefer faith-based/traditional healers as their second point of call. Barriers to accessing healthcare were reported for more than half of the sampled children (52.0%), such as long queues at the health facility, lack of medicines, and the distance to the clinic or hospital; these examples constitute major barriers to obtaining care.[1]

Statistics on Children in South Africa reports that 20% of children are living far from the usual health facility. Distance is measured as the length of time traveled to reach the health facility, by whatever form of transport is typically used. The health facility is regarded as "far" if a child would have to travel more than 30 minutes to reach it, irrespective of mode of transport. This has a limiting impact on children's right of access to health care.[17]

In many of the resource-poor areas in South Africa, differences between provisions for care of adults and for care of children are clearly visible. Many hospitals in South Africa do not employ pediatricians.[21]

Leading Causes of Death

In 2020, average life expectancy in South Africa was 64.9 years (**Figure 1-6**), compared to the global 2020 expectancy of 72.63 years.[27,59]

Despite significant reductions in pediatric mortality, preventable and treatable conditions remain leading causes of death and illness in children in South Africa.[28] The infant mortality rate in 2020 was 23.57 per 1,000 live births, compared to 32.94 per 1,000 live births globally in 2010.[46,59] The under-5 mortality rate significantly declined from 75.3 child deaths per 1,000 live births to 34.1 child deaths per 1,000 live births between 2002 and 2020.[40]

Goga et al. reported in 2019 that although the neonatal mortality rate in South Africa has remained stagnant at 12 deaths per 1,000 live births, the infant and under-5 mortality rates have significantly declined since peaking in 2003.[15] Changes that have influenced this decline include policies to prevent vertical human

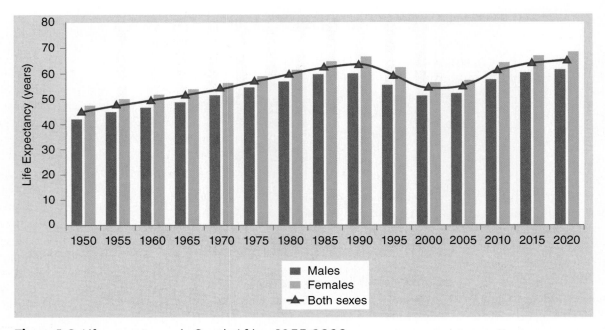

Figure 1-6 *Life expectancy in South Africa, 1955–2020.*
Data from Worldometer. (n.d.). *South Africa demographics.* https://www.worldometers.info/demographics/south-africa-demographics/

immunodeficiency virus (HIV) transmission, earlier treatment of children living with HIV, expanded immunization policies, strengthening breastfeeding practices, and health policies to contain tobacco and sugar use.[15]

Leading Health Problems

Healthcare in South Africa varies from basic primary healthcare offered free by the state, to highly specialized and technological health services available in both the public and private sectors. The public sector has insufficient capacity and is under-resourced in some places. While the state accounts for approximately 40% of all expenditures on health, the public health sector is under pressure to deliver services to about 80% of the country's population. The private sector caters to middle- and high-income earners who tend to be members of medical schemes (plans). The private sector attracts most of the country's health professionals. The government aims to rectify this imbalance through an envisaged national health insurance scheme.

The situation is compounded by public health challenges, including the burden of diseases such as HIV and tuberculosis (TB), and a shortage of key medical personnel. As a result of comprehensive immunization programs, the number of children protected against vaccine-preventable diseases such as measles, TB, cholera, and pertussis has been steadily increasing. Measures to improve child health include expansion and strengthening of school health services and the establishment of district clinical specialist teams that include a pediatrician.

The following issues have a key impact on under-5 and infant morbidity and mortality in South Africa:

- Lower respiratory tract infections, predominantly pneumonia, remain a major cause of morbidity and mortality in children younger than 5 years of age.
- The percentage of households living without any sanitation facilities declined from 12.6% in 2002 to 3.1% in 2017. However, thousands of children still face environmental threats daily, either at home or at school.
- South Africa has a high childhood TB burden, with an estimated 38,000 cases of TB in children younger than 15 years of age in 2017, representing 12% of the country's TB burden.

Malnutrition

The 2016 South African Demographic and Health Survey (SADHS) reported that the prevalence of stunting, wasting, underweight-for-age, and overweight in under-5s as 27.4%, 2.5%, 6%, and 13.3%, respectively. Stunting prevalence had not changed from the 2003 survey. However, wasting decreased from 5% to 3% and underweight-for-age increased from 11.5% to 13%. Although breastfeeding was initiated within 1 hour of delivery in two-thirds of children, only 32% of children younger than 6 months were exclusively breastfed, with only 23% of children between 6 and 23 months being fed a minimum acceptable diet. A double burden of malnutrition in children is emerging, with both undernutrition and overnutrition being associated with short- and long-term disease (such as cardiovascular disease) in adults.[15]

Leading Causes of Emergency Presentations

Pediatric emergencies (injuries and illness) contribute significantly to the patient burden in EDs in South Africa. Approximately 25% of the ED visits are for patients younger than 18 years of age. Despite this significant patient burden, many healthcare facilities are not adequately prepared to deliver effective pediatric emergency care. The variable availability of pediatric expertise, pediatric-specific equipment, appropriately trained staff, and standardized treatment guidelines adversely affects the optimal emergency and trauma care of children in South Africa.[26]

It would appear that there are consistent risk factors globally for children and adolescents to sustain penetrating trauma. However, in certain communities, violence can become endemic and almost impossible to counter. This is a major problem in many areas in South Africa, where the trauma epidemic shows little signs of abating, and the high rate of interpersonal and intentional trauma remains a major cause for concern.[25]

An overall reduction in pediatric emergency center visits was seen during the peak of the COVID-19 pandemic in South Africa and specifically during the Lockdown Level 5 (highest level). This was similar to the experiences associated with the severe acute respiratory syndrome (SARS) and Middle East respiratory syndrome (MERS) pandemics, as people tended to avoid or delay attending hospitals due to the fear of contracting the communicable disease.[2]

Children account for a substantial proportion of ED visits around the world. Exact figures for ED visits by children in Africa, and specifically South Africa, are not available, as South Africa does not have a national database that collects these statistics.

Health Promotion and Injury Prevention Programs

Injuries account for an increasing proportion of child deaths in South Africa and are the leading cause of death among adolescents. In addition, nonfatal injuries contribute to a growing burden of disability in childhood, are concentrated among poor children, and increase in number as children age. Despite this growing and concerning public health problem, a coordinated focus on injury and violence has not been prioritized by the public and/or the private health sectors. Despite extensive global and national policy changes, South Africa's children continue to be threatened by both intentional and unintentional injuries.[34]

While South Africa has adopted various laws, policies, and injury prevention programs in line with international standards, data, and instruments to prevent child violence and injury, the country's response is fragmented due to a lack of coordination and stewardship at the highest levels. At the same time, existing research on child violence and injury is limited in scale, and located within disciplinary and institutional silos, thereby reducing its influence on policy, financing, and intervention decisions.[34]

The large and growing number of child injury deaths, the progressive nature of childhood injuries, and the frequently long-lasting effects of injury on children gave rise to the creation of the nongovernmental organization (NGO) known as "Child Accident Prevention Foundation of Southern Africa" at the Red Cross Children's Hospital. Founded in 1978 by Professor Sid Cywes, it is one of the oldest organizations of its kind in the world. Since July 2008, this NGO has operated under the name and logo of "Childsafe—Keeping kids free from harm." Childsafe South Africa has been working tirelessly over the last four decades to transform South Africa into a safer place for all its children, irrespective of social class, income group, or race, and aims to reduce and prevent intentional and unintentional injuries of all severity through research, education, environmental change, and recommendations for legislation.

Two main focus areas for Childsafe South Africa are child safety education and skills training and creating a child-safe environment. In particular, this organization has specially designed educational and skills training programs for child safety. It has been instrumental in driving legislation in the following areas[10]:

- Manufacturing of South African Bureau of Standards–approved child restraints for use in motor vehicles
- Regulation of children's furniture
- Through written and oral presentations in the South African Parliament, child-friendly legislation, including the New Firearms Bill and Gun Safety and the Prevention of Child Physical and Sexual Abuse bill
- Through presentations made to the Human Rights Commission of South Africa, the Child Safety at Schools program and the National Development Plan and Corporal Punishment

The Netcare Hospital Group launched the "Netcare Trauma Injury Prevention" (NTIP) program in 2012. This program embraces all age groups, from expecting parents, caregivers, and educators to children, adults, and geriatric individuals, while focusing on injury prevention and health promotion topics. Most of the programs and activities start with the pediatric age group in an effort to develop a change in behavior during early childhood development, which will then lead to responsible adults who display safe behavior due to their change of behavior as a young child.

Side-by-Side is a national government-initiated campaign working to ensure that all children younger than age 5 receive the nurturing care they need to develop to the best of their abilities. The Side-by-Side campaign rests on five pillars:

- *Nutrition.* Good nutrition is important for mothers' and children's health. It starts with breastfeeding.
- *Love.* Brain development is spurred by responsive care and love, play, and talk.
- *Protection.* Children can be protected from childhood disease and injury by getting immunized and ensuring safety in the home.
- *Healthcare.* Children need care when they are sick or injured.
- *Extra care.* Some children may need special care or support. Caregivers should know what to do and where to go.

Summary

Since 1994, South Africa has made substantial progress in transforming its health sector, making primary healthcare services available to millions who were previously denied access. Yet access to pediatric-specific healthcare remains a challenge, with vital healthcare interventions not reaching the areas and people who need them.

A persistent focus on prevention of pediatric-specific primary illness and injury, caring for the ill and injured child in the most well-planned manner within an organized healthcare and trauma system (secondary prevention), and ensuring that children are appropriately treated and managed so that they can be reintegrated into society remains the biggest gain related to the daily management of medical and trauma emergencies in the pediatric population. Penetrating trauma in children and adolescents remains a major problem and is associated with significant mortality and morbidity. The general lack of pediatric expertise, pediatric-specific equipment, dedicated pediatric emergency and trauma centers, and appropriately trained staff continues to adversely affect the emergency and trauma care of children in South Africa.

Sweden

Of Sweden's population of more than 10.4 million inhabitants, approximately 22% are children and young people aged 0–19 years. In 1970, this subpopulation numbered 2.23 million. The corresponding figure for 2021 was

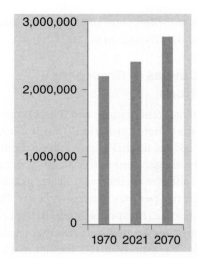

Figure 1-7 *Number of individuals 0–19 years in Sweden—past, present, and future.*

Data from Tortstensson, S. (2022, April 19). *Befolkningsstruktur.* Ekonomifakta [Population structure]. https://www.ekonomifakta.se/Fakta/Arbetsmarknad/Befolkning/Befolkningsstruktur/

2.45 million, and the number of children and young people in Sweden is predicted to increase to 2.82 million by 2070 (**Figure 1-7**).[45]

Emergency departments for children and young people can be found at all seven university hospitals in Sweden. In primary care, access to pediatricians is available at some of the country's more than 1,000 primary care units. Approximately 20 county hospitals and about 40 smaller county hospitals also offer pediatric-specific clinics. In addition, private actors contribute child-specific skills that increase the range of options for children's healthcare. But despite the relatively good access to pediatric emergency care, many acutely ill children are forced to seek emergency care during evenings and weekends at EDs for adults, which, in turn, poses a challenge for these EDs in their effort to provide high-quality pediatric emergency care.

When health and medical care is given to children in Sweden, the best interests of the child are expected to be given special consideration in accordance with Chapter 1 in Section 8 of the Patient Act and Chapter 5 in Section 6 of the Health and Medical Services Act. The best interests of the child should guide the difficult decisions that sometimes need to be made in the course of healthcare activities. The healthcare staff must take into account science and proven experience and—depending on the child's age and maturity—obtain information from guardians. Since January 1, 2020, the Convention on the Rights of the Child has been applied as part of Swedish law. Its incorporation into the national statutes clarifies that Sweden's convention commitments must be secured at all levels in public activities.[36]

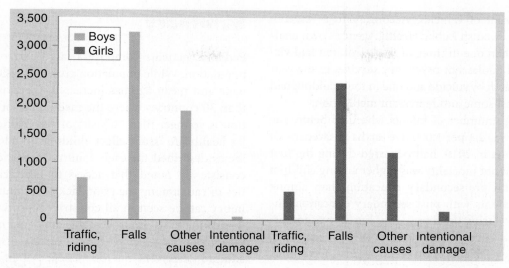

Figure 1-8 *Number of children 0–14 years receiving inpatient care in Sweden due to claims incidents during the years 2018–2020 by sex and type of cause.*

Data from The National Board of Health and Welfare. (2021). *Statistical database for statistics on injuries and damage events in Sweden's municipalities and counties.* https://kib.ki.se/en/databaser/statistical-databases-national-board-health-and-welfare

The National Board of Health and Welfare has produced a guide that is aimed at staff and operations managers in child healthcare, as well as caregivers and decision makers. The intention with this guidance is to achieve the goals for child healthcare outlined by the Health Care Act of 1982 regarding the best possible physical, mental, and social health for children by promoting children's health and development, preventing ill health in children, and ensuring early identification and initiation of measures to address problems in children's health, development, and upbringing.[35] Professional organizations with an interest in child healthcare have also produced a web-based, national handbook that describes content methods and a knowledge base for work in child healthcare. While the National Board of Health and Welfare's guidance provides overall descriptions and frameworks for child healthcare activities, the professional organizations' ambition with the national handbook is to provide concrete advice for the execution of the work.[32]

Statistics for the year 2020 show that respiratory diseases were the most common reason for inpatient care of children. When certain perinatal conditions (e.g., associated with gestational age and fetal growth) were excluded for the youngest age group (0–4 years), acute upper and lower respiratory tract infections were particularly common. In the age groups 5–9 and 10–14 years, symptom diagnoses and diseases of the digestive organs were, respectively, the most common diagnostic groups documented for hospital admission. Mental illness and behavioral disorders were the most common reasons for hospitalization of individuals older than 15 years of age.[37]

Pediatric trauma that leads to care in Swedish hospitals is almost exclusively caused by blunt force. In 2018, approximately 140,000 children sought care in Swedish EDs due to injury, which generated almost 14,000 inpatient care opportunities; 46% were injured by falls and 12% needed care in connection with traffic-related injury events (**Figure 1-8**). The injury mechanism indicates which injuries the child may have suffered, even if initial information from the injury site is often incomplete and, in some cases, misleading.[23,38]

In 2020, 24,700 assaults were reported against children younger than the age of 18, which represented 30% of all reported assault offenses. Of these, 4,280 assault cases were reported against children ages 0–6 years, 13,300 against children ages 7–14 years, and 7,120 against children ages 15–17 years. Abuse crimes against children are reported to a large extent by preschools and schools; thus, fewer crimes are reported during the summer than during school terms. A large part of the increase in reported crimes against children ages 7–14 is also due to reports from school about violence between peers. Solved abuse crimes against children account for only 5% of abuse cases against children 0–6 years of age and 7% of abuse cases against children 7–14 years of age.[6]

In Sweden, about 100 children younger than the age of 18 are injured and killed every year. Injuries are the single most common cause of death. The most common causes of fatal injuries are traffic injuries or suicides.[49] Since the beginning of the decade, an average of 22 children have died by suicide each year in Sweden, about as many girls as boys. The vast majority were between 13 and 17 years old and often used violent methods such as hanging or jumping in front of vehicles. According to a research study and the Swedish Public Health Agency's own analyses,[13] more than one in three of these children had visited child and adolescent psychiatry services in the year before their death by suicide and one in four children had received at least some antidepressant medication.

In 2019, the number of infants who died before the age of 1 year was 2.1 per 1,000 live births in Sweden. Of all infant deaths in 2019, half occurred during the first week of life. Infant mortality was higher among children of parents with pre-secondary education than among children of parents with post-secondary education. Infant mortality during the first year of life decreased during the period 2006–2019 among both girls and boys, regardless of level of education of the parents, and among infants of mothers born in Sweden.[12]

Most school-age children in Sweden report that they feel satisfied with life. But many also state that they have mental and somatic disorders such as difficulty sleeping and headaches. In a 2017–2018 survey, six out of seven school-age children indicated that they felt satisfied with life. This answer was more common among boys than girls, and among younger people compared with older school-age children. The highest proportion who felt satisfied with life was found among 11-year-old boys (93%) and the lowest proportion was found among 15-year-old girls (77%). The proportion of school-age children who state that they feel satisfied with life has been stable since the question began to be asked in 2001–2002, for both girls and boys and for different age groups.[12] A worrying result in the follow-up of Agenda 2030 is that there is a clear tendency toward increased violence and bullying among children and young people in Sweden.[44]

In 2019, 7% of boys and 6% of girls aged 10–17 visited psychiatric care. Attention-deficit/hyperactivity disorder (ADHD) was the most common diagnosis among both sexes, although almost twice as many boys as girls were treated for this condition. The next most common diagnosis among boys was autism spectrum disorder; among girls, it was anxiety syndrome.[12]

Sweden has a long tradition of preventive child safety work, which has contributed to the country having some of the world's lowest incidence rates of children and young people being injured and killed in accidents. Several factors play into this success, but cooperation and collaboration between actors at different levels in society is of crucial importance. Child safety work takes place in all environments. The family, child healthcare, preschool, school, leisure centers, and everyone who works in sports and other leisure activities for children and young people are considered extremely important in creating safe environments for children and young people.[29]

Summary

Pediatric patients compose a large part of the global population. While population growth has slowed worldwide and mean age has increased, there are still more than 30 countries where the median age of the population is younger than 20 years of age. Worldwide, similar healthcare issues affect children. In addition to the issues described for each country in this chapter, it is consistently noted that access to healthcare, disparities in care among the poor, lack of immunization, and injury can be seen in all countries reporting data on a worldwide basis. Improvements are being made to provide greater healthcare access, decrease disparities, and educate caregivers on the benefits of immunizations and injury prevention. However, more education and resources are needed to ensure the health and safety of children around the world.

References

1. Adedini, S. S. (2020). Patterns of healthcare utilisation and barriers affecting access to child healthcare services in low-income urban South African settings. *South African Journal of Child Health, 14*(1), 34–39. http://www.sajch.org.za/index.php/SAJCH/article/view/1541/1001

2. Akuaake, L. M., Hendrikse, C., Spittal, G., Evans, K., & van Hoving, D. J. (2020). Cross-sectional study of paediatric case mix presenting to an emergency centre in Cape Town, South Africa, during COVID-19. *BMJ Paediatrics Open, 4*(1), Article e000801. https://doi.org/10.1136/bmjpo-2020-000801

3. Australian Institute of Health and Welfare. (2022, February 25). *Australia's children.* https://www.aihw.gov.au/reports/children-youth/australias-children/contents/health/the-health-of-australias-children

4. Australian Institute of Health and Welfare. (2022). *Emergency department care.* https://www.aihw.gov.au/reports-data/myhospitals/sectors/emergency-department-care

5. Barrett, M. J., Dalziel, S., Lyttle, M., O'Sullivan, R., & Pediatric Emergency Research Networks. (2022). A bibliometric analysis of global pediatric emergency medicine research networks. *Pediatric Emergency Care, 2022, 38*(4), e1179–e1184. https://doi.org/10.1097/PEC.0000000000002543

6. Brottsförebyggande rådet [Crime Prevention Council]. (2021). *Barnmisshandel.* https://bra.se/statistik/statistik-utifran-brottstyper/barnmisshandel.html

7. Central Bureau of Statistics (n.d.). https://www.cbs.nl/en-gb

8. Central Intelligence Agency. (2022, April 28). *The world factbook.* https://www.cia.gov/the-world-factbook/

9. Cheema, B., & Westwood, A. (Eds.). (2015). *Summary of standards for paediatric emergency care: Expert consensus report for the Western Cape.* http://www.emct.info/uploads/1/4/1/7/14175478/summary_of_standards_for_care_of_children_in_ecs.pdf

10. Department of Paediatrics and Child Health, University of Cape Town. (n.d.). *Childsafe South Africa.* http://www.paediatrics.uct.ac.za/scah/clinicalservices/surgical/trauma/childsafe

11. Folkhälsomyndigheten [Swedish Public Health Agency]. (2021). *Spädbarnsdödlighet.* https://www.folkhalsomyndigheten.se/folkhalsorapportering-statistik/tolkad-rapportering/folkhalsans-utveckling/resultat/halsa/spadbarnsdodlighet/

12. Folkhälsomyndigheten [Swedish Public Health Agency]. (2021). *Statistik om barns psykiska hälsa.* https://www.folkhalsomyndigheten.se/livsvillkor-levnadsvanor/psykisk-halsa-och-suicidprevention/statistik-psykisk-halsa/statistik-om-barns-psykiska-halsa/

13. Folkhälsomyndigheten [Swedish Public Health Agency]. (2021). *Suicid bland barn i Sverige.* Article 21300. https://www.folkhalsomyndigheten.se/contentassets/a0631c7344be413bb4aa754d2770043e/suicid-bland-barn-sverige.pdf

14. Giesen. P. H. J., Stam, D., & Wensing, M. (2010). "You want the certainty that it is all right." *Medisch Contact.* https://www.medischcontact.nl/nieuws/laatste-nieuws/artikel/je-wilt-de-zekerheid-dat-het-goed-zit.htm

15. Goga, A., Feucht, U., Zar, H. J., Vanker, A., Wiysonge, C. S., McKerrow, N., Wright, C. Y., Loveday, M., Odendaal, W., Ramokolo, V., Ramraj, T., Bamford, L., Green, R. J., Pillay, Y., & Nannan, N. (2019). Neonatal, infant and child health in South Africa: Reflecting on the past towards a better future. *South African Medical Journal, 109*(11b), 83–88. https://doi.org/10.7196/SAMJ.2019.v109i11b.14301

16. Hall, K. (2019, November). Children in South Africa. *Statistics on Children in South Africa.* http://childrencount.uct.ac.za/indicator.php?domain=1&indicator=1

17. Hall, K. (2019, November). Children living far from clinics. *Statistics on Children in South Africa.* http://childrencount.uct.ac.za/indicator.php?domain=5&indicator=49

18. IndexMundi. (2021). *Infant mortality rate.* Retrieved April 29, 2022, from https://www.indexmundi.com/factbook/fields/infant-mortality-rate

19. IndexMundi. (2021, September 18). *South Africa age structure.* Retrieved April 29, 2022, from https://www.indexmundi.com/south_africa/age_structure.html

20. IndexMundi. (2021, September 18). *South African population.* Retrieved April 29, 2022, from https://www.indexmundi.com/south_africa/population.html

21. International Federation for Emergency Medicine. (2012). *International standards for care of children in emergency departments.* http://emssa.org.za/wp-content/uploads/2014/10/IFEM-Paediatrics-Standards-of-Care-Document.pdf

22. InternationalInsurance.com. (2021). *Understanding South Africa's healthcare system.* International Citizens Insurance. https://www.internationalinsurance.com/health/systems/south-africa.php

23. Internetmedicin. (2020, September 12). *Barntrauma: Initialt omhändertagande.* https://www.internetmedicin.se/behandlingsoversikter/kirurgi/barntrauma-initialt-omhandertagande/

24. Jobson, M. (2015). *Structure of the health system in South Africa.* Khulumani Support Group.

25. Khumalo-Mugabi, L., Moffatt, S., Bekker, W., Smith, M., Bruce, J. L., Laing, G., Manchev, V., Kong, V., & Clarke, D. L. (2020). Penetrating trauma in children and adolescents in Pietermaritzburg. *South African Journal of Surgery, 58*(1), 33–36.

26. Lai King, L., Cheema, B., & van Hoving, D. J. (2020). A cross sectional study of the availability of paediatric emergency equipment in South African emergency units. *African Journal of Emergency Medicine, 10*(4), 197–202. https://doi.org/10.1016/j.afjem.2020.06.008

27. Macrotrends. (2022). *World life expectancy 1950–2022.* https://www.macrotrends.net/countries/WLD/world/life-expectancy#:~:text=The%20life%20expectancy%20for%20World%20in%202020%20was%2072.63%20years,a%200.24%25%20increase%20from%202018

28. Murdoch, J., Curran, R., Cornick, R., Picken, S., Bachmann, M., Bateman, E., Simelane, M. L., & Fairall, L. (2020). Addressing the quality and scope of paediatric primary care in South Africa: Evaluating contextual impacts of the introduction of the Practical Approach to Care Kit for children (PACK Child). *BMC Health Services Research, 20*(1), Article 479. https://doi.org/10.1186/s12913-020-05201-w

29. Myndigheten för Samhällsskydd och Beredskap; MSB [Swedish Civil Contingencies Agency]. (2011). *Barns och ungas säkerhet* [Publikation MSB307, September 2011]. https://rib.msb.se/filer/pdf/26005.pdf

30. O' Neill, A. (2021, July 15). *South Africa: Age structure from 2010 to 2020.* Statista. https://www.statista.com/statistics/578938/age-structure-in-south-africa/

31. Pediatric Emergency Research Network. (2020). *About PERN.* https://pern-global.com/?page_id=58

32. Rikshandboken [The National Handbook]. (2021). *Barnhälsovård för professionen.* https://www.rikshandboken-bhv.se/

33. Ropers, F., Bossuyt, P., Maconochie, I., Smit, F. J., Alves, C., Greber-Platzer, S., Moll, H. A., & Zacharias, J. (2021). Practice variation across five European paedriatric emergency departments: A prospective observational study. *BMJ Open, 12*, Article e053382. https://doi.org/10.1136/bmjopen-2021-053382

34. Shung-Kiung, M., Lake, L., Sanders, D., & Hendricks, M. (Eds.). (2019). *South African Child Gauge 2019.* Children's Institute, University of Cape Town. http://www.ci.uct.ac.za/sites/default/files/image_tool/images/367/Child_Gauge/South_African_Child_Gauge_2019/ChildGauge_2019_final_print%20%28sm%29.pdf

35. Socialstyrelsen [National Board of Health and Welfare]. (2014). *Vägledning för barnhälsovården.* https://www.socialstyrelsen.se/globalassets/sharepoint-dokument/artikelkatalog/vagledning/2014-4-5.pdf

36. Socialstyrelsen [National Board of Health and Welfare]. (2020). *Barn som söker hälso- och sjukvård.* Meddelandeblad. https://www.socialstyrelsen.se/globalassets/sharepoint-dokument/artikelkatalog/meddelandeblad/2020-12-7117.pdf

37. Socialstyrelsen [National Board of Health and Welfare]. (2021). *Statistik om sjukdomar behandlade i sluten vård 2020.* https://www.socialstyrelsen.se/globalassets/sharepoint-dokument/artikelkatalog/statistik/2021-9-7537.pdf

38. Socialstyrelsen [National Board of Health and Welfare]. (2021). *Statistikdatabas för statistik över skador och skadehändelser i Sveriges kommuner och län.* https://sdb.socialstyrelsen.se/if_skastat/val.aspx

39. South Africa Government. (1996). *The Constitution of South Africa.* https://www.justice.gov.za/legislation/constitution/saconstitution-web-eng.pdf

40. South African Government. (2022). *Health.* https://www.gov.za/about-sa/health#:~:text=By%20September%202020%2C%20there%20were,with%20over%20eight%20million%20beneficiaries

41. Stam, C., & Blatter, B. (2021). *Letsels 2020: Kerncijfers LIS.* VeiligheidNL. https://www.veiligheid.nl/.ibmmodres/domino/OpenAttachment/veiligheid/website.nsf/54F82A64180AEE46C1258718002EC60A/asset/Cijferrapportage%20Letsels%202020.pdf

42. Statistics South Africa. (2015). *Mid-year population estimates: 2015.* Republic of South Africa. https://www.statssa.gov.za/publications/P0302/P03022015.pdf

43. Statistics South Africa. (2020). *Mid-year population estimates: 2019.* Republic of South Africa. https://www.statssa.gov.za/publications/P0302/P03022019.pdf

44. Statistiska Centralbyrån; SCB [Central Bureau of Statistics]. (2020, March). *Genomförandet av Agenda 2030 i Sverige Statistisk lägesbild 2019.* https://www.scb.se/contentassets/632aa89c7076419d8ec71340d738d761/mi1303_2019a01_br_x41br1902.pdf

45. Tortstensson, S. (2022, April 19.). *Befolkningsstruktur.* Ekonomifakta. https://www.ekonomifakta.se/Fakta/Arbetsmarknad/Befolkning/Befolkningsstruktur/

46. UNICEF. (2021, December). *Under-five mortality.* https://data.unicef.org/topic/child-survival/under-five-mortality/

47. United Nations. (1989). *Human rights: Convention on the rights of the child.* https://treaties.un.org/pages/ViewDetails.aspx?src=IND&mtdsg_no=IV-11&chapter=4&clang=_en

48. United Nations, Department of Economic and Social Affairs, Population Division. (2019). *World population prospects 2019: Highlights.* https://population.un.org/wpp/Publications/Files/WPP2019_Highlights.pdf

49. Vårdfokus. (2021). *Trafiken och självmord vanligaste dödsorsakerna bland barn.* Hämtat från. https://www.vardfokus.se/barn-och-ungdom/trafiken-och-sjalvmord-vanligaste-dodsorsakerna-bland-barn/

50. VZinfo.nl. (n.d.). *Letsel informatie system.* https://bronnen.zorggegevens.nl/Bron?naam=Letsel-Informatie-Systeem

51. World Bank Group. (2022). *Life expectancy at birth, total (years).* https://data.worldbank.org/indicator/SP.DYN.LE00.IN

52. World Bank Group. (2022). *Population ages 0–14 (% of total population).* https://data.worldbank.org/indicator/SP.POP.0014.TO.ZS?view=chart

53. World Health Organization. (2019). *Mortality among children aged 5–14 years* [Fact sheet]. https://www.who.int/news-room/fact-sheets/detail/mortality-among-children-aged-5-14-years

54. World Health Organization. (2020). *Children: Improving survival and well-being* [Fact sheet]. https://www.who.int/news-room/fact-sheets/detail/children-reducing-mortality

55. World Health Organization (2020). *Children: New threats to health* [Fact sheet]. https://www.who.int/news-room/fact-sheets/detail/children-new-threats-to-health

56. World Health Organization. (2021). *Childhood cancer* [Fact sheet]. https://www.who.int/news-room/fact-sheets/detail/cancer-in-children

57. World Health Organization (2022). *Child mortality (under 5 years)* [Fact sheet]. https://www.who.int/news-room/fact-sheets/detail/levels-and-trends-in-child-under-5-mortality-in-2020

58. World Health Organization. (2022). *Newborn mortality* [Fact sheet]. https://www.who.int/news-room/fact-sheets/detail/levels-and-trends-in-child-mortality-report-2021

59. Worldometer. (n.d.). *South Africa demographics.* https://www.worldometers.info/demographics/south-africa-demographics/

60. You, D. (2021). Demographic challenges and opportunities for child health programming in Africa and Asia. *BMJ, 372,* Article 19. https://doi.org/10.1136/bmj.n19

Preparing for Pediatric Emergencies

Robin Goodman, MSN, RN, CPEN

OBJECTIVES

Upon completion of this chapter, the learner will be able to:

1. Define *pediatric readiness*.
2. Identify four structural and/or process measures that can be implemented to improve pediatric emergency care.
3. Discuss the role of the pediatric emergency care coordinator and how it can impact pediatric emergency care.
4. Describe two examples of how to incorporate family-centered care.

Introduction

Pediatric patients account for more than 27 million total visits to emergency departments (EDs) each year, which represents approximately 20% of all ED visits in the United States.[7] The majority of these visits occur in community, rural, and critical access EDs that see fewer than 15 pediatric patients per day.[24,56] Children have different developmental, physiologic, anatomic, and medical needs than adults. EDs must integrate these unique pediatric characteristics and considerations into their policies, care guidelines, training, education, supplies, equipment, and quality improvement initiatives to care for children effectively.[58] The vulnerability of children necessitates population-specific, accessible, safe, and high-quality pediatric emergency care.

Background and History

Emergency medical services (EMS) were initially designed to address adult morbidity and mortality.[38] Thus, there was a failure within these systems to recognize the unique needs of ill and injured pediatric patients. Beginning in 1972, pediatric champions such as doctors Calvin Sia and James Seidel and U.S. Senators Daniel Inouye, Orrin Hatch, and Lowell Weicker created increased awareness of the needs of pediatric patients and a lack of pediatric training and equipment within the EMS space. Their work led to the passage of the Emergency Medical Services for Children (EMSC) legislation in 1984. This legislation created funding for state programs to improve emergency care provided to children with life-threatening illness or injury. Administered by the Health Resources and Service Administration's Mother and Child Health Bureau, the EMSC program is the only federally funded program dedicated to ensuring that pediatric patients receive high-quality emergency care throughout the United States and its territories.

Guidelines for Pediatric Care

Following the creation of the EMSC program and efforts to improve pediatric emergency care, disparities in care continued. Published reports in 1993 and 2007 described the variability of pediatric emergency care throughout the United States, with factors such as geographic location, existence of organized trauma systems, and training requirements identified as directly impacting patient outcomes.[38] To improve pediatric patient care and safety, the National Academy of Sciences (formerly called the Institute of Medicine) made recommendations for emergency care systems to implement measures to reduce disparities in pediatric emergency care. These recommendations included incorporating pediatric considerations when developing standards for care and equipment, disaster plans, training programs, and performance measures (**Table 2-1**)[17] and appointing two pediatric emergency care coordinators (PECCs), with one being a physician, to coordinate pediatric-specific activities within an ED.[37]

While the EMSC performance measures evaluate the overall progress of the EMSC program at the state and national levels, pediatric-focused quality improvement (QI) initiatives can be used to measure the safety and efficacy of care provided to pediatric patients presenting to an ED.[26] Pediatric-specific performance measures, such as obtaining and recording weight in kilograms and adhering to evidence-based guidelines when caring for pediatric patients with septic shock, bronchiolitis, asthma, and closed head injury, are examples of metrics that should be included in an ED's overall QI or performance improvement (PI) plan.[58]

Many tools have been developed to improve quality. Some help identify causes of performance issues, whereas others are designed to implement change. Any QI project requires an end evaluation to determine if the changes made actually improved performance. **Table 2-2** provides examples of QI tools.[39]

TABLE 2-1 Summary of 2017 EMSC Performance Measures	
Measure	**Description**
EMSC 01	The degree to which EMS agencies submit data that comply with the National Emergency Medical Services Information System (NEMSIS), version 3.x, to the state EMS office.
EMSC 02	The percentage of EMS agencies in the state or territory that have a designated individual who coordinates pediatric emergency care.
EMSC 03	The percentage of EMS agencies in the state or territory that have a process that requires EMS providers to physically demonstrate the correct use of pediatric-specific equipment.
EMSC 04	The percentage of hospitals with an ED recognized through a statewide, territorial, or regional standardized program that are able to stabilize and/or manage pediatric medical emergencies.
EMSC 05	The percentage of hospitals with an ED recognized through a statewide, territorial, or regional standardized system that are able to stabilize and/or manage pediatric trauma.
EMSC 06	The percentage of hospitals with an ED in the state or territory that have written interfacility transfer guidelines that cover pediatric patients.
EMSC 07	The percentage of hospitals with an ED in the state or territory that have written interfacility transfer agreements that cover pediatric patients.
EMSC 08	The degree to which the state or territory has established permanence of EMSC in the state or territory EMS system.
EMSC 09	The degree to which the state/territory has established permanence of EMSC in the state/territory EMS system by integrating EMSC priorities into statutes/regulations.

Data from Emergency Medical Services for Children Innovation and Improvement Center. (2018). *EMS for children (EMSC) performance measures*. https://dph.illinois.gov/sites/default/files/resources/2018_PM_FactSheet20180110.pdf

The American Academy of Pediatrics (AAP), American College of Emergency Physicians (ACEP), American College of Surgeons Committee on Trauma (ACS COT), Emergency Nurses Association (ENA), National Association of EMS Physicians (NAEMSP), National Association of EMT Professionals (NAEMT), and National Association of State EMS Officials (NASEMSO) have all established sections that work collaboratively and in conjunction with the EMSC program to support pediatric care throughout their broad networks. In addition, AAP, ACEP, and ENA released a joint policy statement, "Guidelines for the Care of Children in the Emergency Department" in 2009 and an updated joint policy statement, "Pediatric Readiness in the Emergency Department," in 2018.[3,58]

TABLE 2-2 Commonly Used Quality Improvement Tools	
Tool	**Use and Characteristics**
Affinity diagrams	Allow for organization and brainstorming of ideas into groupings for confusing or difficult issues.
Checklists	Straightforward but powerful tool to assure consistent implementation of a change.
Control chart	Method to display data over time and determine when variability exceeds the expected randomness based on common probability rules of variation and trends.
DMAIC (define, measure, analyze, improve, control)	Common project structure for a Six Sigma improvement effort that lays out the steps of an improvement process.
Failure mode and effects analysis	Analysis of a process to examine the modes in which an error might occur or a step may fail. Quality improvement work focuses on implementing a mitigation plan based on the analysis.
Fishbone diagram	A graphic representation of the inputs to a particular problem. Common part of a root cause analysis. Each input is broken into possible causes for the input.
Gemba exercise	To "go and see." The direct observation of actual operations in the real-world environment to understand a process. Observations usually have a specific focus (i.e., identifying waste in a process).
Kaizen event	Group working for a fixed time and focusing on a specific improvement while using Lean principles.
Pareto analysis	Typically a bar chart in which items or problems are listed in order of importance of frequency. Based on the principle that 80% of errors are caused by only 20% of all factors.
PDSA cycles	Cycles of improvement focused on small incremental changes. Consists of four steps: Plan, Do, Study, and Act.
Run chart	Graph of data over time to assess the effectiveness of change. Does not use control limits, and cannot make conclusions if the process is stable or if change is from expected or unexpected variation.
Six Sigma approach	Improvement approach using many quantitative tools with an intent focus on quality and reducing variation.
SMART goals	Acronym for effective goals meeting the requirements of being Specific, Measurable, Attainable, Relevant, and Time-Bound.

Reproduced from Iyer, S., & Stone, E. (2018). Pediatric quality improvement in the prehospital and emergency department worlds: Tools and examples to guide change. *Clinical Pediatric Emergency Medicine, 19*(3), 199–205. https://doi.org/10.1016/j.cpem.2018.09.002

These resources provide expanded recommendations to better prepare EDs to care for children. They identify seven pediatric readiness areas of focus:

- Administration and coordination of pediatric care in the ED
- Competencies for physicians, advanced practice providers, nurses, and other ED healthcare providers
- Pediatric emergency care quality improvement and/or performance improvement
- Policies, procedures, and protocols for the ED
- Pediatric patient and medication safety in the ED
- Support services for the ED
- Equipment, supplies, and medications for the care of children

National Pediatric Readiness Projects

The National Pediatric Readiness Project (NPRP) is a QI initiative that was formed between EMSC, AAP, ACEP, and ENA to address needed ED improvements in pediatric readiness.[24] Facilities that are considered "pediatric ready" have the processes, staff, and equipment necessary to care for children and the capability to recognize when a child may benefit from specialized care.[46] The goal of the NPRP is to ensure that all U.S. EDs have the essential guidelines and resources needed to provide effective emergency care

to children.[15] The initial step for the NPRP was an assessment of EDs in all 50 states and U.S. territories to determine compliance with the 2009 Joint Policy Statement,[3] identify gaps in and barriers to implementing pediatric readiness recommendations, and evaluate the effectiveness of nurse and physician PECCs in ensuring pediatric readiness. Since its inception in 2013, the NPRP has grown beyond an assessment tool and now provides open access comprehensive resources and training for EDs to utilize to improve the care of pediatric patients. **Figure 2-1** identifies the components of pediatric readiness.[13]

Research from the 2013 NPRP assessment found the following:

- The national median readiness score was 69 out of 100, indicating that many EDs were lacking key components of pediatric readiness.[5,24]
- A majority of the EDs surveyed did not have policies in place to care for pediatric patients with mental health conditions.[33]
- A majority of children live more than 30 miles from a facility with a high pediatric readiness score, contributing to geographic disparities in care.[55]
- Facilities with a designated PECC were associated with improved pediatric readiness scores and improved patient outcomes.[24,59]
- Children with critical illness had an increased risk of death when they presented to a hospital with a lower pediatric readiness score.[5]

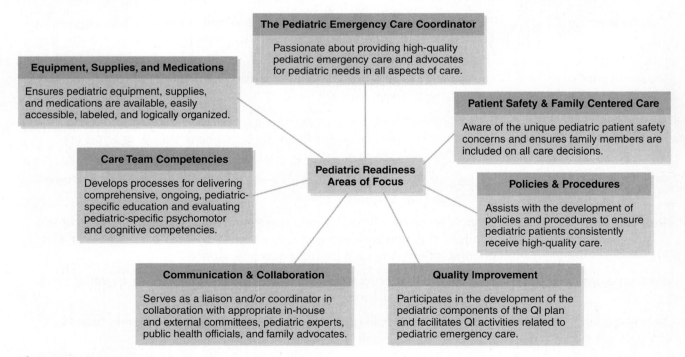

Figure 2-1 *Seven pediatric readiness areas of focus.*

Reproduced from Emergency Medical Services for Children Innovation and Improvement Center. (n.d.). *How it works.* https://emscimprovement.center/collaboratives/pwdc/howitworks/

- Children with critical illness treated in a facility with a high readiness score had a fourfold lower rate of mortality than those treated at facilities with lower readiness scores. Thus, improving pediatric readiness improves outcomes for children and their families.[15]

At the time of this writing, the 2021 NPRP assessment was not yet available but will be able to be found at https://emscimprovement.center/domains/pediatric-readiness-project/.

International Pediatric Emergency Care

Reduction of childhood mortality remains a global priority and has resulted in a reduction in pediatric deaths internationally.[41] Similar to the case in the United States, pediatric emergency care worldwide lags behind the standards of care provided to adult patients.[32,51] In recent years, there has been a shift internationally toward an increase in trauma-related pediatric deaths and a decline in pediatric deaths resulting from poor nutrition and illness. Organizations such as the International Federation of Emergency Medicine (IFEM), the African Federation of Emergency Medicine (AFEM), and the World Health Organization (WHO) have created standards and guidelines for the care of pediatric patients that can be modified based on local resources.[41,51]

A survey assessing pediatric readiness of EDs in 21 European countries found that 95% fulfilled more than 50% of the IFEM essential standards of care. Areas that were scored lower in the survey were linked to inadequate staffing, safety, and quality measures, along with care of pediatric mental health patients and management of major incidents.[44] Association with a multicenter international research network was found to be positively related to level of pediatric preparedness.

Disaster Planning

Incorporating the needs of children into every phase of disaster planning was identified by the National Academy of Sciences as a priority recommendation when addressing the disparities in pediatric emergency care.[4,37] For disaster plans to be successfully operationalized, the unique needs of children call for day-to-day pediatric readiness[43] as a means to ensure overall pediatric patient safety if and when a disaster occurs.[24,27] Disaster triage systems that include the assessment of pediatric patients, resources on the decontamination process of children, and just-in-time resources for care and support of children during a disaster are a few examples of ways that pediatric needs can be integrated into disaster plans.[4] Additionally, since more than 60 million children are separated from their families during the normal course of

a day (e.g., in schools and daycare centers) and disasters can occur at any time, facilities must have a process in place to reconnect children with their families. Facilities should include family information centers, family reunification processes, and policies for care of unaccompanied minors in their disaster planning to successfully reunite children with their families during disasters.[31]

> ### NOTE
>
> **EIIC Pediatric Disaster Preparedness**
>
> The Pediatric Disaster Preparedness Toolkit includes links to a variety of resources for healthcare professionals, families, and caregivers. Sample policy templates, tabletop exercises, articles, and other resources are available from https://emscimprovement.center/domains/preparedness/. The Pediatric Pandemic Network is a new collaborative effort funded by HRSA to improve pediatric disaster care in everyday emergencies, disasters, and global health threats.

Role of the Emergency Nurse and Pediatric Readiness

Emergency nurses care for patients throughout the age continuum and must have resources and clinical competencies to provide emergency stabilization and safe, effective care for pediatric patients.[22] The Emergency Nursing Pediatric Course (ENPC) was launched in 1993 to meet the need for pediatric emergency nursing education. ENPC is taught internationally and continues to be the minimum standard for education for emergency nurses to prepare them to recognize the unique physiologic and anatomical differences that increase the risk of rapid deterioration when a pediatric patient is ill or injured. Key points from ENA's position statement, *The Emergency Nurses Role in Supporting Pediatric Readiness in the Emergency Department*,[22] include the following:

- All EDs have a professional and ethical responsibility to be prepared to deliver life- and limb-saving care and stabilization to pediatric patients just as they do for adult patients.
- Identification of a nurse PECC is central to the readiness of any ED that cares for pediatric patients.
- ED performance improvement plans include pediatric-specific indicators.
- All EDs (hospital based and freestanding) must maintain appropriately sized equipment and supplies to provide quality care for children of all ages.

The Family

A key component of providing high-quality pediatric care is understanding the significant role that the family plays in the pediatric patient's life. Pediatric patient- and family-centered care (PFCC) acknowledges the unique behavioral and developmental needs of children and the fundamental role of the family when caring for the pediatric patient.[11] PFCC creates partnerships between the healthcare team and the patient and family, recognizing that working with patients and families leads to improved patient outcomes, enhanced patient and family experiences, wiser allocation of resources, and heightened clinician and staff satisfaction.[36] Healthcare systems have recognized that increasing patient and family engagement and presence is a central element in ensuring the delivery of high-quality care.[19,54] ENA's *Patient-and Family-Centered Care for Children in the Emergency Department: A Self-Assessment Tool* is an instrument all EDs can use to evaluate their readiness to effectively care for pediatric patients and their families.[20] This tool is based on the integration of PFCC core concepts[20,36]:

- *Dignity and respect.* Patient and family perspectives and choice are honored by the healthcare team. Patient and family knowledge, values, beliefs, and cultural backgrounds are incorporated into the planning and delivery of care.
- *Information sharing.* Healthcare practitioners communicate and share complete and unbiased information with patients and families in ways that are affirming and useful. Patients and families receive timely, complete, and accurate information so that they can effectively participate in care and decision making.
- *Participation.* Patients and families are encouraged and supported in participating in care and decision making at the level they choose.
- *Collaboration.* Patients, families, healthcare practitioners, and healthcare leaders collaborate in policy

---

NOTE

Resources for Patient- and Family-Centered Care

Resources available include the following:

- Institute for Patient- and Family-Centered Care website: https://www.ipfcc.org
- Self-assessment tool for ED PFCC from ENA: https://enau.ena.org/Users/LearningActivityAssetSingleViewer.aspx?LearningActivityAssetID=E6b6limqQg8L6yZTHnbRow%3d%3d

---

and program development, implementation, and evaluation; in facility design; in professional education; in research; as well as in the delivery of care.

Definition of Family

A key principle in PFCC is understanding that "family" is defined by the patient and is their primary source of support. The term *family* has evolved over time to include many different configurations and definitions. Family is ultimately self-defined; it is what each individual considers it to be, and it is the child's primary resource. The structure of a family and the dynamics within it can have long-term influences on a child's health and well-being.

For most families, taking a child to the ED can be a major source of stress, capable of reducing normal coping mechanisms in even the calmest of adults. Children can be affected by how their family members respond to situations. For example, worried caregivers can become emotional, angry, or even confrontational. Children often sense distrust and fear and may also reflect these qualities themselves. Employing a PFCC approach can mitigate some of these negative responses and foster a therapeutic partnership in the child's care.

Recognition of Family Diversity

Identifying a caregiver with the authority to consent to the child's care is a priority in the triage process unless there is an immediate threat to life. The person accompanying the child might not be the child's legal guardian. Asking the simple question "How are you related?" is completely reasonable, especially if asked in an open, nonthreatening manner. Sorting out relationships between the patient and the people accompanying the patient is an important and legally necessary step.

In the United States, 70% of children live in a two-parent household, but 35% also live with other adults who are not their parents, and 4% live with neither parent.[63] In the member countries of the Organisation for Economic Co-operation and Development, the percentage of children living in a two-parent household ranges from 70% to 90%.[49] In the United Kingdom, 79% to 85% of children live in a two-parent household. While multifamily households represent only 1% of U.K. households, they are the fastest-growing type of household.[48]

Grandparents, aunts, uncles, cousins, older siblings, family friends, and nonmarried partners of the child's legal guardian may accompany the child to the ED. The acceptance of family diversity continues to expand. Same-sex marriage is now legal in 29 countries.[34] Same-sex adoption still faces some challenges but is receiving more support.[42] Do not make assumptions about the family structure based on age, gender, skin color, or ethnicity. Understanding the family structure and culture maximizes the nurse's ability to engage the family in the child's care.

Consent

Consent for treatment may be either expressed (communicated verbally or written) or implied (such as in an emergency when the patient is unable to communicate). A parent or legal guardian is usually required to provide consent for a child's treatment. The challenge is to determine if the adult who brought the child to the ED is the patient's legal guardian. If the adult is not the legal guardian, phone consent is often obtained per organizational policy. In addition, in some circumstances minors are legally able to seek care and consent for treatment themselves. **Box 2-1** provides examples of possible allowances for minor consent. Pediatric consent requires the nurse to identify how the adult(s) present are related to the child, have awareness of state and local laws, and comply with facility policies.[62]

BOX 2-1 Possible Allowances for Minor Consent

Minor consent laws vary. Be familiar with the current regional statues and facility policy. Though they are often based on age (12 to 14 years is common), exceptions *may* include the following circumstances:

- Contraceptives
- Emancipation
- Marital status
- Medical care for the minor's child
- Mental health
- Military service
- Pregnancy status (is pregnant or has given birth)
- Prenatal care
- Sexual health
- Substance dependency or use

While dated, this 2013 document from the National District Attorneys Association is a compilation of state statutes for minor consent: https://ndaa.org/wp-content/uploads/Minor-Consent-to-Medical-Treatment-2.pdf. Other lists of pediatric statutes are also available from https://ndaa.org/programs/child-abuse/state-statutes/.

Data from National District Attorneys Association. (2013). *Minor consent to medical treatment laws.* https://ndaa.org/wp-content/uploads/Minor-Consent-to-Medical-Treatment-2.pdf

---

Diversity, Equity, and Inclusion Considerations

Researchers utilizing the PFCC principles of dignity and respect have demonstrated how bias, both implicit and explicit, can contribute to the experience of racism and discrimination in the child or adolescent seeking healthcare.[53] It is crucial that emergency nurses understand the impact that culture has on essential emergency interactions. Providing affirming and inclusive care plays an important role in improving health outcomes and quality. Stereotyping and inequities have been found throughout the continuum of pediatric emergency care, including triage, pain assessment and management, general care, and admission practices.[12,30,65] Housing insecurity, language barriers, reliance on caregivers and healthcare team members to communicate needs, poor access to subspecialist care for persons in rural areas, and reduced access to primary care providers are additional equity considerations the nurse must consider when caring for children and their families.[7] Emergency nurses must work toward creating a culture and environment that welcomes all patients and their families. Creating an evaluation process that includes input from pediatric patients and their families, identifies inequities in care, and encourages advocacy for the inclusion of a patient's cultural beliefs and gender identity will increase an ED's ability to meet this vulnerable population's needs.[11,40]

Nurses are responsible for acknowledging the need to correct bias and inequity that often stem from skin color, socioeconomic status, family structure, language, and many other factors. Physical assessment and nursing interventions should be tailored to best meet the needs of an increasingly diverse patient population. See Chapter 4, "Prioritization," and Chapter 5, "Initial Assessment: The Pediatric Nursing Process," for more specific details about nursing process adaptations to promote equitable care.

Health Promotion and Injury Prevention

Each time a child and their family visit an ED, there is an opportunity to discuss health promotion and injury prevention topics.[61] The 2018 joint policy statement *Pediatric Readiness in the Emergency Department* highlighted the need for these discussions to occur throughout the ED visit as well as to ensure that they are incorporated into quality plans and community outreach and advocacy programs.[58] Despite the work that has been done to decrease injuries in children, injury remains the leading cause of death in children older than 1 year and is a source of significant morbidity and healthcare costs.[6]

Integration of health promotion and child injury prevention strategies, in addition to use of screening tools such as HEAD-ED for adolescent patients[8] (**Table 2-3**), creates a comprehensive approach to the health and development of children and can be completed during various interactions throughout the ED visit.[9,21,29,61] Engaging children in these discussions increases their awareness of healthy practices and injury prevention

TABLE 2-3 The HEADS-ED Screening Tool			
	0 **No action needed**	**1** **Needs action but not immediate/moderate functional impairment**	**2** **Needs immediate action/severe functional impairment**
Home Example: How does your family get along with each other?			
Education, employment Example: How is your school attendance? How are your grades? Are your working?			
Activities and peers Example: What are your relationships like with your friends?			
Drugs and alcohol Example: How often are you using drugs or alcohol?			
Suicidality Example: Do you have any thoughts of wanting to kill yourself?			
Emotions, behaviors, thought disturbance Example: How have you been feeling lately?			
Discharge or current resources Example: Do you have any help or are you waiting to receive help (counseling, other)?			

HEADS-ED is a screening tool and is not intended to replace clinical judgment.

Scoring: Items can be evaluated independently of need for action. To obtain a score, add the value of each item together. Referral for a specialized mental health assessment should be considered if the total sum score is ≥8 and the "Suicidality" item is rated as a 2. See https://www.heads-ed.com/en/home for more details.

Data from Cappelli, M., Gray, C., Zemek, R., Cloutier, P., Kennedy, A., Glennie, E., Doucet, G., & Lyons, J. S. (2012). The HEADS-ED: A rapid mental health screening tool for pediatric patients in the emergency department. *Pediatrics, 130*(2), e321–e327. https://doi.org/10.1542/peds.2011-3798

from an early age and empowers pediatric patients to be participants in their own care. Various modalities for dissemination could include third-party or ED/facility-created videos, discussions, and digital and paper pamphlets that include information and links to vetted resources. Topics to start discussions could include the following:

- Nutrition/food: Ask about favorite foods, with a focus on how options improve health rather than being good or bad choices.
- Activity safety: What color is the child's helmet or how fast do they think they can get their seat belt on? What kind of car seat do they have and where/how is it positioned? Has the parent considered routinely placing an often-used item such as a phone or purse next to the car seat to prevent inadvertently leaving the child in a hot car?
- Home safety: Have the parents anticipated the child's ability to access medications, firearms, candles, or other potential hazards as the child becomes more mobile? Are smoke alarms present and tested? Does the child know two ways to escape from every room in the house if there is a fire?
- Personal safety: For children with special healthcare needs, ask them about their medical condition and medications, if they are able to answer such questions. Ask about personal relationships with family, friends, and partners. What is the safest thing for the child to do if inadvertently separated from their caregivers? Is the child aware of where they live and/or the phone number of a trusted adult?
- Health safety: Review immunization status and overall management of health and/or medical conditions. Promote awareness of safe sleep initiatives for infants.[2]
- Physical activity: Explore activity level, with the understanding that not all patients and families have a safe, outdoor area to be active in, and discuss alternatives. Does the child like to swim or run? What level of supervision and/or protective equipment is recommended based on the child's age and the specific activity?
- Resources: Provide phone numbers for the poison control center and suicide and/or mental health support services. Connect the caregivers with local resources for injury prevention initiatives.

When these conversations occur throughout the visit, it allows for the ED nurse to provide education and information in smaller, more digestible segments rather than just during the patient's discharge, which can overwhelm patients and families. These discussions can also assist the nurse in determining if the patient and family need referrals for housing and/or food insecurity, safety concerns, social and support services, mental health services, establishment of a medical home, or changes in home healthcare needs.

Discharge Planning or Transfer to Definitive Care

Discharge planning or planning for transfer of the patient to definitive care should begin early in the pediatric patient's visit.[21] Most children who visit EDs are discharged home, highlighting the need for high-quality discharge education for this population.[10] Discussions or screening can occur during each patient and family interaction. Topics could include the patient's plan of care, patient/family needs, the ability of the parent to safely care for the patient at home, psychosocial needs, transportation needs, and the need for additional medical equipment and/or medications. Determining the needs of the patient and family early in the visit enables the focus at discharge to be on the discharge instructions and education related to the reason for the ED visit.

Communication strategies such as Ask Me 3[35] (**Box 2-2**) and Teach Back[1] (**Box 2-3**) have been shown to improve parent comprehension of discharge instructions, increase adherence to treatment plans, reduce unnecessary return visits, improve health outcomes for children, and improve health literacy.[10,11] Utilization of pictogram-based instruction sheets has also been shown to decrease error rates.[28]

BOX 2-2 Ask Me 3

The Institute for Healthcare Improvement provides guidance to patients and families intended to increase their participation in their healthcare and improve communications. Complementary educational materials are available.

The three questions are:

1. What is my main problem?
2. What do I need to do?
3. Why is it important for me to do this?

Institute for Healthcare Improvement. (2021). *Ask me 3: Good questions for your good health.* Retrieved September 14, 2021, from http://www.ihi.org/resources/Pages/Tools/Ask-Me-3-Good-Questions-for-Your-Good-Health.aspx

BOX 2-3 Teach Back

Studies have shown that 40% to 80% of the information given to patients is forgotten immediately and nearly 50% is remembered incorrectly. The teach-back method, however, can improve patient comprehension, adherence, satisfaction, and outcomes. After providing the patient and family with any instructions, use variations on the following phrases to help assess their understanding. These can be prefaced with "This was a lot of information. I want to be sure that I explained things well."

- Describe the three things you will do within the next two days.
- Can you show me how you are going to [administer the medication, clean the wound]?
- In your own words, tell me what signs and symptoms you will watch out for.
- When should you come back to the emergency department?

Other techniques include the following:

- Highlight handouts during the teach-back session.
- Use clear, plain language.
- Make eye contact and sit at eye level.
- Use a caring—not testing or judging—tone of voice.

Data from Agency for Healthcare Research and Quality. (2020). Use the teach-back method: Tool #5. *Health literacy universal precautions toolkit* (2nd ed.). https://www.ahrq.gov/health-literacy/improve/precautions/tool5.html

Assessing the patient's discharge readiness includes a review of the discharge instructions for completeness (e.g., clinical condition, new medications and/or changes to home medications, signs and symptoms indicating the need to return to the ED, follow-up appointment information, focused care needs such as dressing/wound care, home health contacts). Ensuring discharge readiness also includes a full reassessment of the patient's primary and focused assessment, pain, and effectiveness of interventions. Vital signs are taken to ensure they are within normal parameters for age. To decrease barriers to continuity of care and adherence to discharge instructions, the patient and family are provided with a paper copy of the discharge instructions to reference once discharged and to share with their primary care or subspecialty providers who may not have access to the ED's electronic medical record system.

Transfer to Definitive Care

Nearly 90% of the children who seek care in EDs throughout the United States are seen in nonpediatric hospitals, where pediatric subspecialty services are not available.[60] To help bridge this gap and maximize positive outcomes for pediatric patients, nonpediatric facilities should have written transfer agreements and relationships with pediatric referral centers. Early recognition of the need to transfer the pediatric patient, effective communication with the receiving center, and establishment of interfacility transfer agreements and guidelines are key components of pediatric readiness.

Regional Transfer Agreements and Guidelines

Interfacility transfer agreements are written contracts between a referring facility (such as a community hospital) and a specialized pediatric center or a facility with a higher level of care and/or appropriate resources for the child. These agreements must formalize arrangements for consultation and transport of a pediatric patient to the facility offering a higher level of care.

Interfacility transfer guidelines are developed between hospitals—including out-of-state/territory facilities—and outline procedural and administrative policies for transferring critically ill pediatric patients to facilities with the resources to provide specialized pediatric care. Specific components of a transfer include the following[14]:

- A defined process for timely initiation of a transfer, including the roles and responsibilities of the referring facility and the referral center (including responsibilities for requesting transfer and communication)
- The process for selecting the appropriate care facility
- Consideration of a verified pediatric center to increase the probability of improved outcomes and survival[45]
- The process for selecting the appropriately staffed transport service to match the patient's acuity level (e.g., level of care required by the patient, equipment needed during the transport)
- The process for patient transfer (including obtaining informed consent)
- Plan for transfer of the patient's medical records, including imaging studies
- Plan for transfer of a copy of the signed transport consent
- Plan for transfer of the patient's personal belongings
- Plan for provision of directions and referral institution information to the family

Transfer Responsibilities

In the United States, transfers of unstable patients must be done in accordance with the provisions in the Emergency Medical Treatment and Active Labor Act (EMTALA), which was passed by Congress in 1986. Under EMTALA, patients who present to an ED for care, including newly born infants, must be provided with a medical screening exam to determine whether a medical emergency exists; the ED must provide care for the patient until either the situation resolves or the patient's condition has been stabilized within the facility's capacity and capabilities. If the patient's condition exceeds the facility's capabilities, the patient can be transferred, as long as this transfer is done in accordance with the EMTALA regulations. EMTALA does not apply to the transfer of stable patients. When transferring an unstable patient, EMTLA requires the referring facility to do the following:

- Ensure a physician, or designee as defined by facility rules or regulations, certifies that the medical benefits expected from the transfer outweigh the risks *or* arranges transfer at the patient's or family's request after being informed of the hospital's obligations under EMTALA and the risks of transfer.
- Continue to provide care within its capabilities until the transfer occurs to minimize transfer risks.
- Provide copies of medical records.
- Confirm that the receiving facility has space and qualified personnel to treat the condition and has agreed to accept the transfer.
- Arrange to transfer the patient with qualified personnel and appropriate medical equipment for the patient's condition. When requesting transport services, special considerations such as the need for a neonatal transport team, use of emergency child restraint systems, ability of the family to accompany the patient, and need for bariatric or mental health transport services should be communicated.

Under EMTALA, hospitals with specialized services are obligated to accept transfers from other U.S. hospitals when the referring facility does not have the capability to treat unstable emergency medical conditions. Internationally, transfer responsibilities and regulations vary widely. Noncitizens might be required to pay before receiving any healthcare services. Travelers may purchase insurance to cover healthcare costs and medical transport back to their home country in the event of injury or illness.

Emerging Trends

Emerging trends in readiness for pediatric emergencies are concerned with pediatric trauma, facility recognition programs, and the Prehospital Pediatric Readiness Project.

Pediatric Trauma

Continued work needs to be done in trauma centers to improve pediatric readiness in these facilities that care for the most critically injured children. A trauma center designation has been found to not equate to a high pediatric readiness score.[47] Gaps in readiness identified in trauma centers include lack of interfacility transfer agreements for pediatric patients, failure to weigh children in kilograms, lack of pediatric-specific QI metrics, and lack of comfort with some pediatric trauma-specific protocols.[26,57] Beginning in 2022, the American College of Surgeons (ACS) required that all ACS-verified adult and pediatric trauma centers complete the NPRP assessment, review their gap analysis, and create improvement plans to address identified gaps in an effort to improve their overall pediatric readiness.[18]

Pediatric Facility Recognition Programs

Pediatric facility recognition is based on national guidelines and identifies those EDs that adhere to a standard level of readiness for children. In the United States, 11 states have established standardized statewide systems to promote pediatric preparedness of EDs.[58] Facilities that have been formally recognized as meeting such standards are associated with higher pediatric readiness.[64] Critical access hospitals that participated in facility recognition programs were found to have higher median readiness scores (84.3) compared to those not participating (59.5) in a facility recognition program.[52]

Prehospital Pediatric Readiness Project

The goal of the Prehospital Pediatric Readiness Project (PPRP) is to integrate pediatric readiness principles into the prehospital care of children to improve the overall system of emergency care. Pediatric patients account for approximately 10% of EMS volume, and the PPRP focuses on ensuring that EMS agencies have the appropriate equipment, supplies, training, education, physician oversight, and policies to effectively provide emergency care to pediatric patients.[16,50] Goals for this program include improving pediatric care outcomes and safety within the prehospital environment.

Summary

Initiatives such as the NPRP continue to demonstrate progress toward improving ED pediatric readiness globally. Continued readiness efforts are needed to ensure that all critically ill and injured children have access to timely, well-resourced, and effective emergency care regardless of where they reside.[5] Identifying an ED nurse PECC can strongly affect pediatric emergency nursing care. The PECC can improve outcomes by overseeing nursing-based aspects of pediatric preparedness such as incorporating principles of PFCC; assessment and care of the pediatric patient; health promotion/injury prevention activities; disaster planning; best practices for the safe disposition of the pediatric patient to include transfer, admission, or discharge; and incorporation of pediatric performance measures into QI plans. Partnering with local emergency medical services and neighboring hospitals to create a community of readiness further improves outcomes for ill and injured children and reduces the fragmented and uneven care that currently exists in some parts of the world.[23,51]

References

1. Agency for Healthcare Research and Quality. (2020). Use the teach-back method: Tool #5. *Health literacy universal precautions toolkit* (2nd ed.). https://www.ahrq.gov/health-literacy/improve/precautions/tool5.html

2. American Academy of Pediatrics. (2016). SIDS and other sleep-related infant deaths: Updated 2016 recommendations for a safe infant sleeping environment. *Pediatrics, 138*(5). https://doi.org/10.1542/peds.2016-2938

3. American Academy of Pediatrics Committee on Pediatric Emergency Medicine, American College of Emergency Physicians Pediatric Committee, & Emergency Nurses Association Pediatric Committee. (2009). Joint policy statement: Guidelines for care of children in the emergency department. *Annals of Emergency Medicine, 54*(4), 543–552. https://doi.org/10.1016/j.annemergmed.2009.08.010

4. American Academy of Pediatrics, Disaster Preparedness Advisory Council, & Committee on Pediatric Emergency Medicine. (2015). Ensuring the health of children in disasters. *Pediatrics, 136*(5). https://doi.org/10.1542/peds.2015-3112

5. Ames, S. G., Davis, B. S., Marin, J. R., Fink, E. L., Olson, L. M., Gausche-Hill, M., & Kahn, J. M. (2019). Emergency department pediatric readiness and mortality in critically ill children. *Pediatrics, 144*(3). https://doi.org/10.1542/peds.2019-0568

6. Attridge, M. M., Holmstrom, S. E., & Sheehan, K. M. (2020). Injury prevention opportunities in the pediatric emergency department. *Clinical Pediatric Emergency Medicine, 21*(1), Article 100761. https://doi.org/10.1016/j.cpem.2020.100761

7. Brown, K. M., Ackerman, A. D., Ruttan, T. K., & Snow, S. K. (2021). Access to optimal emergency care for children. *Pediatrics, 147*(5). https://doi.org/10.1542/peds.2021-050787

8. Cappelli, M., Gray, C., Zemek, R., Cappelli, M., Gray, C., Zemek, R., Cloutier, P., Kennedy, A., Glennie, E., Doucet, G., & Lyons. J. S. (2012). The HEADS-ED: A rapid mental health screening tool for pediatric patients in the emergency department. *Pediatrics, 130*(2), e321–e327._https://doi.org/10.1542/peds.2011-3798

9. Cappelli, M., Zemek, R., Polihronis, C., Thibedeau, N., Kennedy, A., Gray, C., Jabbour, M., Reid, S., & Clouteir, P. (2020). The HEADS-ED: Evaluating the clinical use of a brief, action-oriented, pediatric mental health screening tool. *Pediatric Emergency Care 36*(1), 9–15. https://journals.lww.com/pec-online/Abstract/2020/01000/The_HEADS_ED__Evaluating_the_Clinical_Use_of_a.2.aspx

10. Curran, J. A., Gallant, A. J., Zemek, R., Newton, A. S., Jabbour, M., Chorney, J., Murphy, A., Hartling, L., MacWilliams, K., Plint, A., MacPhee, S., Bishop, A., & Campbell, S. G. (2019). Discharge communication practices in pediatric emergency care: A systematic review and narrative synthesis. *Systematic Reviews, 8*(1). https://doi.org/10.1186/s13643-019-0995-7

11. Dudley, N., Ackerman, A., Brown, K. M., Snow, S. K., American Academy of Pediatrics Committee on Pediatric Emergency Medicine, American College of Emergency Physicians Pediatric Emergency Medicine Committee, & Emergency Nurses Association Pediatric Committee. (2015). Patient- and family-centered care of children in the emergency department. *Pediatrics, 135*(1), e255–e272. https://doi.org/10.1542/peds.2014-3424

12. Earp, B. D., Monrad, J. T., LaFrance, M., Bargh, J. A., Cohen, L. L., & Richeson, J. A. (2019). Featured article: Gender bias in pediatric pain assessment. *Journal of Pediatric Psychology, 44*(4), 403–414. https://doi.org/10.1093/jpepsy/jsy104

13. Emergency Medical Services for Children Innovation and Improvement Center. (n.d.). *How it works.* https://emscimprovement.center/collaboratives/pwdc/howitworks/

14. Emergency Medical Services for Children Innovation and Improvement Center. (n.d.). *Interfacility transfer toolkit.* https://emscimprovement.center/education-and-resources/toolkits/interfacility-transfer-toolbox/

15. Emergency Medical Services for Children Innovation and Improvement Center. (n.d.). *National Pediatric Readiness Project.* https://emscimprovement.center/domains/pediatric-readiness-project/

16. Emergency Medical Services for Children Innovation and Improvement Center. (n.d.). *Prehospital pediatric readiness.* https://emscimprovement.center/domains/prehospital-care/prehospital-pediatric-readiness/

17. Emergency Medical Services for Children Innovation and Improvement Center. (2018). *EMS for children (EMSC) performance measures.* https://media.emscimprovement.center/documents/2018_PM_FactSheet20180110.pdf

18. Emergency Medical Services for Children Innovation and Improvement Center. (2021). *Raising the bar for pediatric trauma care.* https://emscimprovement.center/news/raising-the-bar-for-pediatric-trauma-care-pulse/

19. Emergency Nurses Association. (2017). *Family presence during invasive procedures and resuscitation* [Clinical practice guideline]. https://enau.ena.org/Users/LearningActivityAssetSingleViewer.aspx?LearningActivityAssetID=SJG9pQGDjT3evvUgo5z1uw%3d%3d

20. Emergency Nurses Association. (2019). *Patient- and family-centered care for children in the emergency department: A self-assessment tool.* https://enau.ena.org/Users/LearningActivity

AssetSingleViewer.aspx?LearningActivityAssetID=E6b6limq Qg8L6yZTHnbRow%3d%3d

21. Emergency Nurses Association. (2019). *Safe discharge from the emergency department* [Position statement]. https://enau .ena.org/Users/LearningActivityAssetSingleViewer.aspx?Lear ningActivityAssetID=c2tXTjPFiLwS2ViBtfEVfg%3d%3d

22. Emergency Nurses Association. (2019). *The emergency nurse's role in supporting pediatric readiness* [Position statement]. https://enau.ena.org/Users/LearningActivityAssetSingle Viewer.aspx?LearningActivityAssetID=UlZgbBn2eiJb%2fde qy77q4A%3d%3d

23. Faris, G. W., Marcin, J. P., & Weinstein, E. (2018). The current state of the pediatric emergency medicine workforce and innovations to improve pediatric care. *Clinical Pediatric Emergency Medicine, 19*(3), 272–281. https://doi.org/10.1016/j .cpem.2018.08.003

24. Gausche-Hill, M., Ely, M., Schmuhl, P., Telford, R., Remick, K. E., Edgerton, E. A., & Olson, L. M. (2015). A national assessment of pediatric readiness of emergency departments. *JAMA Pediatrics, 169*(6), 527–534. https://doi.org/10.1001 /jamapediatrics.2015.138

25. Genovese, T. J., Roberts-Santana, C., & Wills, H. (2021). Pediatric trauma readiness: A trauma-specific assessment to complement the National Pediatric Readiness Project. *Pediatric Emergency Care.* https://doi.org/10.1097/PEC.0000000000002144

26. Genovesi, A. L., Edgerton, E. A., Ely, M., Hewes, H., & Olson, L. M. (2018). Getting more performance out of performance measures: The journey and impact of the EMS for Children Program. *Clinical Pediatric Emergency Medicine, 19*(3), 206–215. https://doi.org/10.1016/j.cpem.2018.08.009

27. Gilchrist, N., & Simpson, J. N. (2019). Pediatric disaster preparedness. *Current Opinion in Pediatrics, 31*(3), 306–311. https://doi.org/10.1097/mop.0000000000000750

28. Glick, A. F., Farkas, J. S., Nicholson, J., Dreyer, B. P., Fears, M., Bandera, C., Stolper, T., Gerber, N., & Yin, H. S. (2017). Parental management of discharge instructions: A systematic review. *Pediatrics, 140*(2). https://doi.org/10.1542/peds.2016-4165

29. Goldenring, J., & Cohen, E. (1988). Getting into adolescents heads. *Contemporary Pediatrics, 5*(7), 75–80.

30. Goyal, M. K., Johnson, T. J., Chamberlain, J. M., Cook, L., Webb, M., Drendel, A. L., Alessandrini, E., Bajaj, L., Lorch, S., Grundmeier, R. W., & Alpern, E. R. (2020). Racial and ethnic differences in emergency department pain management of children with fractures. *Pediatrics, 145*(5). https://doi. org/10.1542/peds.2019-3370

31. Gubbins, N., & Kaziny, B. D. (2018). The importance of family reunification in pediatric disaster planning. *Clinical Pediatric Emergency Medicine, 19*(3), 252–259. https://doi .org/10.1016/j.cpem.2018.08.007

32. Gutierrez, C., Gausche-Hill, M., & Lim, R. (2020). Standards of care for children in emergency departments: International Federation of Emergency Medicine Agenda for the Care of Children. *Western Journal of Emergency Medicine, 21*(3), 581–582. https://doi.org/10.5811/westjem.2020.2.46917

33. Hoffmann, J. A., & Foster, A. A. (2020). Ready or not, here I come: Emergency department readiness for pediatric mental health visits. *Pediatrics, 145*(6), Article e20193542. https://doi .org/10.1542/peds.2019-3542

34. Human Rights Campaign. (2021). *Marriage equality around the world.* https://www.hrc.org/resources/marriage-equality -around-the-world

35. Institute for Healthcare Improvement. (2021). *Ask Me 3: Good questions for your good health.* http://www.ihi.org/resources /Pages/Tools/Ask-Me-3-Good-Questions-for-Your-Good -Health.aspx

36. Institute for Patient- and Family-Centered Care. (n.d.). *Patient- and family-centered care.* https://www.ipfcc.org/about /pfcc.html

37. Institute of Medicine. (2006). The future of emergency care in the United States health system. *Academic Emergency Medicine, 13*(10), 1081–1085. https://doi.org/10.1197/j .aem.2006.07.011

38. Institute of Medicine. (2007). *Emergency care for children: Growing pains.* National Academies Press. https://doi.org /10.17226/11655

39. Iyer, S., & Stone, E. (2018). Pediatric quality improvement in the prehospital and emergency department worlds: Tools and examples to guide change. *Clinical Pediatric Emergency Medicine, 19*(3), 199–205. https://doi.org/10.1016/j.cpem.2018.09.002

40. Janeway, H., & Coli, C. J. (2020). Emergency care for transgender and gender-diverse children and adolescents. *Pediatric Emergency Medicine Practice, 17*(9), 1–20. https://www .ebmedicine.net/topics/ethics/transgender-gender-diverse -children

41. Kiragu, A. W., Dunlop, S. J., Mwarumba, N., Gidado, S., Adesina, A., Mwachiro, M., Gbadero, D. A., & Slusher, T. M. (2018). Pediatric trauma care in low resource settings: Challenges, opportunities, and solutions. *Frontiers in Pediatrics, 6*, Article 155. https://doi.org/10.3389/fped.2018.00155

42. Levine, S. (n.d.). *Adoption options overview.* Human Rights Campaign. https://www.hrc.org/resources/adoption-options -overview

43. Macias, C. G., & Remick, K. (2018). Emergency medical services for children: Creating everyday readiness to care for kids. *Clinical Pediatric Emergency Medicine, 19*(3), 193–198. https://doi.org/10.1016/j.cpem.2018.10.001

44. Mintegi, S., Maconochie, I. K., Waisman, Y., Titomanlio, L., Benito, J., Laribi, S., & Moll, H. (2021). Pediatric preparedness of European emergency departments: A multicenter international survey. *Pediatric Emergency Care. 37*(12), e1150–e1153. https://doi.org/10.1097/pec.0000000000001934

45. Myers, S. R., Branas, C. C., French, B., Nance, M. L., & Carr, B. G. (2019). A national analysis of pediatric trauma care utilization and outcomes in the United States. *Pediatric Emergency Care, 35*(1), 1–7. https://doi.org/10.1097/PEC .0000000000000902

46. National Emergency Medical Services for Children Data Analysis Resource Center. (2021, February 18). *Pediatric readiness.* https://www.nedarc.org/pedsReady/index.html

47. Newgard, C. D., Lin, A., Olson, L. M., Cook, J., Gausche-Hill, M., Kuppermann, N., Goldhaber-Fiebert, J. D., Malveau, S., Smith, M., Dai, M., Nathens, A. B., Glass, N. E., Jenkins, P. C.,

McConnell, K. J., Remick, K. E., Hewes, H., Mann, N. C., & Pediatric Readiness Study Group. (2021). Evaluation of emergency department pediatric readiness and outcomes among US trauma centers. *JAMA Pediatrics*, Article e211319. https://doi.org/10.1001/jamapediatrics.2021.1319

48. Office for National Statistics. (2020). *Families and households in the UK: 2020*. https://www.ons.gov.uk/peoplepopulationand community/birthsdeathsandmarriages/families/bulletins /familiesandhouseholds/2020

49. Organisation for Economic Co-operation and Development. (2020, February). SFI.2: Children in families. *OECD family database*. https://oecd.org/els/soc/SF_1_2_Children_in_families .pdf

50. Owusu-Ansah, S., Moore, B., Shah, M. I., Gross, T., Brown, K., Gausche-Hill, M., Remick, K., Adelgais, K., Rapparport, L., Snow, S., Wright-Johnson, C., Leonard, J. C., Lying, J., Fallat, M., Wright, J., Callahan, J., Gonzalez del Rey, J., Joseph, M., Lane, N, Lee, L., . . . Timm, N. (2020). Pediatric readiness in emergency medical services systems. *Pediatrics, 145*(1), e20193308. https://doi.org/10.1542/peds.2019-3308

51. Paediatric Emergency Medicine Special Interest Group. (2019). *Standards of care for children in emergency departments, version 3.0*. International Federation of Emergency Medicine. https://www.ifem.cc/wp-content/uploads/2019/06/Standards -of-Care-for-Children-in-Emergency-Departments-V3-2019. pdf

52. Pilkey, D., Edwards, C., Richards, R., Olson, L. M., Ely, M., & Edgerton, E. A. (2019). Pediatric readiness in critical access hospital emergency departments. *Journal of Rural Health, 35*(4), 480–489. https://doi.org/10.1111/jrh.12317

53. Raphael, J. L., & Oyeku, S. O. (2020). Implicit bias in pediatrics: An emerging focus in healthy equity research. *Pediatrics, 145*(5). https://doi.org/10.1542/peds.2020-0512

54. Raphael, J. L., & Rattler, T. L. (2018). Partnering with families to improve emergency medical services for children. *Clinical Pediatric Emergency Medicine, 19*(3), 289–294. https://doi .org/10.1016/j.cpem.2018.08.004

55. Ray, K. N., Olson, L. M., Edgerton, E. A., Ely, M., Gausche-Hill, M., Schmuhl, P., Wallace, D. J., & Kahn, J. M. (2018). Access to high pediatric-readiness emergency care in the United States. *Journal of Pediatrics, 194*, 225–232.E1. https://doi .org/10.1016/j.jpeds.2017.10.074

56. Remick, K. E. (2019). The time is now: Uncovering the value of pediatric readiness in emergency departments. *Pediatrics, 144*(3). https://doi.org/10.1542/peds.2019-1636

57. Remick, K., Gaines, B., Ely, M., Richards, R., Fendya, D., & Edgerton, E. A. (2019). Pediatric emergency department readiness among US trauma hospitals. *Journal of Trauma and Acute Care Surgery, 86*(5), 803–809. https://doi.org/10.1097 /ta.0000000000002172

58. Remick, K., Gausche-Hill, M., Joseph, M. M., Brown, K., Snow, S. K., Wright, J. L., American Academy of Pediatrics Committee on Pediatric Emergency Medicine and Section on Surgery, American College of Emergency Physicians Pediatric Emergency Medicine Committee, & Emergency Nurses Association Pediatric Committee. (2018). Pediatric readiness in the emergency department. *Pediatrics, 142*(5), Article e20182459. https://doi.org/10.1542/peds.2018-2459

59. Remick, K., Kaji, A. H., Olson, L., Ely, M., Schmuhl, P., McGrath, N., Edgerton, E., & Gausche-Hill, M. (2016). Pediatric readiness and facility verification. *Annals of Emergency Medicine, 67*(3), 320–328.E1. https://doi.org/10.1016/j .annemergmed.2015.07.500

60. Richard, K. R., Glisson, K. L., Shah, N., Aban, I., Pruitt, C. M., Samuy, N., & Wu, C. L. (2020). Predictors of potentially unnecessary transfers to pediatric emergency departments. *Hospital Pediatrics, 10*(5), 424–429. https://doi.org/10.1542 /hpeds.2019-0307

61. Sleet, D. (2018). The global challenge of child injury prevention. *International Journal of Environmental Research and Public Health, 15*(9), 1921. https://doi.org/10.3390/ijerph15091921

62. Szalados, J. E. (2021). The ethics and laws governing informed decision-making in healthcare: Informed, consent, refusal, and discussions regarding resuscitation and life-sustaining treatment. In J. E. Szalados (Ed.), *The medical-legal aspects of acute care medicine: A resource for clinicians, administrators, and risk managers* (pp. 43–74). Springer.

63. U.S. Census Bureau. (2020). Table C3. Living arrangements of children under 18 years and marital status of parents by age, sex, race, and Hispanic origin and selected characteristics of the child for all children: 2020. *America's families and living arrangements: 2020*. https://www.census.gov/data/tables/2020 /demo/families/cps-2020.html

64. Whitfill, T. M., Remick, K. E., Olson, L. M., Richards, R., Brown, K. M., Auerbach, M. A., & Gausche-Hill, M. (2020). Statewide pediatric facility recognition programs and their association with pediatric readiness in emergency departments in the United States. *Journal of Pediatrics, 218*, 210–216. e2. https://doi.org/10.1016/j.jpeds.2019.10.017

65. Zhang, X., Carabello, M., Hill, T., He, K., Friese, C. R., & Mahajan, P. (2019). Racial and ethnic disparities in emergency department care and health outcomes among children in the United States. *Frontiers in Pediatrics, 7*. https://doi .org/10.3389/fped.2019.00525

Pediatric Differences

Kimberly MacKeil-White, MSN, BN, RN, CPEN, NPD-BC

OBJECTIVES

Upon completion of this chapter, the learner will be able to:

1. Describe the anatomic, physiologic, and developmental characteristics of pediatric patients.
2. Incorporate knowledge of physical and cognitive development to optimize patient assessment and employ a more therapeutic approach to children of all ages.
3. Discuss pediatric pain assessment and treatment options for subsets of the pediatric population.
4. Plan interventions to minimize pain and trauma associated with emergency department procedures.
5. Adapt communications and nursing interventions for children in each stage of growth and development to facilitate a trusting relationship with pediatric patients and their families.

Introduction

While some aspects of nursing do not change when working with any population, others change drastically when the patients are not the typical ones providers are used to caring for.[5(Ch29)] The approach to care and sometimes treatment paths differ greatly depending on the child's age and developmental level. Physical and cognitive characteristics are used to describe pediatric patients and adapt nursing care. In this chapter, we explore why children's growth, development, cognition, and emotional responses require specialized knowledge and skills to optimize nursing assessments and interventions.

Growth and Development

When describing *growth* in a pediatric patient, this term refers to physical attributes such as weight, height, and maturation of systems. Growth patterns are predictable, with children developing in both a cephalocaudal (head to tail) and proximodistal (center of the body to the extremities) direction. Care can be planned around this predictability. For example, vital signs measurements, weight, and endotracheal tube sizing formulas will vary with physical growth. Development involves advancing physical, cognitive, emotional, communication, and cognitive capabilities. Mobility, language, potty training, recognition of cause and effect, and other milestones are used to track a child's development. Typically, aspects of both growth and development evolve as the child ages.[28(Ch3),43]

Stages of Development

Division of developmental stages for children is most often based on psychosocial or cognitive development. Most references divide childhood into five stages, identifying characteristics specific to each stage. Awareness of these stages can support the nurse when planning and delivering interventions specific to each subset, thereby providing developmentally appropriate care (**Table 3-1**).[39]

Gender Identity

Experts agree that gender identity is recognized and expressed as early as 2 to 4 years of age.[1,14] There is an increase in social awareness and healthcare presentations of younger gender-diverse children, but gender identity is more commonly an adolescent consideration. This trend continues to evolve as patients present to the emergency department (ED) to seek care and disclose that they identify as a gender other than what they were assigned at birth. Gender-diverse children may appear in previous hospital records under a different name and gender than that with which they present.

TABLE 3-1	Stages of Development			
Age	**Stage**	**Psychosocial Development (Erikson)**	**Cognitive Development (Piaget)**	**Pertinence to Nursing Care**
Birth to 28 days	Neonatal	Trust versus mistrust	Sensorimotor	Need comfort, soft voices; does not matter who holds and soothes them. Should console easily.
1 month to 12 months	Infant	Trust versus mistrust	Sensorimotor	Separation anxiety begins here. Caregivers at the bedside will decrease anxiety.
1 to 3 years	Toddlerhood	Autonomy versus shame and doubt	Sensorimotor/ preoperational	Complete what you can on the caregiver's lap, going from least invasive to most invasive. Distraction is extremely helpful to complete tasks. Prepare for invasive procedures outside of the room.
3 to 6 years	Preschool	Initiative versus guilt	Preoperational (2–7 years)	Give simple explanations; let them play with equipment. Use simple words. Prepare for invasive procedures outside of the room.
6 to 12 years	School age	Industry versus inferiority	Concrete operational (7–11 years)	People pleasers. They want to do well for you and may cover emotions and deny pain to avoid interventions. Give them a job during procedures, such as holding lab tubes or bandages.
13 to 18 years	Adolescence	Identity versus role confusion	Formal operational (11–15 years)	Value honest and straightforward communication. Body image and peer groups are of major concern. Interview away from parents if able to for sensitive issues. Privacy is important.

Data from Prows, C. A., & Hockenberry, M. J. (2022). Developmental and genetic influences on child health promotion. In M. J. Hockenberry, D. Wilson, & C. C. Rodgers (Eds.), *Wong's essentials of pediatric nursing* (11th ed., pp. 38–56). Elsevier.

Gender assignment refers to the gender noted at birth from apparent sex organs, whereas gender identity refers to what the person intimately feels they are. Gender identity may be male, female, both, or neither, and may be the same or different than the gender assignment made at birth. Gender expression refers to how the person expresses their gender in dress, actions, words, and other behaviors. The transitioning individual is pursuing physical alteration of their body so that it affiliates with their identified gender. Gender identity is sometimes confused with sexuality. The two are separate realities, as all people can be heterosexual, homosexual, bisexual, pansexual, or asexual.

It is important for the healthcare team to clarify and respect the patient's name and pronouns. When interacting with any patient, creating a mutually respectful relationship is extremely important to a successful encounter. Demonstrating respect so as to promote trust with the gender-diverse patient is particularly vital. The ED nurse must consider whether discussion about the patient's gender is pertinent to the reason for the visit. For example, it may be important to ask about transitioning treatments that may have been initiated if the patient is presenting with abdominal pain but less pertinent if the chief complaint is ear pain.[17]

Communication Strategies

Communicating with the pediatric patient can be an art in and of itself. Communication efficacy depends on a multitude of factors, such as age, developmental stage, temperament, culture, prior healthcare encounters, expanse of language skills, and the nurse's ability to employ age- and context-specific strategies. Infants are nonverbal and often fearful of strangers. The ability to express their feelings and needs is limited. For infants, crying when uncomfortable, cooing when content, arching the back when upset, and waving the arms when excited are forms of communication. Toddler and preschooler vocabulary expands greatly from 1 to 4 years of age. Communication becomes more verbal and less challenging for the healthcare team. School-age patients are inquisitive, more verbal, and easier to communicate with. Teenagers can be quiet, reserved, and untrusting. However, each child is different, and many techniques can be useful in making communication easier.[5(Ch4),20]

Approach Adaptions

When approaching the pediatric patient, developmental stages are helpful to remember. The neonate, for example, is not yet cognitively aware of their surroundings or who is providing the care. For this patient, warm hands, gentle touch, and a soothing voice are the best approaches. The ED nurse takes care to remember that neonates typically cry when disturbed and should calm easily when consoled.

RED FLAG

Infants who do not soothe easily or are "inconsolable" warrant immediate further assessment.

As they increase in age, infants begin to recognize caregivers, show separation anxiety, and react to strangers. For these reasons, gathering as much information as you can before approaching the child is important. For example, obtain a medical history and count the respiratory rate before touching the patient if possible. Taking vital signs in the order of least invasive (respiratory rate) to most invasive (rectal temperature) will aid the nurse in obtaining accurate results, minimizing the incidence of elevated measurements due to crying.

Younger children interpret language in a very literal fashion (**Table 3-2**).[14,20] Telling them, "I'm going to take your blood pressure," may be interpreted as literally "taking" their blood. It is especially important to talk in terms they can understand and offer choices whenever possible. For instance, "I'm going to give your arm a big hug with this squeezer. It sounds like air in a balloon and feels like a tight hug. You will see the little arm going around the clock right here. Which arm would you like me to squeeze?" In this example, the patient has some control over the choice, and feels involved in care.

School-age patients are typically people-pleasers and want to do well in most things, including a visit to the ED. The truth is important to children of this age and should be presented in simple terms. They are inquisitive and want to know details about what equipment is, what it feels like, and what they will see, hear, and even smell while a procedure is being done as it pertains to their own body. Preparations for invasive procedures such as intravenous (IV) access should be done outside the child's line of vision to decrease the opportunity for anxiety. Giving the school-age child the opportunity to play with the equipment and quick explanations in language they understand satisfies their knowledge need. This might include playing with the stethoscope before measuring vital signs and with the plastic catheter without the needle before establishing IV access.

TABLE 3-2 Considerations When Communicating with Children: Speaking in Their Terms

Common Words and Phrases Used in Hospitals	Possible Interpretation by Child	Child-Friendly Phrases to Use Instead
"I'm going to take your temperature."	What are you going to take from me?	"I'm going to measure your temperature."
"I am going to take your blood pressure."	You're going to take my blood?! I don't want you to do that!	"This cuff is going to give your arm a quick hug and then it will let go. Your job is to be really still." (If the child is old enough to tolerate an oral temperature, obtain the temperature while obtaining the blood pressure, so the child will not talk during the blood pressure measurement.)
"Urine"	What am I in?	Use a term the child understands. (Ask the caregiver which word the child uses.)
"Stool"	A chair	Use a term the child understands. (Ask the caregiver which word the child uses.)
"CAT" scan	Why are they talking about cats? I'm afraid of cats.	"We are going to take you to a room to get a special picture of the inside of your body. It doesn't hurt at all. You just have to be really still for the picture. The camera looks like a big doughnut and sometimes makes an airplane noise."
"You need to get an IV."	Ivy? Is it a plant?	"You're going to get a little straw in your arm so that we can give you medicine to help you feel better." Show the child a catheter without the needle, if possible, and allow the child to touch it.
"The medicine may burn."	Does it burn me like fire? Is it dangerous?	"The medicine may feel warm. How do you think it feels?"
"This part is going to hurt."	Why would I let you hurt me? I better leave now!	"Some kids say this part feels like a pinch. Tell me how it feels to you."
"Now I am going to flush your IV."	Are you going to put it down the toilet?	"I'm going to put some special water through your straw."
"I am going to give you a shot."	With a gun? Why are you going to shoot/hurt me?	"I need to give you some medicine in your arm (or leg) that will help you get better." Be honest and say it may pinch.
"The [medicine] is going to make you go to sleep."	They put my dog to sleep. He died.	"This medicine will help you feel relaxed, and you may even start feeling silly."
"The doctor is going to make an incision in your stomach."	Are my insides going to come out?	"The doctor is going to make a small opening in your stomach."
"We are going to move you to the pediatric floor."	Why are you going to take away my bed? Why do you want me to get on the floor?	"We are going to move to the room where you will stay overnight."
"You are going to get some sutures."	What are sutures? Do they hurt?	"We are going to give you some string bandages for your boo-boo [owie, cut, or wound]."
"You need a dressing change."	Why are you going to undress me?	"I'm going to put a clean bandage on your boo-boo."

Data from Deering, C. G., & Cody, D. J. (2002). Communicating with children and adolescents. *American Journal of Nursing, 102,* 34–41; Foote, J. M. (2019). Communication, physical, and developmental assessment of the child and family. In M. J. Hockenberry, D. Wilson, & C. C. Rodgers (Eds.), *Wong's nursing care of infants and children* (11th ed., pp. 57–113). Elsevier.

Adolescent patients value honest, sincere communication that includes them directly. They respond best when rapport is established with the nurse and uninterrupted attention can be given. It may be necessary to speak without the presence of caregivers in the room to gather honest information pertinent to the ED visit with the teenage patient, as caregivers are not always aware of sensitive details in certain circumstances. These may include sexual health, behavioral health, or substance abuse issues. Parental presence may inhibit adolescent communication due to privacy concerns. Regional statutes and policies often permit adolescents to provide consent for their own treatment for these concerns, thereby safeguarding their privacy and facilitating access to care. See Chapter 2, "Preparing for Pediatric Emergencies," for more information. **Table 3-3** summarizes some important communication considerations.

Infant, Child, and Adolescent Anatomy and Physiology

Children are not just little adults, having the same physiology as adults on a smaller scale. They have important mental and physical differences from adults that change throughout childhood. In addition to the cognitive differences mentioned in the previous section, awareness of expected anatomic and physiologic differences further improves nurses' ability to tailor assessments and interventions to best meet children's healthcare needs. Understanding what is normal and abnormal in the context of the child's development in the pediatric assessment is vital to recognizing alarming variations and providing quality care that leads to optimal pediatric outcomes.

Vital Signs

Vital signs measurements for the pediatric patient typically include blood pressure, heart rate, respiratory rate, temperature, pulse oximetry, and weight in the ED setting. Most pediatric dosing is based on kilograms, so the measurement of weight in kilograms—as opposed to pounds—is considered an area of high risk. Doubling the dose of some medications can be lethal if calculated based on the patient's weight in pounds instead of kilograms. Most EDs use pediatric scales that are locked to kilograms and cannot be changed to pounds to avoid this risk.

RED FLAG

Most pediatric medication calculation systems refer to the patient weight in kilograms. This is a high-risk area for those facilities that have scales that change from pounds to kilograms. EDs must be diligent in ensuring weights are documented appropriately.

Due to the immaturity of the cardiorespiratory systems and a higher metabolic rate in the pediatric patient, normal ranges for vital signs for children are typically different from those for adults. For example, a fixed stroke volume (due to lack of myocardial stretch) but increased need for cardiac output makes the child's heart rate run higher than the adult rate according to their age. As the infant develops, stroke volume and heart size increase, causing heart rate to decrease as they grow. Likewise, the younger the patient, the faster the respiratory rate will be due to the increased oxygen consumption and lack of tidal reserves. **Table 3-4** identifies normal vital signs by age range.[2(P4),18,31] Consider the child's clinical condition and context when interpreting the vital signs. The heart and respiratory rate will be slower when the child is calm or sleeping and faster when the child is active, in pain, or febrile.

Appropriate equipment for pediatric vital signs measurement is important to obtain accurate readings as well. Blood pressure cuffs that are too small for the patient will result in inaccurately high readings, whereas cuffs that are too large for the patient will result in inaccurately low

TABLE 3-3 General Communication Considerations
› Maintain eye contact with the child as much as possible.
› Use child-friendly language.
› Speak with the child as well as the adults in the room.
› Use play as a tool to help educate.
› Use "one voice" in the room when procedures are being done, to decrease anxiety. (This means one person is assigned to do the talking in the room. "One voice" lessens the stimulation and helps create a nonthreatening environment.)
› Be honest.
› Do not use threats ("If you don't take your medicine, you can't have an ice pop").
› Respect privacy (especially with the adolescent group).

TABLE 3-4   Normal Vital Signs for Pediatric Patients

Age	Heart Rate (beats/min)	Respiratory Rate (breaths/min)	Systolic Blood Pressure (mm Hg)
Term neonate to <1 month	90–190	35–60	67–84
Infant, 1–12 months	90–180	30–55	72–104
Toddler, 1–3 years	80–140	22–40	86–104
Preschooler, 3–5 years	65–120	18–35	89–112
School-age, 5–12 years	70–120	16–30	90–115
Adolescent, 12–18 years	60–100	12–20	100–130

Data from American Heart Association. (2020). Part 4: Systematic approach to the seriously ill or injured child. *Pediatric advanced life support provider manual*; Ernst, G. (2020). Pediatric trauma. In J. E. Tintinalli, O. J. Ma, D. M. Yealy, G. D. Meckler, J. S. Stapczynski, D. M. Cline, & S. H. Thomas (Eds.), *Tintinalli's emergency medicine: A comprehensive study guide* (9th ed., pp. 689–697). McGraw Hill; and Lucia, D., & Glenn, J. (2017). Pediatric emergencies. In C. K. Stone & R. L. Humphries (Eds.), *Current diagnosis and treatment: Emergency medicine* (8th ed., pp. 964–1016). McGraw Hill.

BOX 3-1   Pediatric Advanced Life Support (PALS) Guidelines for Hypotension

PALS defines hypotension by systolic blood pressure (SBP) as follows:

- Neonate (0 to 28 days old): SPB <60 mm Hg
- Infants (1 month to 12 months): SBP <70 mm Hg
- Children (1 year to 10 years): SBP <[70 + (2 × age in years)] mm Hg
- Children (older than 10 years): SBP <90 mm Hg

These blood pressures defining hypotension commonly overlap with the lower-normal SBP value spectrum.

Data from American Heart Association. (2020). Part 4: Systematic approach to the seriously ill or injured child. *Pediatric advanced life support provider manual*.

such as hypoxia, infection, and shock. Thus, when the patient's heart rate is high for their age group, further investigation is required as to the source. Fever, irritability, anxiety, and pain are also reasons why a heart rate can be high in a pediatric patient. However, it is important to first consider less benign reasons for abnormal vital signs during the assessment.

RED FLAG

Just a Fever or Something More?

It is dangerous to attribute tachycardia to a fever. Catch perfusion issues by evaluating tachycardia quickly! Blood pressure will not drop in children until 25% to 50% of volume is lost or depleted.[48]

System Differences

Pediatric-related system differences include those in the respiratory, cardiovascular, musculoskeletal, neurologic, gastrointestinal, genitourinary, and integumentary systems.

Respiratory

The respiratory system continues to develop after the fetal physiologic changes occur at birth and is fully developed by the age of 8, where it is comparable to the adult system.[12,13] Until then, several factors affect the child's oxygenation and ventilation needs. The respiratory rate, depth, and regularity all continue to change in the first year of life, making respiratory assessment different than that in older children. Infants breathe faster and

readings. Both cases may require further investigation and prompt unneeded treatment, or worse, could miss actual hypotension/hypertension that could have been addressed. The "just right" blood pressure cuff will be two-thirds the width of the patient's arm and fall within the indicators on the cuff itself. **Box 3-1** provides guidelines for blood pressure levels corresponding to hypotension in children.[2(P4)]

As further discussed in Chapter 7, "The Child in Need of Stabilization," the need for increased cardiac output in the pediatric patient is often a result of physiologic insults

less regularly, with apnea not considered as such until 20 seconds without a breath or associated with other physiologic effects such as bradycardia.[33(Ch14)] Infants are typically obligate nose breathers, only developing the ability to breathe through their mouths at about 4 to 6 months of age.[29] This can make obstructive issues such as secretions or blankets an extra risk.

The length from the eustachian tubes to the pharynx is shortened and straighter in children, sending inhaled pathogens to the ear more readily and causing infections. The tongue and epiglottis are larger in relation to the oropharynx. The narrowest part of the pediatric airway may not be the cricoid cartilage (as previously believed), but rather the area above it. This may increase focus on the glottic region during intubation.[24,47] The laryngeal and tracheal cartilage is more pliable, increasing the potential for airway collapse. The smaller airway diameter increases airflow resistance and is more susceptible to obstruction. The trachea is shorter than that of an adult, making right mainstem intubation common. Alveoli are fewer and smaller, diminishing gas exchange capacity and reserves.[29]

The diaphragm is more horizontal in children, and is the principal muscle used for inspiration. The chest wall is also shorter with more horizontal ribs, limiting chest expansion. The chest and abdominal muscles are used to increase chest expansion, but these accessory muscles are less developed in children and will fatigue quickly. Retractions are visible on assessment and indicate increased respiratory effort. Compensation for hypoxia with signs of respiratory distress is extremely concerning for impending respiratory failure.[29]

CLINICAL PEARL

Assessing Respiratory Rate

When assessing a respiratory rate, be sure to count for a full minute in infants and those patients presenting with respiratory complaints or symptoms. This will help account for the irregularity in pattern for smaller children—for example, infant apnea that is normal if less than 20 seconds in duration.

Cardiovascular

Fetal circulation evolves into infant circulation over the first 2 weeks of life (see Chapter 6, "The Neonate") and continues to mature in size over the span of childhood. As the left ventricle gains more ability to increase stroke volume with growth and myocardial stretch, the heart rate decreases and the blood pressure increases. (Normal ranges for age are listed in Table 3-4.) Higher metabolic rates and oxygen demand are required to support the infant, and decompensation can be triggered by subtle stressors.[40] The parasympathetic nervous system is more pronounced in the younger child and can be triggered quite easily with suction, rectal temperature measurement, or intubation, causing the heart rate to drop fairly quickly. Because of the ability to compensate for long periods, blood pressures in pediatric patients with shock are maintained past the typical time frames seen in adult shock. Hypotension manifests much later when children are in shock. Refer to Chapter 7, "The Child in Need of Stabilization," for more detailed cardiovascular information.

CLINICAL PEARL

Heart Disease?

Neonates with respiratory or shock symptoms and no fever or exposure to ill contacts may be exhibiting signs of congenital heart disease. A quick screening tool that can help identify patients with congenital heart disease is the preductal and postductal saturation measurements. Measuring a pulse oximetry on the right hand and comparing it to the measurement of either foot can indicate an issue with the heart when the difference in the two measurements is more than 3% or the oxygen saturation is less than 90% in either site.[10,35]

Musculoskeletal

As the infant grows into a child, bone ossifies, making it stronger and denser. Bone growth occurs at the epiphyseal (growth) plates near the end of the bones themselves. Until they close at approximately 14 years of age, fractures across these plates can affect how the bone will grow in the future unless appropriate treatment is given and care is given to monitor the fracture site until then.[5]

Due to incomplete ossification, fractures are common in children and a frequent reason for ED visits. Ligaments and tendons are stronger than bone until ossification is complete, but sprains and strains are common in the child as well. Muscles are fully formed in infancy but continue to increase in length and circumference until adolescence.[5]

Neurologic

The brain more than doubles its size by the end of the first year of life and accounts for between one-fourth and one-third of the infant's entire mass. The fontanelles close by 18 months of age, but fibrous membranes called sutures connect the skull plates to allow room for brain development.[6] Approximately 90% of brain growth is complete by the age of 6. Sutures are usually fused by the age of 12.[9]

As infants begin to become mobile, their large head size causes a shift in the center of gravity and puts the child at risk for head injuries. The thin infant skull does not protect against traumatic injury very well, so skull fractures and intracranial bleeds are common in this age group. To give the brain room to grow, the cranial sutures do not seal until the child is approximately 2 years of age. Fontanelles are excellent points of assessment. The anterior fontanelle closes last, by 18 months of age. A sunken fontanelle can indicate dehydration, whereas a bulging fontanelle may indicate increased intracranial pressure.[10]

Infants begin to process information from the time they are born, and this ability increases as they age. Primitive reflexes, such as the rooting, Moro, and Babinski reflexes, begin to disappear as the infant begins to control its movement with development. See Chapter 6, "The Neonate," for more information on neonatal reflexes.

Gastrointestinal

The gastrointestinal system of the infant is immature, and is unable to break down certain proteins until toddlerhood. The lower esophageal sphincter develops in the first month of life but may be weak for the first year. The infant's stomach is smaller and empties quickly, requiring small and frequent feedings.[25] The liver is able to conjugate bilirubin and perform other basic functions (such as production of bile) within a few weeks of life. In contrast, other functions, such as gluconeogenesis and production of certain enzymes needed for digestion, are delayed for approximately 12 months. The abdomen is at increased risk of trauma due to the protuberant positioning, thin musculature, and shortness of the ribs, which translates into less protection for vital organs.[41]

Genitourinary

At birth, the urinary system, including the kidneys, ureters, bladder, and urethra, are all present, but they continue to grow and develop functionality until puberty. During infancy, the ability to concentrate urine is limited, so the infant can easily become dehydrated if the intake of fluids cannot be managed to balance the output. Bladder capacity is limited in young children as well, so frequency of urination is increased. Bladder training increases capacity as children become physiologically capable of holding their urine. The length of the urethra is short in the very young and puts these patients at an increased risk for urinary tract infections. This factor, along with the urethra's close proximity to the anus, creates pathways for bacteria to enter the bladder. Uncircumcised males have an increased risk of urinary tract infections as well. Urinary tract infections are the leading cause of fever in patients younger than 3 years of age.[13,21]

The reproductive systems in both males and females are also mostly present at birth and continue to grow and mature into puberty. Sperm begin to develop in males during puberty, and the onset and regulation of menstrual cycles for females begin during this stage as well. Hormones associated with this developmental stage regulate themselves and may prompt visits to the ED for concerns about pubertal changes that are either actually or perceived as abnormal. Sometimes only education is required, but it is safest to approach the presentation as abnormal until a full evaluation has been completed.

Integumentary

At birth, the infant skin is particularly thin, and vernix covers it to protect it from insult and infection. During the first month after birth, the skin matures and becomes more protective, continuing to develop throughout the first year of life. During infancy, the greater opportunities for loss of heat and fluids through this thinner skin may make it difficult to keep infants warm and hydrated. By the end of the first year of life, the skin develops the ability to contract to protect from heat loss, and the infant develops the ability to shiver to produce energy. Brown fat that is burned for energy is replaced with subcutaneous tissue that can store glucose more efficiently.[28(Ch3)]

CLINICAL PEARL

Warm and Sweet

Keeping the infant "warm and sweet" is a good rule to follow to support this patient's metabolic and cardiovascular needs. Hypothermia and hypoglycemia are dangerous but preventable conditions.

Vascular Access

Obtaining vascular access can be tricky in a pediatric patient, as the circulatory system tends to be smaller, and anxiety tends to constrict the vessels. The patients are often scared and/or nervous and may be unable to control their movements during the procedure. Hypovolemia also makes it difficult to locate veins. All these issues can make the process of obtaining IV access challenging in the infant and child.

The technique for pediatric IV access is not altogether different than in an adult, with the following exceptions[3]:

- Help is needed to secure the patient during the procedure to limit movement.
- Education for the procedure and why it is necessary is presented in simpler terms.
- Caregivers are encouraged to be present both for patient support and to encourage family-centered care.
- The equipment used is typically smaller than that for an adult.

Optimal site selection for IV access is based on several factors, including age, soothing habits such as thumb sucking, ability to walk, parental preference, and hand dominance. Some considerations include the following:

- Prepare the equipment and supplies outside of the room to reduce the anxiety level for the younger child.
- Use the "one voice" principle when performing any procedure, deciding beforehand who will do the communicating in the room. Less verbal stimulation will mean less anxiety for the child.[34]

- Use child life techniques to educate and help the patient cope. These include simple words such as "a drinking straw [IV catheter] in your blue line [vein]" and "quick pinch" instead of "shot."
- Provide distraction with toys, books, and conversation during the procedure, and reward the child with praise and stickers when it is complete.
- Avoiding placing peripheral intravenous lines over joints in infants (like the antecubital joint) unless absolutely necessary.
- Dorsal hands in younger children work well for IV access, but avoid them if the patient self-soothes with a thumb or fingers, if possible.
- Scalp veins have no valves and can easily be accessed if needed in infants younger than 9 months. The IV catheter is inserted toward the heart in a superficial vessel after checking for arterial pulsation. Do not access this vessel if pulsation is present. Scalp vein access is contraindicated if the patient has a skull fracture, ventricular shunt, hydrocephalus, or anencephaly.
- Avoid placing an IV in the feet if the patient is learning to ambulate or is ambulating.
- Never wrap an IV line circumferentially or with a pressure dressing. Signs of infiltration may be subtle in children due to increased subcutaneous fat, and tissue damage may incur before the infiltrate is recognized. Use a dressing with a transparent window over the site itself and assess the site often.

Figure 3-1 identifies the locations of pediatric veins.

Intraosseous (IO) access is an option if the situation warrants, such as cardiac arrest, impending arrest, or inability to gain venous access in a timely manner when the patient's condition demands quick treatment (e.g., burns or septic shock). Viable IO sites include the medial tibia just below the tuberosity, the distal tibia, the femur, and the humerus. Contraindications include bone fracture or a previous IO attempt in that bone. IO access should be removed as soon as other reliable venous access is obtained to decrease the risk of osteomyelitis or fracture of the bone. Ideally, it will be removed as soon as other access can be established, but no more than 24 hours after insertion.[37,38]

IO site infiltration may look different than an infiltrated IV line. IO infiltration tends to present as swelling behind the site instead of at the insertion site. For example, a tibial IO infiltration will create a shiny, taut calf that is easy to miss if the IO access point is wrapped circumferentially (which may occur in the prehospital environment for transport stability) or not appropriately assessed. All staff who may encounter IO access should have training and competency assessment specific to the device used at their facility.

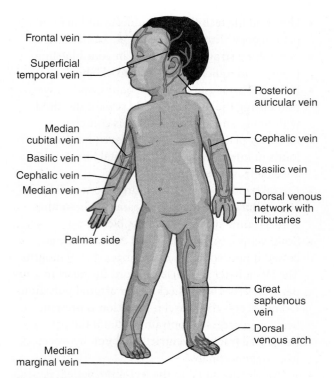

Frontal vein
Superficial temporal vein
Posterior auricular vein
Median cubital vein
Cephalic vein
Basilic vein
Cephalic vein
Basilic vein
Median vein
Dorsal venous network with tributaries
Palmar side
Great saphenous vein
Dorsal venous arch
Median marginal vein

Figure 3-1 *Pediatric vein locations.*

Insertion of central venous access in the ED has been limited in practice since the IO route was introduced. With the ease of insertion and capabilities that IO access brings, central access is a third-line option in the race for emergent line placement. Providers may opt for central venous access if necessary, and ED nursing staff are needed to support the provider with this procedure.

In those patients who have chronic needs, central lines such as tunneled catheters, implanted ports, and peripherally inserted central catheters (PICC lines) are seen quite often. Access to and usage of these specialty vascular access devices is performed by a nurse with adequate training. Improper use can cause infection and device damage. Refer to the facility policies and evidence-based practice guidelines specific to the device.

Medication Administration

Pediatric medication administration is based on the principles derived from anatomy and physiology, the child's developmental stage, and the focused assessment of the child. For example, as the child grows, so does the body mass and ability to hold volume (such as for an intramuscular injection). The body fat in a child may be increased, and lipid-soluble medications may be stored in the body versus being processed and excreted. Developmentally, children may have the ability to weigh the options of oral versus intramuscular administration to promote autonomy and acceptance of the therapy.

Weight-based dosing for medications is necessary in the infant/child weighs less than 50 kg. Accounting for variations in muscle mass, lipid stores, height, and body mass index necessitates a more precise method than simply adjusting an adult dose of a medication by cutting it in half or in fourths. Length-based resuscitation tapes are used with critical patients to determine an estimated weight based on height when it is not possible to obtain an exact weight via scale. This method is preferred over the parent "guesstimate." Length-based resuscitation tapes often include weight-based equipment sizes and critical medication dose references for use in emergencies.

Oral administration tends to be the most common route for children, with antipyretics and antibiotics being most frequently used. Liquid formulations are often flavored to make them more palatable to children, but this also may lead to unintentional overdoses or ingestions of medications disguised as a sweet treat. Caution caregivers to avoid calling any medication "candy" and help them determine where medications can be safely stored in their home. Older children can swallow a pill or tablet, and parents are generally able to inform the nurse whether their child can swallow pills. Flavored syrup can be helpful when the liquid form of a medicine is not available and the tablet form can be crushed. It is not recommended that extended-release medications be crushed in this way. Giving ice pops just before administration slightly numbs the tastebuds and may help dull the patient's sense of taste. The reluctant child may need syringe administration of liquid medication into the buccal cavity to help promote swallowing of the dose. Instilling it behind the tongue makes it less likely the child will be able to push it out of their mouth. Administering smaller amounts at a time will help the swallowing reflex do its job.

Intranasal (IN) administration of certain medications has gained popularity in recent years. The IN route is utilized when IV access is unavailable and the patient's condition does not warrant IO access. This easy administration route is proving to be effective in early management of frequently seen conditions in children, such as fracture pain or seizure activity. Often, IN medication administration can be used in place of IV or IM administration, avoiding a painful needle stick. IN administration of medications can quickly and effectively manage pain, anxiety, and seizures.[16] **Figure 3-2** is an illustration of an IN medication administration device.

Tips for IN medication administration include the following:

- Consider allowing the child to hold the device, play with it, insert it, and practice sniffing before actual administration of medication.

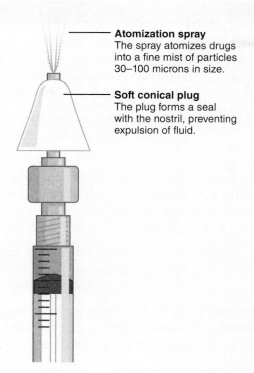

Atomization spray
The spray atomizes drugs into a fine mist of particles 30–100 microns in size.

Soft conical plug
The plug forms a seal with the nostril, preventing expulsion of fluid.

Figure 3-2 *Intranasal device.*

- Ensure the medication is approved for IN administration.
- The volume amount is limited to 1 mL per nare, but 0.2–0.3 mL volumes are ideal. Add 0.1 mL of medication for dead space if recommended by the manufacturer.
- Divide the volume between each nare. Some sources advise obstructing the opposite nare during administration, but others do not.[16,28]
- Ensure head stability before administration. One or more assistants who maintain firm physical control of the child, providing distraction and reassurance, is key to the success of many pediatric procedures. Anticipate young children coughing or gagging from the sensation.

After oxygen, asthma medications are the most commonly administered inhaled medications in the ED. Nebulizers mix the ordered medicine with saline, allowing for a diluted administration over a period of time, and can be driven by either pressurized air or oxygen depending on the need. Several child-friendly devices are commercially available to make the administration effective for children, including dinosaur masks for younger patients and breath-activated nebulizers with a mouthpiece for older children who can perform the proper technique consistently.[8]

Just as common, due to its ability to deliver concentrated amounts of medicine to target areas in a shorter

RED FLAG

All patients who receive opioid or sedative medications are monitored, per facility policy, for cardiovascular and respiratory compromise. Initiate precautions for increased fall risk.

amount of time, is the metered-dose inhaler (MDI) delivery method. In some cases, MDIs have proved more effective than nebulizers in providing timely delivery of prescribed medicine, including bronchodilators and inhaled steroids. MDIs are most effective when paired with a spacer device that traps the aerosol until the patient breathes the dose in completely. Spacers are recommended for patients of all ages who require MDI medications. The mask-spacer devices work best for infants and young children. When children are able to create a seal around a mouthpiece and inhale, they can use a traditional spacer. Use of a spacer ensures the dose is delivered in full. Without a spacer, much of the medication is deposited on the tongue and hypopharynx, diminishing the amount that is inhaled into the lungs.[36]

Pain, Procedures, and Sedation

This section discusses how to handle pain, procedures, and sedation for the pediatric patient.

Pain

Pain is frequently the reason patients seek ED care. Many variables impact pediatric pain evaluation and require assessment adaptions based on the patient's ability to communicate and their developmental experience of pain. Pain assessment is an initial part of the triage process and should then be performed at regular intervals. Uncontrolled pain can be a red flag for a high-risk issue (e.g., inconsolable infants), as well as somewhat diagnostic in nature (e.g., abdominal pain with palpation of the right lower quadrant or rebound tenderness for appendicitis). In addition, untreated pain can alter vital signs measurements and make it difficult to obtain physical findings (e.g., abdominal guarding upon palpation). For patients with chest injuries, increased pain on inhalation can impair their respiratory status, creating the inability to breathe deeply enough for adequate air exchange.

For many years, it was generally believed that the neonatal population did not feel pain with procedures due to the immaturity of their nervous systems. Pain medicine and scales were not considered as important for them until this myth was debunked. Pain has since been proven

TABLE 3-5 Revised FLACC Scale

Variable	0	+1	+2
Face	No expression or smile	Occasional grimace, frown; withdrawn or disinterested. *Appears sad or worried.*	Consistent grimace, quivering chin, clenched jaw, *distressed-looking face, expression of fright or panic*
Legs	Normal position, relaxed, *usual tone and motion to limbs*	Uneasy, restless, tense, *occasional tremors*	Kicking, drawn up, *marked increase in spasticity, constant tremors or jerking*
Activity	Lying quietly, normal position, moves easily, *regular and rhythmic respirations*	Squirming, shifting back and forth, *tense or guarded movements, shallow splinting respirations*	Arched, rigid or jerking, *head banging, breath holding, gasping or severe splinting*
Cry	None	Moans or whimpers, occasional complaint, *occasional verbal outburst or grunt*	Crying steadily, screams or sobs, frequent complaints, *repeated outbursts, constant grunting*
Consolability	Content and relaxed	Reassured by occasional touching/hugging or being talked to, distractible	Difficult to console or comfort, *pushing away, resisting care or comfort measures*

Note: The areas where the revised scale differs from the original FLACC scale appear in italics.

Data from Kjeldgaard Pendersen, L., Rahbek, O., Nikolajsen, L., & Møller-Madsen, B. (2015). The revised FLACC score: Reliability and validation for pain assessment in children with cerebral palsy. *Scandinavian Journal of Pain, 9,* 57–61. https://doi.org/10.1016/j.sjpain.2015.06.007

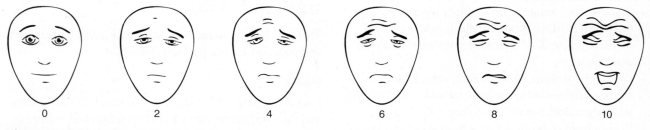

Figure 3-3 *FACES Pain Scale—Revised.*

to be very real in neonates; it is just their reaction and expression of that pain that are different. Neonates have more of a behavioral and physiological type of response that can be measured using a pain scale concentrating on those factors, such as the revised Face, Legs, Activity, Cry, Consolability (rFLACC) scale[26] (**Table 3-5**); the Neonatal Pain, Agitation and Sedation Scale (N-PASS); or the Neonatal Infant Pain Scale (NIPS). The rFLACC is also an appropriate scale for nonverbal patients with chronic conditions who present for care, as communication regarding pain is not specific and responses to pain tend to be behavioral and physiological. For example, a child with severe cerebral palsy who cannot express pain verbally will sometimes moan, grimace, and exhibit increased heart and respiratory rates when uncomfortable.

Objective pain scales take these responses into account and score them accordingly.[28(Ch14)]

For young children, faces-based pain scales, such as Wong-Baker FACES pain rating scale or the Faces Pain Scale—Revised (**Figure 3-3**), are alternatives that have been validated as helpful self-report tools for the pediatric patient to rate their own pain. Young children are generally able to relate to a "happiest with no pain" to "very sad with a lot of pain" scale when a simple explanation is given. Some studies have also validated caregivers as an acceptable proxy for these options.[23,30] It is important to note that the healthcare worker is not an acceptable proxy for self-assessment tools such as the FACES scale for pain. At approximately age 8, the child has the ability to understand the concept of numbers being smaller to bigger (not just the memorization of the numbers themselves) and can accurately use a number-based scale to rate their own pain as a comparative measure.

Nonpharmacologic Interventions

Once assessed, treatments of pediatric pain are similar to treatments for adults, and are divided into nonpharmacologic and pharmacologic categories. Nonpharmacologic pain management includes such interventions as repositioning, allowing the patient to assume a position of comfort, physical stabilization of the affected area, distraction techniques (e.g., blowing bubbles, games, singing, guided imagery, books, video), warm blankets, caregiver presence, massage, and pressure. Ice is a useful adjunct for musculoskeletal pain, but be aware of the risk for hypothermia. Studies have shown anxiety to be directly related to reported pain, and lessened anxiety with caregiver presence alone. Also, infants have shown to exhibit decreased pain behaviors during procedures when sucrose is added to a pacifier for non-nutritive sucking. Nonpharmacologic techniques do not replace the need for pharmacologic pain management but are an extremely useful supplement to analgesic medications.[29]

> **RED FLAG**
>
> While non-nutritive sucking is encouraged for comfort, never attempt to feed an infant during a painful procedure, as aspiration may ensue.

Pharmacologic Interventions

When pharmacology is the option of choice, children are treated based on their pain rating, source of pain, and chronicity of pain. Mild to moderate pain is treated with acetaminophen or nonsteroidal anti-inflammatory drugs (NSAIDs). Opioids are used for moderate to severe pain. Coanalgesic drugs (also known as adjuvant analgesics) are medications that are typically indicated for other conditions, such as depression, anxiety, and seizures, but also help manage pain.[4,22] Ketamine, in subanesthetic doses as an infusion, intramuscularly, or intranasally, is gaining favor for pediatric pain management.[32,44] **Table 3-6** lists some common pediatric pain medications[49] but is not all-inclusive. Be aware of precautions based on age, renal or hepatic pharmacokinetics, and side effects such as bleeding and central nervous system depression. An

TABLE 3-6 Analgesic Medications for Children

Drug Name	Route	Pain	Notes
Acetaminophen	Oral	Mild/moderate	Be aware of combination formulations containing acetaminophen. Use the recommended dose per kg weight and do not exceed 5 doses in 24 hours.
	Rectal	Mild/moderate	
	Intravenous	Moderate/severe	Avoid use in patients with hepatic impairment.
Ibuprofen	Oral	Mild/moderate	Dosing interval is every 6 hours. Maximum dose: 2,400 mg/day.
	Intravenous	Moderate/severe	Take with food. Relative contraindication for patients younger than 6 months due in part to their underdeveloped renal system.
Ketorolac	Oral	Mild/moderate	Serious risk of increased bleeding. Not to be used before surgery (e.g., appendectomy).
	Intramuscular	Moderate/severe	
	Intravenous	Moderate/severe	
Oxycodone	Oral	Moderate/severe	Serious respiratory depression is possible; monitor closely.
			Increased fall risk.
Morphine	Oral	Moderate/severe	Severe respiratory depression is possible, especially in higher doses or with rapid parenteral administration.
	Intramuscular	Severe	Infuse slowly over 3 to 5 minutes.
	Intravenous		Do not crush or chew tablets.

(continues)

TABLE 3-6   Analgesic Medications for Children (*continued*)

Drug Name	Route	Pain	Notes
Hydromorphone	Oral Intravenous	Moderate/severe Severe	Severe respiratory depression is possible, especially in higher doses or with rapid parenteral administration. Infuse slowly over 3 to 5 minutes. Do not crush or chew tablets.
Fentanyl	Intravenous Intranasal	Severe Severe	Severe respiratory depression is possible, especially in higher doses or with rapid parenteral administration. Infuse slowly over 3 to 5 minutes. Intranasal administration may be associated with higher rates of respiratory depression.

Data from Wolters Kluwer. (n.d.). *Lexicomp*. https://www.wolterskluwer.com/en/solutions/lexicomp

altered mental status increases the risk for falls and hypoventilation. Close monitoring for respiratory depression is indicated for many pharmacologic interventions.

Procedural pain in the ED can be approached by using nonpharmacologic and pharmacologic techniques as well. When inserting IV lines, giving intramuscular injections, or preparing to repair lacerations, approaches such as distraction coupled with numbing adjuncts can reduce pain. Cold and vibration have been shown to decrease needle-related pain.[42,46] Topical medicines can be applied to prepare an area for procedure by numbing the skin and making the invasive portion less painful. **Table 3-7** lists topical anesthetics, their intended uses, and onset of action.[27]

Child life specialists are not universally available. When they are, they can enhance patient- and family-centered care to an extent above and beyond what most busy ED nurses can provide due to competing priorities. The specialist can prepare the patient for what is to come and keep them engaged in activities aimed at distraction during the procedure. Nurses without the benefit of child life specialists can incorporate their strategies as time allows with a bit of education.

Procedural Sedation

Procedural sedation is used frequently in the ED to control pain and minimize movement during procedures that are appropriately carried out in this setting. Orthopedic reductions and other uncomfortable procedures such as laceration repairs or incision and drainages commonly use sedation for optimal success, as do some diagnostic procedures such as magnetic resonance imaging (MRI) and lumbar punctures.[7] Sedation is typically used for urgent procedures when the department can afford focus to its completion. Procedural sedation carries a high risk, requiring preparation and the presence of dedicated and trained staff for patient monitoring without distraction.

The child's overall status is evaluated to determine eligibility for sedation, with last oral intake, sedation history, and airway anatomy being key components of this assessment. **Table 3-8** presents one system, from the American Society of Anesthesiologists (ASA), that is used to assess sedation risk.[11,19] Parental consent and education includes the procedure benefits, alternatives and risks, medication effects, and postprocedure/home monitoring. While the provider is responsible for obtaining the consent, the nurse supports the entire process and ensures patient and parental understanding.

Appropriate staff for both the procedure and the sedation should be present in the room, including dedicated staff who are familiar with the medication's administration, its effects, and cardiopulmonary compromise and its treatment. Documentation of vital signs every 5 minutes is recommended by most governing bodies. Along with appropriate staff being present in the sedation room, equipment required includes a bag-mask device with the correct size of mask for the patient; cardiopulmonary monitoring equipment, including pulse oximetry and capnography; suction equipment; and intubation supplies. Reversal agents should be available if needed.

Once the procedure is completed, sedated patients should be monitored until discharge criteria are met

TABLE 3-7   Topical, Spray, and Oral Anesthetics

Anesthetic	Use	Onset of Action
EMLA (lidocaine 2.5% and prilocaine 2.5%)	Intact skin (typically applied at home)	60 minutes
LMX (lidocaine 4%)	Intact skin	20–30 minutes
Tetracaine 4%	Intact skin	30–45 minutes
LET (lidocaine, epinephrine, and tetracaine solution)	Open wounds	20 minutes
Vapocoolant sprays	Intravenous, intramuscular, or scalpel lances Intact skin	Immediate
Needle-free injection system	Intravenous or intramuscular injection	Immediate
Benzocaine sprays	Oral procedures	Immediate

Data from Krauss, B. S., Calligaris, L., Green, S. M., & Barbi, E. (2016). Current concepts in management of pain in children in the emergency department. *The Lancet, 387*, 83–92. https://doi.org/10.1016/S0140-6736(14)61686-X; and Wolters Kluwer. (n.d.). *Lexicomp.* https://www.wolterskluwer.com/en/solutions/lexicomp

TABLE 3-8   ASA Physical Status Classification

ASA Class	Description	Examples
I	Normal, healthy patient	—
II	Patient with mild systemic disease	Mild controlled asthma, patient with seizures and adequate seizure control
III	Patient with severe systemic disease	Moderate to severe asthma, pneumonia, moderate obesity, poorly controlled seizures or diabetes
IV	Patient with severe systemic disease that is a constant threat to life	Severe bronchopulmonary dysplasia; advanced pulmonary, cardiac, hepatic, renal, or endocrine disease
V	A moribund patient who is not expected to live through the procedure	Severe trauma, septic shock, and multisystem failure

Data from Committee on Economics. (2020, December 13). ASA physical classification system. *American Society of Anesthesiologists.* https://www.asahq.org/standards-and-guidelines/asa-physical-status-classification-system; and Evidence-Based Outcomes Center. (2020). *Procedural sedation: Evidence-based guideline.* Texas Children's Hospital. https://www.texaschildrens.org/sites/default/files/uploads/documents/outcomes/standards/Procedural%20Sedation%20Guideline%2011.24.20.pdf

based on facility policy. Policies include common regulatory recommendations such as those listed in **Table 3-9**.[19]

Discharge education for the family of a patient after procedural sedation is vital, as medicinal effects may last for some time after leaving the ED. This information is included with the standard condition-specific discharge instructions. Ensure that the caregivers understand the importance of monitoring the patient for medication effects and which symptoms warrant a return to the ED or call for emergency medical services. Such symptoms may include difficulty arousing the patient, respiratory issues, and excessive vomiting.

Positioning for Procedures

While much can be done to decrease procedural pain, the reality is that many ED interventions will cause fear, anxiety, and discomfort. A variety of techniques have been employed to prevent patient movement while minimizing restraint-induced distress. The patient can be held on an adult's lap, facing forward or backward, using the

TABLE 3-9 Sedation Discharge Criteria
Stable cardiopulmonary status
Ability to sit up and talk
Ability to control head
Able to maintain hydration status
Returned to sedation baseline regarding communication, mobility, and alertness

Data from Evidence-Based Outcomes Center. (2020). *Procedural sedation: Evidence-based guideline.* Texas Children's Hospital. https://www.texaschildrens.org/sites/default/files/uploads /documents/outcomes/standards/Procedural%20Sedation% 20Guideline%2011.24.20.pdf

---

BOX 3-2 Positioning Techniques

One example of a position of comfort is the two-person hold for nasal swabs or intramuscular injections:

- The caregiver can provide a hugging hold to control the patient's arms and head.
- If double nasal swabs or injections are needed, it is preferable to use a second staff member and perform both at the same time.

Another example is the infant swaddle for starting intravenous access:

- Use a warm blanket to swaddle the infant.
- Hold the child in your arms or lay the child on the bed with the caregiver holding the infant from the side.

---

adult's arms, torso, and legs to provide stability. This is often called a "hugging hold" (see **Box 3-2** for two examples). Physical safety is the priority, as some positioning techniques have the potential to compromise the airway. Psychological safety must also be considered. Medical procedures requiring restraint, while intended to help the patient, may be traumatic enough to be considered an adverse childhood experience. See Chapter 17, "The Child, Family, and Healthcare Team in Crisis," for more information on adverse childhood experiences.

Summary

Pediatric patients have their own specific needs, warranting a knowledge base and skill set that varies between age groups and is much different than what is needed for adults.

Acquiring the knowledge needed to adapt the nurse's approach to infant, toddler, preschool, school-age, and adolescent patients will arm the healthcare provider with the tools needed to create a therapeutic encounter with the patient and family. This may also positively impact future healthcare encounters and lessen the stress associated with medical care. The pediatric patient exists within the family. It is important to remember to involve the caregivers by communicating with and educating them, thereby supporting them as partners in the child's care.

References

1. Alderman, E. M., & Breuner, C. C. (2019). Unique needs of the adolescent. *Pediatrics, 144*(6), 1–12. https://doi-org.proxy .library.vanderbilt.edu/10.1542/peds.2019-3150

2. American Heart Association. (2020). *Pediatric advanced life support provider manual.*

3. Anderson, C. E., & Herring, R. A. (2022). Pediatric nursing interventions and skills. In M. J. Hockenberry, C. C. Rogers, & D. Wilson (Eds.), *Wong's essentials of pediatric nursing* (11th ed., pp. 551–618). Elsevier.

4. Anekar, A. A., & Cascella, M. (2021). *WHO analgesic ladder.* StatPearls Publishing. https://pubmed.ncbi.nlm.nih .gov/32119322/

5. Ball, J., Bindler, R., Cowen, K. & Shaw, M. (2017). *Principles of pediatric nursing: Caring for children* (7th ed., pp. 821–860). Pearson.

6. Banta-Wright, S. A. (2020). Developmental management of infants. In *Burns' pediatric primary care* (7th ed., pp. 92–108). Elsevier.

7. Ben-Yakov, M., & Bhatt, M. (2020). Emergency procedural sedation in children. *CMAJ, 192*(40), Article E1162. https://doi .org/10.1503/cmaj.200332

8. Bryant, R. (2022). The child with respiratory dysfunction. In M. J. Hockenberry, C. C. Rogers, & D. Wilson (Eds.), *Wong's essentials of pediatric nursing* (11th ed., pp. 619–679). Elsevier.

9. Butterfield, R. J., & Huether, S. E. (2019). Alterations of neurologic function in children. In K. L. McCance & S. E. Huether (Eds.), *Pathophysiology* (8th ed, pp. 619–643). Elsevier.

10. Cleveland, L. M. (2022). Health promotion of the newborn and family. In M. J. Hockenberry, C. C. Rogers, & D. Wilson (Eds.), *Wong's essentials of pediatric nursing* (11th ed., pp. 175–212). Elsevier.

11. Committee on Economics. (2020, December 13). *ASA physical classification system.* American Society of Anesthesiologists. https://www.asahq.org/standards-and-guidelines/asa-physical -status-classification-system

12. Crawford, D., & Davies, K. (2020). Biological basis of child health 5: Development of the respiratory system and elements of respiratory assessment. *Nursing Children & Young People, 32*(6), 33–42. https://doi.org/10.7748/ncyp.2020.e1246

13. Davies, K. (2021). Biological basis of child health 7: Growth, development, and the reproductive system. *Nursing Children & Young People, 33*(2), 33–43. https://journals.rcni.com

/nursing-children-and-young-people/cpd/biological-basis
-of-child-health-7-growth-development-and-the-reproductive
-system-ncyp.2020.e1308/abs

14. Deering, C. G., & Cody, D. J. (2002). Communicating with children and adolescents. *American Journal of Nursing, 102,* 34–41.

15. Duffy, E. A. (2022). Health promotion of the toddler and family. In M. J. Hockenberry, C. C. Rogers, & D. Wilson (Eds.), *Wong's essentials of pediatric nursing* (11th ed., pp. 339–364). Elsevier.

16. Elsevier. (n.d.). *Medication administration: Nasal instillation.* Elsevier Clinical Skills. http://Point-of-care.elsevierperformance manager.com/skills/893/quick-sheet?skilled=CPP_161

17. Emergency Nurses Association. (2016). *Care of the gender expansive and transgender patient in the emergency care setting* [Topic brief]. https://enau.ena.org/Users/LearningActivityAsset SingleViewer.aspx?LearningActivityAssetID=IXPw3nKaNB% 2fjQw%2baCD7sQg%3d%3d

18. Ernst, G. (2020). Pediatric trauma. In J. E. Tintinalli, O. J. Ma, D. M. Yealy, G. D. Meckler, J. S. Stapczynski, D. M. Cline, & S. H. Thomas (Eds.), *Tintinalli's emergency medicine: A comprehensive study guide* (9th ed., pp. 689–697). McGraw Hill.

19. Evidence-Based Outcomes Center. (2020). *Procedural sedation: Evidence-based guideline.* Texas Children's Hospital. https://www.texaschildrens.org/sites/default/files/uploads /documents/outcomes/standards/Procedural%20Sedation% 20Guideline%2011.24.20.pdf

20. Foote, J. M. (2019). Communication, physical, and developmental assessment of the child and family. In M. J. Hockenberry, D. Wilson, & C. C. Rodgers (Eds.), *Wong's nursing care of infants and children* (11th ed., pp. 57–113). Elsevier.

21. Hamilton, J. L., Evans, S. G., & Bakshi, M. (2020). Management of fever in infants and young children. *American Family Physician, 101*(12), 721–729. https://www.aafp.org/afp/2020/0615 /p721.html

22. Hellsten, M. (2022). Pain assessment and management in children. In M. J. Hockenberry, C. C. Rogers, & D. Wilson (Eds.), *Wong's essentials of pediatric nursing* (11th ed., pp. 114–147). Elsevier.

23. Herr, K., Coyne, P. J., Ely, E., Gélinas, C., & Manworren, R. C. B. (2019). Pain assessment in the patient unable to self-report: Clinical practice recommendations in support of the ASPMN 2019 position statement. *Pain Management Nursing, 20*(5), 404–417. https://doi.org/10.1016/j.pmn.2019.07.005

24. Holzki, J., Brown, K. A., Carroll, R. G., & Coté, C. J. (2018). The anatomy of the pediatric airway: Has our knowledge changed in 120 years? A review of historic and recent investigations of the anatomy of the pediatric larynx. *Paediatric Anaesthesia, 28*(1), 13–22. https://doi.org/10.1111/pan.13281

25. Keeton, V. F. (2019). Abdomen and rectum. In K. G. Duderstadt (Ed.), *Pediatric physical examination: An illustrated handbook* (3rd ed., pp. 239–254). Elsevier.

26. Kjeldgaard Pendersen, L., Rahbek, O., Nikolajsen, L., & Møller-Madsen, B. (2015). The revised FLACC score: Reliability and validation for pain assessment in children with cerebral palsy. *Scandinavian Journal of Pain, 9,* 57–61. https://doi .org/10.1016/j.sjpain.2015.06.007

27. Krauss, B. S., Calligaris, L., Green, S. M., & Barbi, E. (2016). Current concepts in management of pain in children in the emergency department. *Lancet, 387,* 83–92. https://doi .org/10.1016/S0140-6736(14)61686-X

28. Kyle, T., & Carman, S. (2020). *Essentials of pediatric nursing* (4th ed., pp. 807–838). Lippincott Williams & Wilkins.

29. Lewis, C. A. (2022). The pediatric patient. In L. D. Urden, K. M. Stacey, & M. E. Lough (Eds.), *Critical care nursing: Diagnosis and management* (9th ed., pp. 974–996). Elsevier.

30. Lifland, B. E., Mangione-Smith, R., Palermo, T. M., & Rabbitts, J. A. (2018). Agreement between parent proxy report and child self-report of pain intensity and health-related quality of life after surgery. *Academic Pediatrics, 18*(4), 376–383. https://doi .org/10.1016/j.acap.2017.12.001

31. Lucia, D., & Glenn, J. (2017). Pediatric emergencies. In C. K. Stone & R. L. Humphries (Eds.), *Current diagnosis and treatment: Emergency medicine* (8th ed., pp. 964–1016). McGraw Hill.

32. Masaracchia, M. M., Sites, B. D., Lee, J., Thomas, J. J., & Fernandez, P. G. (2019). Subanesthetic ketamine infusions for the management of pediatric pain in non-critical care settings: An observational analysis. *Acta Anasthesiologica Scandinavica, 63*(9), 1225–1230. https://doi.org/10.1111/aas.13429

33. Ngo, T. L. (2021). Apnea. In K. N. Shaw & R. G. Bachur (Eds.), *Fleisher & Ludwig's textbook of pediatric medicine* (8th ed., pp. 102–106). Wolters Kluwer.

34. Olsen, A. (2019, January 9). *One Voice helps children stay calm during procedures.* University of Kentucky Healthcare. https://ukhealthcare.uky.edu/wellness-community/blog/one -voice-helps-children-stay-calm-during-procedures

35. Oster, M. (2019). Newborn screening for critical congenital heart disease using pulse oximetry. *UpToDate.* Retrieved August 19, 2021, from https://www.uptodate.com/contents /newborn-screening-for-critical-congenital-heart-disease -using-pulse-oximetry

36. Percy, A. (2021). Procedures. In K. Kleinman, L. McDaniel, & M. Molloy (Eds.), *Harriet Lane handbook* (22nd ed., pp. 61–97). Elsevier.

37. Perron, C. E. (2021). Intraosseous infusion. *UpToDate.* Retrieved October 24, 2021, from https://www.uptodate.com /contents/intraosseous-infusion?search=intraosseous%20 access&source=search_result&selectedTitle=1~150&usa ge_type=default&display_rank=1

38. Perth Children's Hospital. (2020). *Intraosseous access.* https:// pch.health.wa.gov.au/For-health-professionals/Emergency -Department-Guidelines/Intraosseous-access

39. Prows, C. A., & Hockenberry, M. J. (2022). Developmental and genetic influences on child health promotion. In M. J. Hockenberry, C. C. Rodgers, & D. Wilson (Eds.), *Wong's essentials of pediatric nursing* (11th ed., pp. 38–56). Elsevier.

40. Saikia, D., & Mahanta, B. (2019). Cardiovascular and respiratory physiology in children. *Indian Journal of Anaesthesia, 63*(9), 690–697. https://doi.org/10.4103/ija.IJA_490_19

41. Saladino, R. A. & Gaines, B. A. (2021). Abdominal trauma. In K. N. Shaw & R. G. Bachur (Eds.), *Fleisher & Ludwig's textbook of pediatric medicine* (8th ed., pp. 1084–1094). Wolters Kluwer.

42. Sapci, E., Kocamaz, E. B., & Gungormus, Z. (2021). Effects of applying external cold and vibration to children during vaccination on pain, fear, and anxiety. *Complementary Therapies in Medicine, 58.* https://doi.org/10.1016/j.ctim.2021.102688

43. Sheldrick, R. C., Schlichting, L. E., Berger, B., Clyne, A., Pensheng Ni, Perrin, E. C., & Vivier, P. M. (2019). Establishing new norms for developmental milestones. *Pediatrics, 144*(6), 1–10. https://doi.org/10.1542/peds.2019-0374

44. Silva, L. O. J. E., Lee, J. Y., Bellolio, F., Homme, J. L., & Anderson, J. L. (2020). Intranasal ketamine for acute pain management in children: A systematic review and meta-analysis. *American Journal of Emergency Medicine, 38*(9), 1860–1866. https://doi.org/10.1016/j.ajem.2020.05.094

45. Steinkrauss, L. J. (2021). Defense against hypoglycemia: Normal fasting adaptation in children. *Journal of Pediatric Nursing, 58,* 110–111. https://doi.org/10.1016/j.pedn.2021.01.024

46. Su, H., Hsieh, C., Lai, N. M., Chou, P., Lin, P., & Chen, K. (2021). Using vibrating and cold device for pain relief in children: A systematic review and meta-analysis of randomized controlled trials. *Journal of Pediatric Nursing, 61,* 22–33.

47. Wani, T. M., Bissonnette, B., Engelhardt, T., Buchh, B., Arnous, H., AlGhamdi, F., & Tobias, J. D. (2019). The pediatric airway: Historical concepts, new findings, and what matters. *International Journal of Pediatric Otorhinolaryngology, 121,* 29–33. https://doi.org/10.1016/j.ijporl.2019.02.041

48. Weiss, A. K., Lavoie, M. E. & Khoon-Yen, E. T. (2021). A general approach to the ill or injured child. In K. N. Shaw & R. G. Bachur (Eds.), *Fleisher & Ludwig's textbook of pediatric medicine* (8th ed., pp. 26–33). Wolters Kluwer.

49. Wolters Kluwer. (n.d.). *Lexicomp.* https://www.wolterskluwer.com/en/solutions/lexicomp

CHAPTER

4

Prioritization

Robin Powers-Jarvis, PhD, RNC, CEN, CCRN, TCRN, CPEN

OBJECTIVES

Upon completion of this chapter, the learner will be able to:

1. Integrate Pediatric Assessment Triangle findings into a categorization of "sick, sicker, or sickest."
2. Identify pediatric considerations within common triage systems.
3. Recognize pediatric red flags.

Introduction

Making decisions regarding the order in which patients are seen and/or which assessments and interventions are most important, more simply referred to as prioritization, is an essential skill for nurses. Prioritization encompasses the initial formal triage, which assigns a patient acuity when the patient enters the department, and the ongoing triage of patient care based on patient workload and condition. The ability to prioritize accurately requires experience and a level of skill often not attained until the nurse has achieved a level of experience and competence equivalent to what Benner[9] would classify as proficiency. However, nurses in the emergency department (ED) are called upon to make these decisions on a daily basis, often long before they have had sufficient experience to have reached the proficient stage of nursing practice. It is essential that the nurse, who is often the first healthcare provider a pediatric patient encounters,

be able to identify the often-subtle signs of pediatric distress or illness.

A study done by Ageron et al. demonstrated that the under-triage rate for pediatric patients in general EDs can be as high as 33%.[1] Providing a relatively simple, clear-cut process to assist in determining the urgency of a pediatric patient's need for care and thereby aiding in assigning an acuity level and the ongoing prioritization of patient care is the goal of this chapter. It is essential knowledge needed to assist in triaging patients, especially pediatric patients.

The art of triaging was initially practiced on the battlefield, where limited resources had to be allocated to provide the best possible outcomes for the greatest number of casualties. The word *triage* means "to sort" in French, and this sorting was initially used in the early 1800s on the French battlefields during the Napoleonic Wars to quickly assess and determine the level of injury sustained by the soldiers and the urgency of their need for care. This practice has evolved into the triage systems used in today's EDs throughout the world to establish patient acuity and the order in which patents are seen, as well as to control the flow of the ED.[37]

It is important to remember that triage is *not* a place and is *not* solely confined to EDs. Triage is an ongoing process, and the prioritization of patients can occur anywhere that patients and their families go to seek medical care. It could occur in an ED, but it could also occur in a doctor's office, an urgent care or freestanding clinic, a school clinic, or any other out-of-hospital setting. Triage is also used during disaster management and mass-casualty incidents and events to facilitate the greatest good for the greatest number of injured. Additionally, it is important to consider prioritization when transferring a patient from one department to another within a hospital or from one facility to another. Moreover, the patient needs to be continually reevaluated as the situation warrants. A patient's condition and order of priority can change based on these ongoing assessments.

> ### NOTE
>
> **Triage Is a Process, Not a Place**
>
> Triage is an ongoing process that can occur anywhere, not just in the ED.

Research regarding triage decision making highlights the importance of nursing expertise in accurate prioritization and stresses the need for good critical thinking ability, intuition, and multiple levels of knowledge on the part of the nurse. Hassani et al. demonstrated the importance of nursing intuition when caring for critically ill patients.[22] Intuition is more than a feeling: Rather, intuition "is a process based on knowledge and care experience" and uses sensory perceptions embedded in the nurse's assessment.[30] The nurse needs to accurately determine acuity and urgency of the need for care by interpreting subjective data, including a history provided by the patient and/or parent, combined with objective physical assessment data.

A literature review done by Recznik and Simko regarding pediatric triage indicates that, despite their additional training, general ED nurses tend to under-triage pediatric patients.[35] Pediatric patients as a whole tend to deteriorate very quickly. Such patients have the ability to compensate, compensate, compensate—until they suddenly can no longer do so, and then they crash. An old adage is "Adult patients roll down a hill, but pediatric patients fall off a cliff." In view of this, it is essential that the nurse accurately prioritizes the pediatric patient initially and then consistently reevaluates the patient's condition. The nurse needs to be able to detect subtle signs of decompensation and deterioration and to be aware that the patient's physiologic condition can change at any time.

Using a consistent assessment tool assists in the initial and ongoing pediatric assessments, thereby helping to ensure proper placement of the pediatric patient in the queue for care. The Pediatric Assessment Triangle (PAT) is such a tool (**Figure 4-1**).[25] As nurses are responsible for the ongoing care and assessment of patients after the triage encounter and initial assessment, this tool is also vital to identifying deterioration and the need for reprioritization.

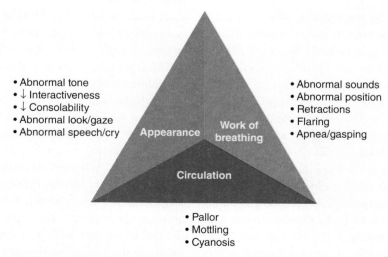

Figure 4-1 *The Pediatric Assessment Triangle.*

Data from Horeczko, T., Enriquez, B., McGrath, N. E., Gausche-Hill, M., & Lewis, R. J. (2013). The Pediatric Assessment Triangle: Accuracy of its application by nurses in the triage of children. *Journal of Emergency Nursing, 39*(2), 182–189. https://doi.org/10.1016/j.jen.2011.12.020

The Pediatric Assessment Triangle

The PAT is a relatively simple tool that enables the nurse to obtain a quick general impression of the patient's physiologic status. Its validity as a first step in the assessment process for pediatric emergency patients has been supported by research.[19,25,27] The PAT provides a rapid assessment of the pediatric patient's general physiologic stability and can be performed before engaging in direct physical contact with the patient. The PAT, which uses visual and auditory cues, has been found to be a reliable tool for identification of acutely ill and injured infants and children. Its use enables the nurse to quickly determine the patient's general condition and decide whether the child is "sick," "sicker," or "sickest," and thus determine which patient receives the highest priority and gets first in line in the queue for care.

The PAT consists of three components:

- Appearance
- Work of breathing
- Circulation to the skin

These three components are somewhat reminiscent of the ABCs from basic life support (BLS), advanced cardiovascular life support (ACLS), and pediatric advanced life support (PALS). One major difference is that the PAT components are quickly assessed without touching the patient.

CLINICAL PEARL

Utility of the PAT

Whether the nurse is faced with multiple pediatric patients who need to be triaged upon arrival to the ED or is running around during a patient assignment and peeking in to see if the patients are okay, the PAT can help. The PAT is not always related to ED triage or priority. It is simply an effective tool that calls out critical physical assessments the nurse can see or hear in a moment.

Appearance

The child's general appearance is the first thing that the nurse sees when looking at the child and is paramount when determining how critical the illness or injury is and, therefore, how emergent the need for care is. The child's interaction with the caregiver or the environment reveals much information regarding adequacy of ventilation and

---

BOX 4-1 TICLS Mnemonic

T Tone: Is the muscle tone demonstrated by the child appropriate? Is the child moving arms and legs, or does the child appear limp or flaccid?

I Interactiveness: Does the child appear to interact appropriately with the environment and/or the caregiver? If age appropriate, does the child play with toys and/or interact with others?

C Consolability: Is the child easily consoled or comforted by the caregiver or a blanket, toy, pacifier, or is there no consoling the child?

L Look/gaze: If the eyes are open, does the child appear to be alert or is the child staring into space? If the child's eyes are closed, do they open to noise or sound, or is the child just sleeping?

S Speech/cry: Is the child's speech appropriate or the cry loud, strong, and vigorous, or is the speech or cry weak or listless?

---

oxygenation and perfusion to the brain and central nervous system. Any alteration in general appearance may indicate a significant underlying problem.

The mnemonic TICLS is helpful in remembering what to look for when assessing appearance (**Box 4-1**). A quick assessment of appearance, using these five TICLS parameters, tells a lot about the child's overall condition.

Work of Breathing

The second component of the PAT is work of breathing, or how much effort the child is exerting to breathe. The work of breathing reflects the child's oxygenation and ventilatory status. Looking and listening for any abnormalities in respiratory effort will help the healthcare provider identify a possible attempt to compensate for other physiologic abnormalities. Observe the child's respiratory rate and effort.

Increased work of breathing may be seen as a change in rate from what would be normal for the child's age—either tachypnea or bradypnea. Observe the child for abnormal positioning (tripoding or leaning forward with hands on knees to breathe), retractions (intercostal, clavicular, sternal, tracheal, or abdominal), nasal flaring, or head-bobbing, any or all of which can indicate increased work of breathing. Listen for any abnormal audible breath sounds such as stridor; wheezing; or a barky, prolonged, or persistent cough. All of these are telltale signs of increased work of breathing and may be suggestive of significant illness or injury.

Circulation to the Skin

The third parameter in the PAT is circulation to the skin. Look at the child's skin color in central areas, such as the lips and mucous membranes. The palms of the hands and the soles of the feet are also good indicators of circulation. Changes from the patient's normal color are a strong indicator of insufficiency of cardiac output and core perfusion. Is the child's skin color normal, or is it pale, mottled, ashen, gray, dusky, or cyanotic? In children with darker skin tones, it is especially important to look at the lips, tongue, conjunctiva, mucous membranes, gums, nail beds, palms of the hands, and soles of the feet to identify problems with circulation.[32,34] Although mottling can be a normal response to cold that is caused by vasoconstriction,[25] err on the side of caution and assume that any mottling is indicative of poor cardiac output until proven otherwise. At this juncture, the nurse should also look for any unusual redness or obvious rashes on the skin, which might indicate significant temperature elevation or the need to isolate the child from the rest of the general population.

Sick, Sicker, or Sickest

This section discusses more specifically what is meant by the concepts of sick, sicker, or sickest.

Sick

Simply by virtue of the fact that the patient presents for medical care, the child is classified as "sick." Someone—whether it was the child, parent, caregiver, teacher, police officer, or other individual—felt that "something was not right." The child needs to be evaluated by a healthcare professional. This child can be placed in the queue for care, and a more thorough evaluation and focused assessment can be done at a somewhat later time. The focused assessment would include additional parameters requiring direct hands-on assessment of the child, such as obtaining vital signs, history taking, and other more in-depth assessments, which are discussed in greater detail in Chapter 5, "Initial Assessment."

Sicker

Any child who exhibits a deviation or abnormality in *any one* of the three components of the PAT is automatically considered "sicker." This single abnormality in any one of the three components increases the child's acuity

rating and pushes the child ahead of a "sick" child in the queue for care. Depending on the severity of the deviation, the child may be elevated to a level requiring rapid intervention.

Sickest

If there is a deviation from normal in *two or more* of the components of the PAT, the child is considered "sickest" and often warrants a high acuity level rating. A child determined to be sickest is placed in an area where rapid treatment, including resuscitation (if indicated), can be initiated. However, a "sick" or "sicker" child may take priority after a more thorough assessment is completed.

Triage Assessment Tools

While the PAT can be used with every pediatric patient encounter, it is also the first step of a more formalized triage assessment to determine order of priority when children present to the ED. A number of assessment tools are employed in EDs around the world that are designed to rapidly determine a patient's acuity and urgency of need for care beyond the PAT. Zachariasse et al. found that performance of 33 established triage systems was variable but validity for emergent and less urgent patients was moderate to good.[43] Some of these systems have been used and modified for use in the pediatric population. A study done by Ebrahimim et al. explored the reliability of pediatric triage systems in the ED.[16] These researchers concluded that the Australasian Triage Scale (ATS), Canadian Triage and Acuity Scale (CTAS), Emergency Severity Index (ESI), and Manchester Triage System (MTS) are substantially reliable and acceptable for pediatric ED triage. Hinson et al. found that an "opportunity to improve interrater reliability and triage performance in identifying patients at risk of adverse outcome exists"[24(P24)] with established triage systems. No matter the triage tool used, ongoing quality monitoring and performance improvement are needed to increase triage accuracy. **Table 4-1** compares a variety of triage systems.[6,10,21,28,42]

Disaster Triage

In disaster situations involving a massive number of casualties, triaging of patients takes an entirely different approach. The PAT can still be used to form a general impression, but the "sick, sicker, sickest" determination may not always govern priority of care. Disaster triage uses the axiom "The greatest good for the greatest number."

TABLE 4-1 Triage System Comparison

Triage System	Description	Maximum Waiting Time	Examples of Conditions/Triage Categories
Australasian Triage Scale (ATS) Used in Australia and New Zealand	**Category 1:** RED Immediately life threatening	Immediate	Cardiac or respiratory arrest Multiple trauma Unconscious (Glasgow Coma Scale [GCS] score < 9) Systolic blood pressure (SBP) < 80 mm Hg in adult, severe shock in infant/child Intravenous overdose Severe behavioral disorder
	Category 2: ORANGE Imminently life threatening	10 minutes	Airway risk (stridor) Severe dyspnea Heart rate < 50 or >150 beats/minute Severe blood loss Poor perfusion Cardiac chest pain Acute stroke Sepsis Major fracture/dislocation Febrile neutropenia Fever with lethargy GCS score < 13 High-risk history Severe pain
	Category 3: GREEN Potentially life threatening or important time-critical treatment	30 minutes	Severe hypertension Moderate blood loss Moderate shortness of breath Severe/projectile vomiting Dehydration Seizure/post-ictal Moderate to severe pain Potential child abuse Behavioral/psychiatric patient very distressed, risk of self-harm or aggression toward others

(continues)

TABLE 4-1 Triage System Comparison (*continued*)

Triage System	Description	Maximum Waiting Time	Examples of Conditions/Triage Categories
	Category 4: BLUE Potentially life threatening, serious, or situational urgency or significant complexity	60 minutes	Mild blood loss Minor limb injury Vomiting and diarrhea without dehydration Moderate pain Semi-urgent mental health issue
	Category 5: WHITE Less urgent	120 minutes	Mild pain with no risk Minor wounds Low risk history Minor symptoms of low-risk conditions
Canadian Triage Acuity Scale (CTAS) Most commonly used in Canada. Multiple decision trees based on patient presentation and/or condition. Has specific modifiers for pediatric patients, including concern for patient's welfare, disruptive behavior, floppy child, gait disorder or painful walk, stridor, apneic spells in infants, inconsolable crying in infants, and congenital problems in children.	**Level I:** BLUE Resuscitation: conditions that are threats to life or limb requiring aggressive interventions	Immediate	Unstable vital signs with any of the following complaints: cardiac/respiratory arrest, major trauma (in shock), severe respiratory distress, altered level of consciousness (GCS score 3–9) **Pediatric-specific modifiers:** Cardiac/respiratory arrest, conflict or unstable situation, airway compromise, apneic episodes on presentation

Level II: RED

15 minutes

Emergent: conditions that are a potential threat to life, limb, or function requiring rapid medical intervention

One abnormal vital sign with any of the following complaints: shortness of breath (moderate respiratory distress), vomiting blood (dizzy on sitting up), hypertension (SBP > 220 mm Hg or diastolic blood pressure [DBP] > 130 mm Hg with symptoms), altered level of consciousness (GCS score 10–13), fever (temperature > 38°C [100.4°F]), looks septic (with three positive systemic inflammatory response syndrome [SIRS] criteria), chest pain with cardiac features, chest pain and noncardiac features, severe abdominal pain (pain: 8/10), headache (sudden, severe, worst ever), major trauma not in check

Pediatric-specific modifiers: Risk of flight or ongoing abuse, uncertain flight or safety risk/family distress, no tone, unable to support head, marked stridor, recent spell consistent with apnea or respiratory compromise, inconsolable infant with abnormal vital signs, conditions and protocol letters identifying concerns for rapid deterioration or need for immediate therapy, vomiting/diarrhea in child with known inherited metabolic disease, type 1 diabetes, or adrenal insufficiency

Level III: YELLOW

30 minutes

Urgent: conditions that could potentially progress to a serious problem requiring emergency interventions

Vital signs usually normal or near upper or lower ends of normal limits with any of the following complaints: shortness of breath (mild respiratory distress), hypertension (SBP > 220 mm Hg or DBP > 130 mm Hg without symptoms), vomiting and/or diarrhea (mild dehydration), abdominal pain (pain: 4–7/10), headache (moderate pain: 4–7/10), diarrhea (uncontrolled bloody diarrhea)

Pediatric-specific modifiers: Physical or sexual assault more than 48 hours prior, acute difficulties with others/environment, limited/less than expected muscle tone, gait or limp problems with fever, audible stridor, history of spell consistent with apnea, inconsolable infant with stable vital signs, caregivers identifying need for care

Level IV: GREEN

60 minutes

Less urgent: conditions that relate to patient age, distress, or potential for deterioration that would benefit from intervention or reassurance within 1 to 2 hours

Normal vital signs with any of the following complaints: confusion (chronic, no change from usual state), urinary tract infection (UTI) complaints/symptoms (mild dysuria), constipation (mild pain: < 4/10)

Pediatric-specific modifiers: History/signs of abuse or maltreatment, persistent problematic behavior, walking with difficulty, irritable but consolable, stable child with known congenital disease with potential for problems

(continues)

TABLE 4-1 Triage System Comparison (continued)

Triage System	Description	Maximum Waiting Time	Examples of Conditions/Triage Categories
	Level V: WHITE Non-urgent: conditions that may be acute but non-urgent, as well as conditions that may be part of a chronic problem with or without evidence of deterioration	120 minutes	Normal vital signs with any of the following complaints: diarrhea (mild, no dehydration), minor bites or injuries (+/- mild acute peripheral pain), dressing change (uncomplicated), medication request **Pediatric-specific modifiers:** Chronic unchanged behavior
Emergency Severity Index (ESI) Most commonly used in the United States and gaining favor elsewhere. Uses decision tree to determine acuity and triage coding. Handbook contains separate chapter[21(Ch6)] regarding use of the ESI for pediatric patients.	**Level 1:** Requires immediate life-saving interventions	Immediate	Cardiac/respiratory arrest, major multiple trauma, intubated, apneic, pulseless, severe respiratory distress, pulse oximetry (SpO_2) < 90%, acute mental status changes, unresponsive (not following commands or reacting to noxious stimulus), overdose with respiratory rate ≤ 6 breaths/min, severe bradycardia or tachycardia with hypoperfusion, chest pain, pale, diaphoretic, SBP 70 mm Hg palpated, weak and dizzy, heart rate ≤ 30 beats/min, anaphylactic shock, flaccid baby, hypoglycemia with changes in mental status, head injury with unequal pupils, acute signs of stroke **Pediatric-specific modifiers:** Petechial rash with altered mental status, alteration in capillary refill (> 3 seconds), persistent gastrointestinal symptoms with signs of dehydration
	Level 2: High-risk situation, confused, lethargic, disoriented, severe pain or distress	No set time frame, but continuous re-assessments required to watch for deterioration and need to increase acuity level	Active chest pain with suspicion of acute coronary syndrome, signs of stroke, possible ectopic pregnancy, hemodynamically stable, possibly immunocompromised patient with fever, suicidal or homicidal patient, overdose, new-onset confusion/lethargy/disorientation, severe pain (≥ 7/10) Patient with any of above complaints and ≥ 2 abnormal vital signs should be moved to Level 1. **Pediatric-specific modifiers:** Temperature > 38°C (100.4°F) in child < 1-3 months old, syncope, seizures (not actively seizing), sepsis or dehydration, diabetic ketoacidosis, suspected child abuse, head trauma, ingestion or overdose including vitamins, sickle cell crisis, hemophilia with possible acute bleeding, hypothermic infants < 90 days old with temperature < 36.5°C (97.7°F) rectally, moderate to severe croup, lower airway obstruction (moderate to severe) from bronchiolitis, reactive airway disease (asthma), signs of respiratory distress

Pediatric Danger Zone Vital Signs

Age	Heart Rate (beats/min)	Respiratory Rate (breaths/min)	O₂ Saturation
< 3 months	>180/< 60	> 50/< 20	< 92%
3 months–3 years	>160/< 60	> 40/< 20	
3–8 years	>140/< 60	> 30/< 16	
>8 years	>100/< 60	> 20/< 12	

Level 3: Two or more resources required for care

Not applicable. Frequent reassessments recommended to identify deterioration and need to increase acuity level.

These patients may have a significant level of pain (pain: 4–7/10) and their presenting complaints require further investigation. Unanticipated or unusual responses to the complaint-specific questions, concerning vital signs, or identification of a high-risk comorbidity may increase the patient's level of acuity.

Also, the level of distress experienced by the patient may increase the patient's level of acuity.

Pediatric-specific modifiers: Temperature > 39°C (102.2°F) in child 3 months–3 years old; incomplete immunizations or no obvious source of fever. Danger zones for pediatric vital signs will increase the level of acuity to Level 2.

Level 4: One resource required for care

Not applicable. Reassessments recommended to identify deterioration and need to increase acuity level.

Any patient who presents with normal vital signs and a chief complaint that the triage nurse estimates will utilize only one resource while in the ED will receive a Level 4 ESI acuity score.

Pediatric-specific modifiers: Medication refills, ear pain in healthy school-age children, contusions and abrasions, upper respiratory symptoms with normal vital signs

(continues)

TABLE 4-1 Triage System Comparison (continued)

Triage System	Description	Maximum Waiting Time	Examples of Conditions/Triage Categories
	Level 5: No resources required for care	Not applicable. Reassessments recommended to identify deterioration and need to increase acuity level.	Any patient who presents with normal vital signs and a chief complaint that the triage nurse estimates will utilize no resources while in the ED will receive a Level 5 ESI acuity score.
Manchester Triage System (MTS) Most commonly used in Europe; special caveats for children and elderly patients	**Group 1:** RED Immediate	Immediate	Airway compromise, stridor or drooling, inadequate breathing, shock, actively seizing, (unresponsive children), exsanguinating hemorrhage
	Group 2: ORANGE Very urgent	10 minutes	Altered level of consciousness; children who score V or P on the AVPU scale, uncontrollable major hemorrhage, hot baby (<12 months old with temperature ≥ 101.3°F [38.5°C]); any age very hot (temperature ≥ 105.8°F [41°C]) or cold (temperature < 95°F [35°C]); severe pain (≥ 8/10)
	Group 3: YELLOW Urgent	1 hour	History of unconsciousness, uncontrollable minor hemorrhage, temperature > 101.3°F (38.5°C) but < 41°C in patient older than 12 months, moderate pain (5–7/10)
	Group 4: GREEN Standard	2 hours	Normothermic, recent mild pain (1–4/10), recent onset of complaint (< 7 days)
	Group 5: BLUE Non-urgent	4 hours	Minimal pain (≤ 1/10), chronic complaint with no acute changes

Note: AVPU = Alert, Verbal, Pain, Unresponsive.

Data from Australasian College for Emergency Medicine. (2016). *Guidelines on the implementation of the Australasian triage scale in emergency departments.* https://acem.org.au/getmedia/51dc74f7-9ff0-42ce-872a-0437f3db640a/C24_04_Guidelines_on_Implementation_of_ATS_Jul-16.aspx; Bullard, M. J., Musgrave, E., Warren, D., Unger, B., Skeldon, T., Grierson, R., van der Linde, E., & Swain, J. (2016). *Revisions to the Canadian Emergency Department Triage and Acuity Scale (CTAS) guidelines 2016* [Position statement]. Canadian Association of Emergency Physicians. http://ctas-phctas.ca/wp-content/uploads/2018/05/revisions_to_the_canadian_emergency_department_triage_and_acuity_scale_ctas_guidelines_2016.pdf; Gilboy, N., Tanabe, P., Travers, F., & Rosenau, A. M. (2020). Use of the ESI for pediatric triage. In *Emergency Severity Index implementation handbook 2020 edition: A triage tool for emergency department care—version 4* (pp. 39–48). Emergency Nurses Association. https://www.ena.org/docs/default-source/education-document-library/esi-implementation-handbook-2020.pdf?sfvrsn=fdc327df_2; Mackway-Jones, K., Marsden, J., & Windle, J. (Eds.). (2014). *Emergency triage: Manchester Triage Group* (3rd ed.). Wiley Blackwell; and Warren, D. W., Jarvis, A., LeBlanc, L., Gravel, J., CTAS National Working Group, Canadian Association of Emergency Physicians, National Emergency Nurses Affiliation, Association des Médecins d'Urgence du Québec, Canadian Paediatric Society, & Society of Rural Physicians of Canada. (2008). Revisions to the Canadian Triage and Acuity Scale Paediatric Guidelines (PaedCTAS). *Canadian Journal of Emergency Medicine, 10*(3), 224–232. https://doi.org/10.1017/S1481803500010149

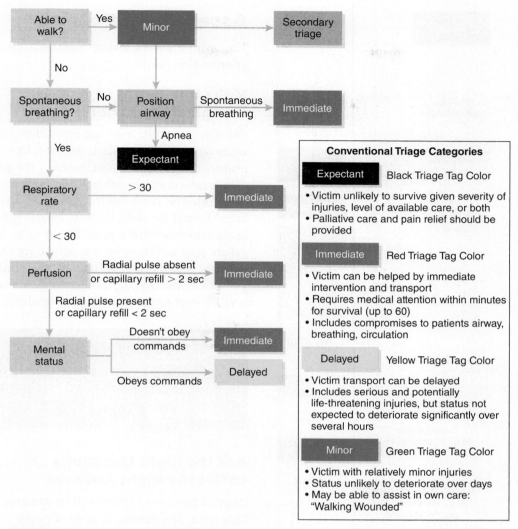

Figure 4-2 *The START algorithm.*

Reproduced from U.S. Department of Health and Human Services. (2021, August 16). *START adult triage algorithm.* https://chemm.hhs.gov/startadult.htm

A decision tree called START (**Figure 4-2**) is used to facilitate rapid patient assessment in patients older than age 8.[40] The JumpSTART[39] (**Figure 4-3**) and SALT[38] (**Figure 4-4**) algorithms are used for younger casualties. Patients are color-coded (**Table 4-2**) based on the decision tree assessments.[3(AppD)]

Reevaluation

It is important to remember that triage acuity (regardless of which system is used) reflects only the patient's initial presentation to the ED. Acuity is a determination that is often made prior to the patient being placed in a treatment room to be seen. The assigned acuity level is simply a tool to guide the healthcare provider in establishing the sequence of care (i.e., which patient gets seen first). Acuity can change if the patient deteriorates or decompensates, requiring increased and more rapid care. This does not necessarily mean the

triage acuity level changes. ESI, for example, was studied only for patients' initial presentation to the ED. If a patient's condition deteriorates before being seen by the physician or advanced practice provider, the acuity level may be upgraded. The ESI acuity level is never downgraded.

As previously stated, triage is not a place, but rather an ongoing process. Because pediatric patients can deteriorate rapidly, frequent reevaluations are warranted. Many institutions have set standards regarding the frequency of reevaluation of patients based on their assigned triage acuity rating. Any patient who has not received definitive care and/or placement in a treatment room within the prescribed maximum waiting time for the assigned triage acuity rating (using ATS, CTAS, or MTS) is reassessed. Institutions using ESI may develop reevaluation standards based on a more in-depth assessment after the triage acuity assignment is made, as there are no prescribed

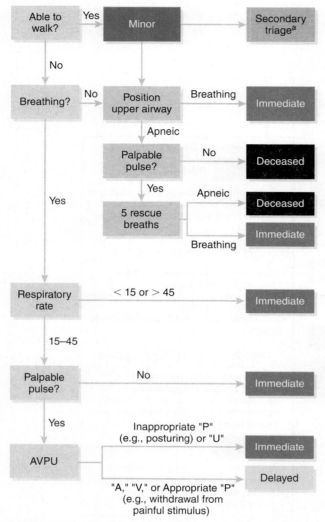

Figure 4-3 *JumpSTART pediatric mass-casualty incident triage algorithm.*

* Nonambulatory children (infants who cannot walk yet, children with preexisting conditions) are evaluated beginning with Breathing.

Reproduced from U.S. Department of Health and Human Services. (2021, August 16). *JumpSTART pediatric triage algorithm.* https://chemm.hhs.gov/startpediatric .htm

waiting times for this tool. Additionally, anytime an intervention is instituted, a reevaluation of the patient's status is performed to determine the effectiveness of that intervention.

CLINICAL PEARL

Recruit the Caregivers

Recruit the patient's caregivers to assist with ongoing patient reassessment. Teach the caregivers which signs and symptoms are concerning and warrant immediate notification of the healthcare team. This intervention can also relieve anxiety while waiting for treatment or results.

Assessment Pearls

This section covers several additional assessment and prioritization pearls.

Make the Parent or Primary Caregiver Your Friend

Probably one of the most important things to remember when caring for the pediatric patient is that the parent or primary caregiver is, in most instances, the greatest source of information and an invaluable assessment aide. If a parent or caregiver states that the child is not acting normally, *listen!* Even if the child seems to be acting perfectly normally, remember that a nurse who is unfamiliar with the patient does not know what is normal for that child. The parent or primary caregiver does. A basic understanding of pediatric norms and the most common disease processes is vitally important when assessing a pediatric patient.

RED FLAG

Any alteration in mental status in a pediatric patient should be considered to be the result of decreased cerebral perfusion or hypoglycemia until proven otherwise.

Ask the Right Questions to Get the Right Answers

Another pearl that applies to all assessments, but particularly when determining priority of care is "You *must* ask the right questions to get the right answers!" Avoidance of yes-and-no questions and asking open-ended questions can be of significant value, especially during a focused assessment of a pediatric patient. Two commonly used mnemonics to assist the nurse with which questions to ask are SAMPLE (**Box 4-2**; appropriate for patients of any age) and CIAMPEDS (**Box 4-3**; slightly more in-depth and focused on the pediatric population).

The SAMPLE mnemonic is more commonly used. The version in Box 4-2 is slightly adapted to include immunizations and last output. Decreased urination is a way to assess dehydration and is apparent if the parent describes fewer diapers that seem less heavy in the past day. This information is lost if the nurse does not ask about output. Older children can be asked about the last time they used the bathroom, the color of their urine, or the frequency of loose stools.

The use of one or both of these mnemonics will assist the nurse in remembering which questions to ask when doing a focused assessment to aid in prioritizing the pediatric patient beyond "sick, sicker, or sickest." It is also becoming

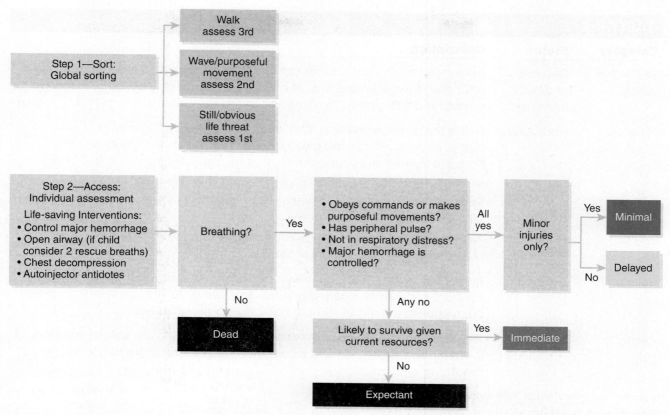

Figure 4-4 *The SALT algorithm.*

Reproduced from SALT Mass Casualty Triage: Concept Endorsed by the American College of Emergency Physicians, American College of Surgeons Committee on Trauma, American Trauma Society, National Association of EMS Physicians, National Disaster Life Support Education Consortium, and State and Territorial Injury Prevention Directors Association. (2008). *Disaster Medicine and Public Health Preparedness, 2*(4), 245–246. https://doi.org/10.1097/DMP.0b013e31818d191e

increasingly important to perform maltreatment, violence, substance use, suicide risk, and other safety screenings at some point during the assessment of pediatric patients.[7,13] These evaluations can often be initiated during the triage process after it is determined that the child is in stable condition. Health promotion and injury prevention assessments and interventions ideally will occur multiple times during a pediatric patient encounter.

Vital Signs: Now or Later?

There has been much debate and discussion regarding obtaining vital signs as a necessary part of prioritization and acuity assignment. If the child needs immediate care based on the PAT or other findings, obtaining vital signs may delay potentially life-saving interventions. If the child appears to be physiologically stable based on the PAT and other findings, obtaining a complete set of vital signs aids in determining the patient's triage acuity level. Some emergency acuity indices use abnormalities in vital signs as a parameter for determining acuity. The challenge then becomes getting accurate vital signs, especially for children younger than 2 years of age. Attempting to get vital signs for a child who is crying, whether from pain, discomfort, or fear, is challenging. Having the

appropriately sized blood pressure cuff and finger probe for assessment of pulse oximetry readings also helps to ensure the accuracy of the measurements.

Learning to count respirations from afar, before the young pediatric patient even sees you, is a valuable skill. Also, remember that when measuring vital signs in an alert pediatric patient, especially a younger patient, the nurse should start with the *least* invasive vital sign first and then proceed to the most invasive last. In other words, start with respiratory rate first, then heart rate, then blood pressure (giving the child's arm a "hug" with the cuff), and finally temperature, especially if it will be a rectal temperature.

Normal ranges for pediatric vital signs are quite different from what nurses are accustomed to seeing in adults. Quick access to a pediatric vital signs reference based on age is also of tremendous value. A posted chart or normal vital signs reference embedded into an electronic health record is critical in determining whether the vital signs are abnormal.

Table 4-3 identifies normal vital signs for specific age ranges.[4(P4),18,26,31] Consider the child's clinical condition and context when interpreting vital signs. The heart and respiratory rate will be slower when the child is calm or sleeping and faster when the child is active, in pain, or febrile.

TABLE 4-2	Disaster Triage	
Category	**Status**	**Description**
Black (black/white)	Deceased or death imminent	Persons who are apneic (after opening the airway and, if a pediatric patient, after giving 5 rescue breaths) or are pulseless or who will require extensive resuscitation. Designed to conserve limited resources.
Red	Immediate	Persons who are breathing after establishing an open airway (or if a pediatric patient, after being given rescue breaths), or respiratory rate is > 30 breaths/min, or if younger than 8 years respiratory rate is < 15 or > 45 breaths/min; OR
		Persons who are breathing within normal limits but who have a capillary refill > 2 seconds OR
		AVPU assessment is = P (inappropriate posturing in response to Pain) or U = Unresponsive
Yellow	Delayed	Persons who are breathing within normal limits and who have a capillary refill ≤ 2 seconds or a palpable pulse and whose AVPU is A, V, or P (appropriate response to painful stimuli) but who are nonambulatory
Green	Minor	Persons who are able to walk without difficulty or who are able to ambulate with minimal assistance and who have no significant anomalies in airway, breathing, or circulation

Note: AVPU = Alert, Verbal, Pain, Unresponsive.

Used in the United States and some international disaster arenas for mass-casualty triage.

Uses the START decision tree to determine acuity code.

For pediatric patients younger than 8 years, use the JumpSTART decision tree to determine acuity code (Figure 4-3).

Data from American College of Surgeons. (2018). *Advanced trauma life support: Student course manual* (10th ed., pp. 289–300). Author.

BOX 4-2 SAMPLE Mnemonic

S Signs/Symptoms
A Allergies
M Medications (routine and given for this illness/injury)
P Past medical history/Past immunizations
L Last meal/Last output/Last menstrual period
E Events leading up to the current illness/injury

BOX 4-3 CIAMPEDS Mnemonic

The CIAMPEDS mnemonic is pronounced C-I-AM-PEEDS.

C Chief Complaint
I Immunizations/need for isolation
A Allergies
M Medications (routine and given for this illness/injury)
P Past medical history/Parent's perception of illness or injury
E Events leading up to/surrounding the current illness/injury
D Diet (last meal—when and what), Diapers (last elimination—when and what)
S Symptoms associated with illness/injury

Size Is Everything!

A pediatric patient's weight is vitally important because all pediatric medication doses and fluid replacements are based on the patient's weight in *kilograms*. A scale that is locked in kilograms is an essential tool in any healthcare setting where pediatric patients receive care. Length-based resuscitation tapes can be useful in lieu of accurate weights but should be used only if the child is too critically ill to obtain an exact weight measurement. Obtaining an accurate weight in kilograms for all pediatric patients as soon as possible is a best practice.[17]

Crying Is Good—to a Point

An old adage in EDs is "A crying child is a good child!" This is true up to a point, because a child who is crying is usually a child who is responsive to the environment, which is one of the components of the PAT. But a crying

TABLE 4-3 Normal Vital Signs for Pediatric Patients

Age	Heart Rate (beats/min)	Respiratory Rate (breaths/min)	Systolic Blood Pressure (mm Hg)
Term neonate to < 1 month	90–190	35–60	67–84
Infant, 1–12 months	90–180	30–55	72–104
Toddler, 1–3 years	80–140	22–40	86–104
Preschooler, 3–5 years	65–120	18–35	89–112
School-age, 5–12 years	70–120	16–30	90–115
Adolescent, 12–18 years	60–100	12–20	100–130

Data from American Heart Association. (2020). Part 4: Systematic approach to the seriously ill or injured child. *Pediatric advanced life support provider manual*; Ernst, G. (2020). Pediatric trauma. In J. E. Tintinalli, O. J. Ma, D. M. Yealy, G. D. Meckler, J. S. Stapczynski, D. M. Cline, & S. H. Thomas (Eds.), *Tintinalli's emergency medicine: A comprehensive study guide* (9th ed., pp. 689–697). McGraw Hill; and Lucia, D., & Glenn, J. (2017). Pediatric emergencies. In C. K. Stone & R. L. Humphries (Eds.), *Current diagnosis and treatment: Emergency medicine* (8th ed., pp. 964–1016). McGraw Hill.

BOX 4-4 AH! IF IT CRIESS Mnemonic

A Anger

H Hunger

I Infection

F Fear/Frustration

I Increased intracranial pressure

T Trauma (intentional or nonintentional)/Testicular torsion

C Cardiac issues

R Reflux (GERD)/Reaction to medication/formula

I Immunizations/Insect bites

E Eye-corneal abrasions/ocular foreign body

S Surgical needs (intussusception, inguinal hernia, malrotation/volvulus)

S Strangulation—hair tourniquet on digits, penis, or clitoris

Data from Herman, M., & Le, A. (2007). The crying infant. *Emergency Medicine Clinics of North America, 25*(4), 1137–1159. https://doi.org/10.1016/j.emc.2007.07.008

child also presents a multitude of challenges for the nurse, especially when attempting to obtain accurate vital signs.

The most important element is the *quality* of the cry and whether the child is consolable. In younger, preverbal children, crying is the only way the child has to communicate needs, and younger children are often not able to accurately localize pain.[23] Crying or fussiness can be indicative of discomfort caused by pain, hunger, frustration, or tiredness. An estimated 5% of crying results from organic (e.g., cardiac, gastrointestinal, infectious, traumatic) causes.[11] The list of threats to a child that can cause crying is extensive; some of these can be identified with the AH! IF IT CRIESS mnemonic (**Box 4-4**).[23]

The nurse assessing the crying child should consider the characteristics of the cry in relation to the child's general appearance and ability to be comforted. A quick head-to-toe assessment (explained in detail in Chapter 5, "Initial Assessment: The Pediatric Nursing Process") and a brief history can often help to identify the cause of the crying. If the crying is weak, it can be a sign of serious illness. A high-pitched, screeching, catlike cry in an infant can be indicative of increased intracranial pressure[2] or a chromosomal disorder (cri du chat syndrome).[33] A low-pitched, hoarse-sounding cry can be indicative of an upper respiratory illness.[23] Otherwise, if the crying is strong and robust, and is appropriate for the situation, it can be reassuring that the child is breathing adequately.[2]

RED FLAG

If a parent or caregiver uses the term "fussy" or "fussiness" to describe difficulty in consoling the child, consider this a red flag for serious illness or injury. Other red flags in triage are discussed later in this chapter.

Fever, Pain, and Rashes, Oh My!

Assessment of the pediatric patient for fever, pain, and rashes is an integral part of the initial triage of the patient beyond the PAT. Sometimes, partial assessment of these parameters can be done while doing the PAT. A child who is crying during the assessment of the general appearance and breathing portions of the PAT may be crying due to pain. A child who appears flushed when assessing the color of the skin may have a fever, and some assessment for the presence of skin rashes may also be done as part of the PAT. Evidence of any of these three parameters during the PAT warrants additional focused assessment.

Fever

Temperature greater than 39°C (102.2°F) in a child of any age is concerning. Temperature greater than 38°C (100.4°F) in an infant younger than 90 days is also concerning and is considered a red flag in triage. Hypothermia is also of concern. Temperature less than 35°C (95°F) in a child of any age is concerning. In neonates and young infants, temperatures less than 36.1°C (97°F) are considered a red flag for early sepsis.[41]

Pain

Studies continue to indicate that pediatric pain assessment and management by nurses in all areas of patient care are inadequate.[5,8,14,20,36] Gender bias has been noted in pediatric pain assessment and management, with male patients being more adequately treated for pain than are female patients.[15] Using an age-appropriate pain scale is essential when assessing pain in any patient. Assessment of the pediatric patient's pain is a significant consideration when prioritizing care. Standing orders are often used to facilitate prompt pain management. Refer to Chapter 3, "Pediatric Differences," for acceptable age-appropriate pain scales and pain management strategies.

Skin Rashes

Identification of the presence of a skin rash may be accomplished during the PAT determination. If a rash is not identified initially, then its presence should be determined during the focused assessment. Presence of a skin rash, accompanied by an abnormal PAT, should be considered life threatening until proven otherwise. A child with an abnormal PAT and a skin rash should be prophylactically isolated until the cause of the rash is identified. Obtaining a vaccination and exposure history can be helpful in determining the etiology of the skin rash.

Infection Prevention and Immunizations

Knowledge of the potential for spread of communicable diseases to or by the pediatric patient is an important consideration. Infection control practices are evolving. It is the nurse's responsibility to identify risks and implement precautions in accordance with the most current guidelines.

Isolation has always been a challenge with the pediatric population. Younger children are not cognitively able to comply with infection control measures and may require special attention to limit disease transmission. The use of appropriate personal protective equipment by the nurse, the patient, and the family members is essential, along with easily accessible hand sanitizer, handwashing facilities, tissues, emesis containers, and appropriate disposal receptacles in the triage and waiting areas.

Determining the patient's immunization status early is essential to protect the child and promote the well-being of all. Under-vaccinated children might warrant isolation for their own protection or be at higher risk for significant illness than fully vaccinated children. Familiarity with regional immunization recommendations and resources enables the nurse to assess and manage the risks involved with under-vaccination as well as to provide education.

NOTE

Immunization Schedules

The Centers for Disease Control and Prevention's Immunization Schedule can be found at https://www.cdc.gov/vaccines/schedules/hcp/imz/child-adolescent.html and the World Health Organization's schedule at https://www.who.int/immunization/policy/Immunization_routine_table2.pdf?ua=1 for further information.

Children with Special Needs Require Special Attention

It goes without saying that children with special needs require extra diligence and consideration during the prioritization and triaging process. Often these children arrive with their primary caregiver, who can be your best source of information regarding what is abnormal for the child. Attention to detail regarding the etiology of the special need(s) and the concern that prompted the ED visit can dramatically improve the accuracy of the determination of acuity. Awareness of the possibility that these children may not be fully vaccinated due to contraindications or immunosuppression related to their condition is also an important factor. Isolation may be warranted to protect the child if any immunocompromise is suspected. See Chapter 18, "The Child with Special Health Care Needs," for more in-depth information.

Pediatric Red Flags

Certain abnormalities identified during either the PAT or the focused assessment of the pediatric patient should be considered red flags that require immediate attention and intervention. These red flags are identified in **Table 4-4**.

Case Examples

Table 4-5 profiles a few patients and considers how they would be categorized based on the PAT.

TABLE 4-4	Red Flags of Pediatric Triage
General Area of Concern	**Specific Symptoms**
Alertness and Airway	Patient is not alert
	Choking, drooling
	Severe, uncontrolled, and persistent cough (consider the need for isolation)
	Audible airway sounds (gurgling, snoring, or stridor)
	Swelling of the mouth, face, or neck
	Positioning to assist breathing (tripod position or head bent forward)
Breathing	Apnea or irregular respiratory pattern with periods of apnea
	Respiratory rate > 60 or < 20 breaths/min in children younger than 6 years
	Audible respiratory sounds (wheezing, grunting)
	Increased work of breathing
	Absence of breath sounds in any lung field
Circulation	Cyanosis or marked pallor to skin
	Heart rate significantly above or below what is normal for age; any heart rate > 200 or < 60 beats/min
	Capillary refill > 2 seconds
	Presence of uncontrolled bleeding
	Hypotension (late sign of shock in pediatric patient)
	Systolic blood pressure < 70 + (2 × child's age in years) mm Hg for children 1 to 10 years old is considered hypotension[4(P4)]
	Signs of dehydration (dry/cracked mucous membranes, crying without tears, sunken fontanel or eyes, poor skin turgor)
Disability	Altered Glasgow Coma Scale score
	Child described as "irritable," "fussy," or "inconsolable" by caregiver
	Lethargy or poor muscle tone
	Bulging fontanelle
	Alteration in pupillary response
	Seizure activity
	Check blood glucose if *any* abnormality is noted in the assessment of disability
Exposure	Petechiae or purpura (consider the need for isolation)
	Any signs of trauma
	Rash (consider the need for isolation)
	Indications of unintentional injury or maltreatment
	Indication of possible human trafficking (physical injuries, abuse, tattoos, malnourished, poor hygiene, other)
	Hives or severe itching
Full set of vital signs	Anything significantly above or below normal for child's age.
	Temperature > 38°C (100.4°F) in child 3 months or younger or temperature > 40°C (104°F) in child older than 3 months

(continues)

TABLE 4-4	Red Flags of Pediatric Triage (*continued*)
General Area of Concern	**Specific Symptoms**
Get adjuncts and Give comfort	Pulse oximetry < 94% End-tidal CO_2 > 45 or < 35 mm Hg (> 6 or < 4.7 kilopascals) Moderate to severe pain (as assessed using an age-appropriate pain scale)
History	History of chronic disease or immunosuppression History of family crisis Unscheduled return to the ED within 24 hours Actual or potential threat to self or others

TABLE 4-5	Case Examples	
Patient	**Observations Made Using the PAT**	**Categorization and Rationale**
1	Adult arrives in the ED carrying a toddler and states, "He was horsing around with his older brother on the top of the bunk beds and fell off." **Appearance:** Child is limp in the adult's arms. **Work of breathing:** Breathing is regular; appears slower than normal with no increased respiratory effort. **Circulation to skin:** Color is normal.	Child is categorized as **Sickest**. Child's general appearance is abnormal, and breathing is slower than normal. The two abnormalities in the PAT classify this child as *sickest*, despite the color of the skin being normal.
2	Teacher arrives with an ambulatory young school-age child, stating, "She was running on the playground and fell and cut her forehead." **Appearance:** Child is alert and looking around, holding a wet cloth to her forehead. **Work of breathing:** Breathing is regular, normal rate; no increased work of breathing. **Circulation to skin:** Color is normal.	Child is categorized as **Sick**. All parameters of the PAT are within normal limits. A focused assessment reveals the child has an approximately 3-cm laceration to the right side of her forehead above her right eyebrow, oozing small amount of blood that will require suturing.
3	Adult arrives with an older school-age child who is audibly wheezing and states, "She was at the neighbors, and they just got a new kitten. She has a history of asthma, and has used her inhaler, but she is still wheezing." **Appearance:** Child is awake and interactive, holding her inhaler in her hand. **Work of breathing:** Audible wheezing noted; breathing is somewhat labored and faster than normal; some accessory muscle use noted. **Circulation to skin:** Color is normal.	Child is categorized as **Sicker**. Her appearance is appropriate, and she is interactive with her environment. She has audible wheezing and increased work of breathing. Her circulation to the skin is normal. She has one abnormality in the PAT; therefore, she is *sicker*.
4	Adult arrives carrying an infant tightly wrapped in a blanket and states, "This is my first child, and she cries all the time. She is 3 weeks old, and now she feels hot."	Child is categorized as **Sickest**. Her appearance is abnormal—she appears distressed and not easily comforted. Her breathing demonstrates increased work of breathing (sternal retractions), and her color is abnormal (bright red).

Patient	Observations Made Using the PAT	Categorization and Rationale
	Appearance: Child is crying loudly despite the mother's attempts to comfort her, and appears to be flailing inside blanket (assume "fussiness"; in a neonate, considered a red flag). **Work of breathing:** Crying loudly with evident sternal retractions (perhaps due to crying, but assume due to illness or injury) **Circulation to skin:** Color of face is bright red (perhaps due to crying but assume due to elevated temperature).	Although all those abnormalities may be due to her crying, based on her age and the chief complaint as verbalized by the mother, she warrants the *sickest* category. Especially with neonates and preverbal children, always err on the side of caution and assume that the abnormalities in the PAT are the result of serious illness or injury until proven otherwise.
5	Adolescent male arrives with an adult. Child states, "My left ball hurts really bad!" **Appearance:** Alert and interactive, but facial expression and grimacing indicate severe pain. **Work of breathing:** Respiratory rate within normal limits and no evidence of increased respiratory effort. **Circulation to skin:** Skin color is normal.	Child is categorized as **Sick**. Appearance, breathing, and circulation to skin are all normal. A focused assessment reveals sudden onset of severe (10/10) left testicular and groin pain about 30 minutes prior to arrival with no known injury. However, this child should be brought back immediately despite being categorized as *sick* based on the PAT. His symptoms are suggestive of testicular torsion, for which treatment is time sensitive.
6	Crying toddler arrives in an adult's arms. Adult states, "He has been pulling at his left ear for the past two days and now he won't stop crying." **Appearance:** Child is crying loudly and pulling at his left ear. **Work of breathing:** Respiratory rate is within normal limits when not crying; no increased work of breathing. **Circulation to skin:** Skin color is normal.	Child is categorized as **Sicker**. His appearance is abnormal. Severe crying may be due to pain, but always err on the side of caution. Breathing and circulation to the skin are normal. There is one abnormality in the PAT, so the child is categorized as *sicker*.
7	Adolescent in a wheelchair is brought to the ED by his mother, who states, "He has been acting strangely for the past couple of days, he isn't sleeping well at night, and I think he may have taken something. He has seemed really depressed lately." **Appearance:** Child is awake and interactive, lower extremities appear atrophied. States, "I'm fine. I just don't want to live like this anymore." **Work of breathing:** Respiratory rate is within normal limits with no increased work of breathing. Child answers questions in complete sentences. **Circulation to skin:** Skin color is normal.	Child is categorized as **Sick**. However, due to the potential overdose, further investigation with a focused assessment including a complete history is warranted. This child should be given a higher acuity rating and immediately placed for rapid assessment and interventions due to possible ingestion and suicidal ideation.

Emerging Trends

Staffing shortages, ED overcrowding, throughput delays, and inpatient boarding have been long-standing obstacles to quality emergency care. Providing complete care in the ED without ever bringing the patient back to a room is not uncommon. This adds to the complexity of the triage nurse role and prioritization of patients presenting for care. The COVID-19 pandemic worsened many of these issues, but also made them more public. This public scrutiny may prompt further analysis, leading to changes and improvements in healthcare delivery systems.

Bias that impacts triage accuracy is often the result of long-standing structures in both medicine and nursing, affecting people of color, people with disabilities, people with language barriers, and members of the LGBTQ+ community. To prevent patient harm, it is critical that nurses examine their assumptions about patients and appraise evidence with an understanding of these structures. Racism, ableism, and bias against the LGBTQ+ community can be understood clinically as a cognitive error and can impede safe and effective nursing care.

Summary

Appropriately prioritizing a pediatric patient's need for care and the severity of their illness or injury can be challenging. The Pediatric Assessment Triangle is an essential tool in the nurse's arsenal when faced with having to rapidly and accurately determine how sick the child is and how urgent the need is for care. Because the PAT is relatively easy to use and is done from across the room, it enables the nurse to make a quick assessment of the patient's overall physiologic status prior to coming in direct contact with the patient. Determination of sick–sicker–sickest status aids in implementation of interventions as required and enables further investigation if the child's condition permits.

A focused assessment of the presenting complaint helps to further identify the severity of the illness or injury and facilitate proper assignment of triage acuity. As with all skills, practice makes perfect, and the more nurses practice their prioritization and triage skills, the better they will be at determining patient acuity and the urgency of the need for care. Most importantly, the nurse must always remember that the pediatric patient's condition can change rapidly, requiring ongoing reassessment for early identification of decompensation and the need to reprioritize the patient.

References

1. Ageron, F., Porteaud, J., Evain, J., Millet, A., Greze, J., Vallot, C., Levrat, A., Mortamet, G., Bouzat, P., & TRENAU Group. (2021). Effect of under triage on early mortality after major pediatric trauma: A registry-based propensity score matching analysis. *World Journal of Emergency Surgery, 16*, Article 1. https://doi.org/10.1186/s13017-020-00345-w

2. Akhnikh, S., Engelberts, A. C., van Sleuwen, B. E., & Bennings, M. A. (2014). The excessively crying infant: Etiology and treatment. *Pediatric Annals, 43*(4), e69–e75. https://doi.org/10.3928/00904481-20140325-07

3. American College of Surgeons. (2018). *Advanced trauma life support: Student course manual* (10th ed.).

4. American Heart Association. (2020). *Pediatric advanced life support provider manual.*

5. Amponsah, A. K., Bjorn, A., Bam., V., & Axelin, A. (2019). The effect of educational strategies targeted for nurses in pain assessment and management in children: An integrative review. *Pain Management Nursing, 20*(6), 604–613. https://doi.org/10.1016/j.pmn.2019.03.005

6. Australasian College for Emergency Medicine. (2016). *Guidelines on the implementation of the Australasian Triage Scale in emergency departments.* https://acem.org.au/getmedia/51dc74f7-9ff0-42ce-872a-0437f3db640a/G24_04_Guidelines_on_Implementation_of_ATS_Jul-16.aspx

7. Ballard, E. D., Cwik, M., Van Eck, K., Goldstein, M., Alfes, C., Wilson, M. E., Virden, J. M., Horowitz, L. M., & Wilcox, H. C. (2017). Identification of at-risk youth by suicide screening in a pediatric emergency department. *Prevention Science, 18*, 174–182. https://doi.org/10.1007/s11121-016-0717-5

8. Beltramini, A., Kilojevic, K., & Pateron, D. (2017). Pain assessment in newborns, infants, and children. *Pediatric Annals, 46*(10), e387–e395. https://doi.org/10.3928/19382359-20170921-03

9. Benner, P. (2001). *From novice to expert: Excellence and power in clinical nursing practice* (Commemorative ed). Prentice Hall Health.

10. Bullard, M. J., Musgrave, E., Warren, D., Unger, B., Skeldon, T., Grierson, R., van der Linde, E., & Swain, J. (2016). *Revisions to the Canadian Emergency Department Triage and Acuity Scale (CTAS) guidelines 2016* [Position statement]. Canadian Association of Emergency Physicians. http://ctas-phctas.ca/wp-content/uploads/2018/05/revisions_to_the_canadian_emergency_department_triage_and_acuity_scale_ctas_guidelines_2016.pdf

11. Consolini, D. M. (2020). Crying. *Merck Manual professional version.* Retrieved January 15, 2022, from https://www.merckmanuals.com/professional/pediatrics/symptoms-in-infants-and-children/crying

12. Corneli, H. M., & Kadish, H. (2020), June 5). Hypothermia in children: Clinical manifestations and diagnosis. *UpToDate.* Retrieved September 12, 2021, from https://www.uptodate.com/contents/hypothermia-in-children-clinical-manifestations-and-diagnosis

13. Coulton, S., M. Alam, M. F., Boniface, S., Deluca, P., Donoghue, K., Gilvarry, E., Kaner, E., Lynch, E., Maconochie, I., McArdle, P., McGovern, R., Newbury-Birch, D., Patton, R., Phillips, C. J., Phillips, T., Rose, H., Russell, I., Strang, J., & Drummond, C. (2018). Opportunistic screening for alcohol use problems in adolescents attending emergency departments: An evaluation of screening tools. *Journal of Public Health, 41*(1), e53–e60. https://doi.org/10.1093/pubmed/fdy049

14. Crellin, D. J., Harrison, D., Santamaria, N., Huque, H., & Babl, F. E. (2018). The psychometric properties of the FLACC Scale to assess procedural pain. *Journal of Pain, 19*(8), 862–872. https://doi.org/10.1016/j.jpain.2018.02.013

15. Earp, B. D., Monrad, J. T., LaFrance, M., Bargh, J. A., Cohen, L. L., & Richeson, J. A. (2019). Gender bias in pediatric pain assessment. *Journal of Pediatric Psychology, 44*(4), 1–12. https://doi.org/10.1093/jpepsy/jsy104

16. Ebrahimi, M., Mirhaghi, A., Najafi, Z., Shafaee, H., & Roudi, M. H. (2020). Are pediatric triage systems reliable in the emergency department? *Emergency Medicine International*, Article 9825730. https://doi.org/10.1155/2020/9825730

17. Emergency Nurses Association. (2016). *Weighing all patients in kilograms* [Position statement]. https://enau.ena.org/Users/LearningActivityAssetSingleViewer.aspx?LearningActivityAssetID=mEigQMFxphlUI%2fEvoRx8Fg%3d%3d

18. Ernst, G. (2020). Pediatric trauma. In J. E. Tintinalli, O. J. Ma, D. M. Yealy, G. D. Meckler, J. S. Stapczynski, D. M. Cline, & S. H. Thomas (Eds.), *Tintinalli's emergency medicine: A comprehensive study guide* (9th ed., pp. 698–697). McGraw Hill.

19. Fernandez, A., Ares, M. I., Garcia, S., Martinez0Indart, L., Mintegi, S., & Benito, J. (2017). The validity of the Pediatric Assessment Triangle as the first step in the triage process in a pediatric emergency department. *Pediatric Emergency Care, 33*(4), 234–238. https://doi.org/10.1097/PEC.0000000000000717

20. Franck, L. S., Greenberg, C. S., & Stevens, B. (2000). Pain assessment in infants and children. *Pediatric Clinics of North America, 47*(3), 487–512. https://doi.org/10.1016/S0031-3955(05)70222-4

21. Gilboy, N., Tanabe, P., Travers, F., & Rosenau, A. M. (2020). Use of the ESI for pediatric triage. In *Emergency Severity Index implementation handbook 2020 edition: A triage tool for emergency department care—version 4* (pp. 39–48). Emergency Nurses Association. https://www.ena.org/docs/default-source/education-document-library/esi-implementation-handbook-2020.pdf?sfvrsn=fdc327df_2

22. Hassani, P., Abdi, A., Jalali, R., & Salari, N. (2016). The intuitive nurse in critical care practice: A phenomenological study. *Nursing Reports, 6*(1). https://doi.org/10.4081/nursrep.2016.5665

23. Herman, M., & Le, A. (2007). The crying infant. *Emergency Medicine Clinics of North America, 25*(4), 1137–1159. https://doi.org/10.1016/j.emc.2007.07.008

24. Hinson, J. S., Martinez, D. A., Cabral, S., George, K., Whalen, M., Hansoti, B., & Levin, S. (2018). Triage performance in emergency medicine: A systematic review. *Annals of Emergency Medicine, 74*(1) 140–152. https://doi.org/10.1016/j.annemergmed.2018.09.022

25. Horeczko, T., Enriques, B., McGrath, N., Gausche-Hill, M., & Lewis, R. (2013). The Pediatric Assessment Triangle: Accuracy of its application by nurses in the triage of children. *Journal of Emergency Nursing, 39*(2), 182–189. https://doi.org/10.1016%2Fj.jen.2011.12.020.

26. Lucia, D., & Glenn, J. (2017). Pediatric emergencies. In C. K. Stone & R. L. Humphries (Eds.), *Current diagnosis and treatment: Emergency medicine* (8th ed., pp. 964–1016). McGraw Hill.

27. Ma, X., Liu, Y., Du, M., Ojo, O., Huang, L., Feng, X., Gao, Q., & Wang, X. (2021). The accuracy of the pediatric assessment triangle in assessing triage of critically ill patients in emergency pediatric department. *International Emergency Nursing, 58*. https://doi.org/10.1016/j.ienj.2021.101041

28. Mackway-Jones, K., Marsden, J., & Windle, J. (Eds.). (2014). *Emergency triage: Manchester Triage Group* (3rd ed.). Wiley Blackwell.

29. Marett, B. (2019). Emergency nursing review questions: July 2019. *Journal of Emergency Nursing, 45*(4), 450–451. https://doi.org/10.1016/j.jen.2019.04.002

30. Melin-Johansson, C., Palmqvist, R., & Rönnberg, L. (2017). Clinical intuition in the nursing process and decision making: A mixed-studies review. *Journal of Clinical Nursing, 26*(23–24), 3936–3949. https://doi.org/10.1111/jocn.13814

31. Mersch, J. (2020). *Pediatric vital signs ranges and charts*. https://www.emedicinehealth.com/pediatric_vital_signs/article_em.htm

32. Mukwende, M., Tamonyh, P., & Turner, M. (2020). *Mind the gap* (1st ed.). St. George's University of London. https://www.blackandbrownskin.co.uk/mindthegap

33. National Institute of Health, National Human Genome Research Institute. (2017). *About cri du chat syndrome*. https://www.genome.gov/Genetic-Disorders/Cri-du-Chat

34. Nnedu, C. C. (2021). Nigerian Americans. In J. N. Giger & L. G. Haddad (Eds.), *Transcultural nursing* (8th ed., pp. 589–611). Elsevier.

35. Recznik, C. T., & Simko, L. M. (2018). Pediatric triage education: An integrative literature review. *Journal of Emergency Nursing, 44*(6), 605–613.e9. https://doi.org/10.1016/j.jen.2018.01.003

36. Recznik, C. T., Simko, L. C., Travers, D., & Devido, J. (2019). Pediatric triage education for the general emergency nurse: A randomized crossover trial comparing simulation with paper-case studies. *Journal of Emergency Nursing, 45*(4), 394–402. https://doi.org/10.1016/j.jen.2019.01.009

37. Robertson-Steel, I. (2006). Evolution of triage systems. *Emergency Medicine Journal, 23*(2), 154–155. https://doi.org/10.1136/emj.2005.030270

38. SALT mass casualty triage: Concept endorsed by the American College of Emergency Physicians, American College of Surgeons Committee on Trauma, American Trauma Society, National Association of EMS Physicians, National Disaster Life Support Education Consortium, and State and Territorial Injury Prevention Directors Association. (2008).

Disaster Medicine and Public Health Preparedness, 2(4), 245–246. https://doi.org/10.1097/DMP.0b013e31818d191e

39. U.S. Department of Health and Human Services. (2021, August 16). *JumpSTART pediatric triage algorithm.* https://chemm.hhs.gov/startpediatric.htm

40. U.S. Department of Health and Human Services. (2021, August 16). *START adult triage algorithm.* https://chemm.hhs.gov/startadult.htm

41. Ward, M. A. (2020, March 25). Fever in infants and children: Pathophysiology and management. *UpToDate.* Retrieved September 12, 2021, from_https://www.uptodate.com/contents/fever-in-infants-and-children-pathophysiology-and-management

42. Warren, D. W., Jarvis. A., LeBlanc, L., Gravel, J., CTAs National Working Group, Canadian Association of Emergency Physicians, National Emergency Nurses Affiliation, Association des Médecins d'Urgence du Québec, Canadian Paediatric Society, & Society of Rural Physicians of Canada. (2008). Revisions to the Canadian Triage and Acuity Scale Paediatric Guidelines (PaedCTAS). *Canadian Journal of Emergency Medicine, 10*(3), 224–232. https://doi.org/10.1017/S1481803500010149

43. Zachariasse, J. M., van der Hagen, V., Seiger, N., Mackway-Jones, K., van Veen, M., & Moll, H.A. (2019). Performance of triage systems in emergency care: A systematic review and meta-analysis. *BMJ Open, 9*(5), Article e026471. https://doi.org/10.1136/bmjopen-2018-026471

Initial Assessment

Lisa Jamerson, DNP, RN, CNE, CPEN, NRP

OBJECTIVES

Upon completion of this chapter, the learner will be able to:

1. Implement a systematic approach to the initial assessment of the pediatric patient with an emphasis on recognizing life-threatening abnormalities and anticipating life-saving interventions.
2. Identify options for definitive care considering facility and regional resources.
3. Prioritize ongoing reassessments and interventions while awaiting transfer to definitive care or discharge.

Introduction

Amidst the chaos of the emergency department (ED), pediatric patients present with a variety of conditions. A systematic approach to the initial assessment of each child is necessary to recognize and address life threats, discern signs and symptoms of injuries or illness, and prioritize the patient's needs. The systematic approach taught in this course is called the Pediatric Nursing Process (PNP).

An alphabetical mnemonic is used to delineate the steps in this process. The initial assessment begins with preparation and triage, which may occur upon patient arrival if there is no prenotification. A general impression is formed, sometimes from across the room, using the Pediatric Assessment Triangle (PAT). Control of external hemorrhage or initiation of cardiopulmonary resuscitation may be required at this point.

The primary survey (ABCDE), with corresponding interventions (FG) as required, is used to rapidly identify life-threatening abnormalities and necessary interventions. Consideration of the need for transfer to a higher level of care is paramount throughout the initial assessment. Transfer may be initiated by ancillary staff by coordinating facility communication during the primary survey. The secondary survey (HI) includes a thorough history and head-to-toe assessment. Reevaluation (J) is vital while awaiting definitive care.

The A–J mnemonic delineates the components of the initial assessment (**Box 5-1**).

The primary survey portion of the initial assessment is performed in a stepwise fashion. Generally, it is not appropriate to move on to the next skill step before addressing life-threatening abnormalities. There are some exceptions, such as when obtaining the child's weight and intravenous access is required to facilitate medication administration for endotracheal intubation. In "real life," however, assessments and interventions do happen simultaneously. This does not alter the assessment and intervention priorities in the primary survey. A team member focused on assessing pupils when they could be assisting ventilations is one example of why the stepwise prioritization is vital. The effectiveness of each intervention is assessed.

Preparation and Triage

The approach to pediatric care may begin with a notification that the patient is or will soon be arriving in the ED. The nurse may then have time to activate necessary members of the healthcare team and assign roles. Triage is used to determine whether it is necessary to relocate a patient who is occupying a pediatric resuscitation room or reprioritize care of other patients in the department. Some facilities maintain a pediatric-specific cart that is stocked with a length-based resuscitation tape, pediatric-sized equipment such as blood pressure cuffs and blood collection tubes, pediatric protocols with dosing guidelines, and other vital supplies. This cart can easily be brought into any room. Preplanning helps ensure necessary resources are available. Failure to have the appropriate resources for the pediatric patient can delay care and impact patient outcomes.[13,15,32] See Chapter 2, "Preparing for Pediatric Emergencies," for more detailed information.

With or without prior notification of such issues, the team needs to consider potential safety threats or the need for decontamination. Safety threats may include violence, weapons, and infectious or toxic agents that can harm the team if inhaled or touched. Donning personal protective equipment is necessary for any patient encounter. Decontamination may be the priority patient intervention because patient care is compromised if a toxic exposure incapacitates the healthcare team. Additionally, the toxin may be harming the patient. Security or law enforcement involvement might minimize the potential for workplace violence in some patient presentations.

General Impression

Listen to the prehospital report upon patient arrival. The PAT is used upon initially seeing the pediatric patient to form a general impression of the patient's condition. See Chapter 4, "Prioritization," for more information on this valuable assessment tool. The nurse determines whether the patient is "sick, sicker, or sickest." As this quick assessment is performed, note the presence of uncontrolled hemorrhage or signs of cardiopulmonary arrest (unresponsiveness/apnea), which would alter the priorities from ABC to C-ABC, with circulation assuming the highest priority.[2(Ch1),4(P4)] Cardiopulmonary resuscitation with pediatric advanced life support measures is initiated if the patient is pulseless. See Chapter 7, "The Child in Need of Stabilization," for more information on resuscitation.

The Stop the Bleed course from the American College of Surgeons[3] teaches the lay public to control external bleeding with (in this order) direct pressure, wound packing, and tourniquets. In a hospital setting, other options are available to the physician or advanced practice provider. Throughout the initial assessment, assure that interventions are effective before proceeding to the next step. Continue to reassess life-saving interventions throughout the patient's care.

Primary Survey

Once the determination of sick, sicker, or sickest has been made using the PAT, the next step in the initial assessment is the primary survey. The primary survey includes the ABCDE components of the mnemonic and is designed to quickly identify life-threatening conditions and implement life-saving interventions. If any life-threatening abnormalities are noted, interventions must take place quickly.[40] More than one intervention may be required to improve the patient's condition. Reassessment to determine the effectiveness of these life-saving interventions and the need for additional measures is crucial.

A: Alertness and Airway

Determine the child's level of alertness using the AVPU mnemonic. Each letter used to quickly describe the child's mental status in this mnemonic is the answer to one of the following questions:

- Is the child **A**lert?
- Does the child require a **V**erbal stimulus to respond?
- Is the child only responding to **P**ainful stimulation?
- Is the child **U**nresponsive?

Consider the need for cervical spinal motion restriction. If the child was subjected to kinetic forces that could cause spinal injury, manual cervical spine stabilization can be provided by another team member while the assessment continues.[1] Spinal precautions will affect maneuvers needed to open the patient's airway.

Vocalization may be noted when assessing the child's alertness and is a positive finding during the airway assessment. If the patient is alert and developmentally capable, ask them to open their mouth so that you can assess the oropharynx. If the patient is unresponsive or unable to open their mouth, open the airway using an appropriate method such as the head tilt–chin lift maneuver or the jaw-thrust maneuver. The head tilt–chin lift maneuver is contraindicated in patients with suspected injury to the cervical spine.[4(P4)] Assess for tongue obstruction, loose or missing teeth, foreign objects, fluids (blood, vomit, secretions), edema, sounds (snoring, gurgling, stridor), and bony deformity. In children with large occiputs, place padding beneath the child's shoulders and torso to facilitate a sniffing position, as shown in **Figure 5-1**.

Other airway interventions include suctioning the airway, patient positioning, removing foreign objects, inserting an oral or nasopharyngeal airway, and anticipating the need for endotracheal intubation. In many conditions, a supine position would not be optimal for the patient. A child with difficulty breathing may assume a tripod position to improve air entry and chest

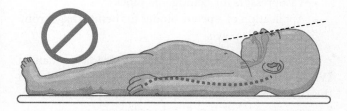
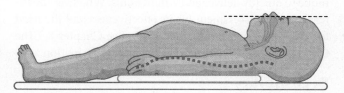

Figure 5-1 *Padding under the patient with a large occiput.*

expansion. The child's preferred position may be encouraged if it does not obstruct the airway.

The oral airway is measured from the corner of the mouth to the angle of the jaw. An oral airway cannot be used if the gag reflex is present. A tongue depressor or tonsil-tip suction device may be used to assess for a gag reflex and stabilize the tongue during oral airway insertion. Insert the oral airway anatomically, sliding it over the tongue, using care not to push the tongue back into the airway, until the flange meets the patient's lips. The rotation insertion technique for an oral airway is not recommended. A nasopharyngeal airway is measured from the naris to the top of the patient's earlobe. The nasopharyngeal airway is contraindicated when facial trauma is evident. If the patient is unable to maintain an open airway, prepare for endotracheal intubation by gathering supplies, preoxygenating the patient, and administering medications as ordered.[2(ApG),4(P8),43]

NOTE

Size Matters

Pediatric airway adjuncts are available in various sizes. Length-based resuscitation tapes and other pediatric emergency references include sizes based on patient weight. Consider the diameter, width, and length of the airway adjunct in comparison to the patient.

The child's fifth digit (little finger) may be used to approximate endotracheal tube size.[25]

B: Breathing and Ventilation

Once airway patency is assured, move on to the breathing and ventilation assessment. Breathing effectiveness is assessed by inspecting for spontaneous breathing; symmetrical chest rise; the depth, pattern, and general rate of respirations; skin color; open wounds or deformities; and signs of increased work of breathing. Signs of increased work of breathing include abnormal positioning, grunting, retractions or accessory muscle use, head bobbing, and nasal flaring. Auscultate breath sounds and palpate for deformities or subcutaneous emphysema.

Pallor, cyanosis, and mottling are concerning findings, but are easily missed in patients with darker skin tones. Conjunctival, mucus membrane, and nail bed pallor may be more evident in patients of color.[21,29] Midaxillary breath sounds are more likely to confirm bilateral breath sounds, as referred breath sounds are common in the child's small chest.[25] Abnormalities in the breathing assessment should be addressed before progressing to the circulation assessment. Interventions for inadequate breathing and ventilation include oxygen administration and assisting ventilations with a bag-mask device. Anticipate the need for medications such as epinephrine, noninvasive positive-pressure ventilation, or intubation. Needle decompression or tube thoracostomy (chest tube) may be required for a pneumothorax or hemothorax. The effectiveness of any intervention should be reassessed periodically.

If the child is intubated, it is important to assure that the endotracheal tube is properly placed. Verify endotracheal tube placement by first attaching an end-tidal CO_2 detector. Observe for rise and fall of the chest with assisted ventilations. Auscultate over the epigastrium and bilateral lungs. After five to six breaths, assess for evidence of exhaled CO_2. The rise and fall of the chest with each breath, an absence of sounds over the epigastrium, the presence of equal bilateral lung sounds, and the presence of exhaled CO_2 help confirm proper endotracheal tube placement. After placement is confirmed, secure the tube, noting the measurement at the gums or lips, and initiate controlled ventilatory support. A chest radiograph and continuous end-tidal CO_2 monitoring will provide further confirmation of appropriate tube placement.[25]

If the placement of the endotracheal tube is not confirmed, immediate intervention is necessary. If breath sounds are unilateral, and only one side of the chest rises and falls, the tube may be too deep and ventilating only one lung, or the patient may have a pneumothorax or hemothorax. If no breath sounds are heard, no rise and fall of the chest is observed, and there is no evidence of exhaled CO_2, the endotracheal tube should be removed and bag-mask ventilation resumed. Anticipate regurgitation of stomach contents due to esophageal insufflation and be ready with suction. Prepare for another intubation attempt or use of an alternative airway adjunct.

C: Circulation and Control of Hemorrhage

After any life-threatening conditions related to breathing or ventilation are addressed, assess the child's circulation. In trauma patients, it is important to consider any sources of external or internal hemorrhage. Circulation is assessed by palpating a pulse. A carotid or femoral pulse is acceptable for children. Assess the brachial pulse in infants. Note the quality (strong, weak) and the rate of the central pulse and compare it to the peripheral pulses. A slow or weak central pulse is an ominous finding, while weak peripheral pulses as compared to central pulses are a sign of compensation for shock. Tachycardia may be an early indication of compensated shock. If the pulse is absent or slower than 60 beats per minute and the patient

has signs of poor perfusion, initiate pediatric life support measures.[4(P4),38]

The color, temperature, and moisture of the skin provide additional cues about circulatory status. Skin that is cool, diaphoretic, pale, mottled, gray, or cyanotic indicates poor perfusion. These cues can be difficult to appreciate in patients with darker skin tones. Capillary refill is assessed by applying brief pressure over a nailbed, palmar surface, or sternum and watching for the perfusion to return to that area. Capillary refill of 2 seconds or less is normal. Delayed capillary refill is indicative of vasoconstriction and is an important sign of circulatory compromise. If the child is cold, the capillary refill may be artificially delayed.[4(P4),20,25]

Signs of inadequate circulation require immediate attention. Intravenous (IV) access is established to provide fluid boluses and medications if necessary. In some cases, two IV lines may be needed. If the child arrives with vascular access in place, confirm the patency of the IV access. If IV access cannot be obtained quickly and urgent intervention is required, intraosseous (IO) access is recommended.

At this point, it is important to consider the cause of circulatory compromise so as to initiate goal-directed therapy for shock. Attaching the patient to a cardiac monitor is appropriate if the palpated pulse suggests the patient has a life-threatening dysrhythmia. Depending on the cause of circulatory compromise, interventions will vary.[4(P4),5] Here are some examples:

- 20 mL/kg isotonic crystalloid bolus for hypovolemic shock
- 10 mL/kg of blood for hemorrhage
- 10 mL/kg of isotonic crystalloids for neonates or cardiogenic shock
- Epinephrine for anaphylactic shock
- Antidysrhythmics or cardioversion for dysrhythmias
- Vasopressors for neurogenic shock
- Application of a pelvic binder for hemorrhage from an unstable pelvis

In many cases, the IV fluids are needed faster than an IV pump or pressure bag can deliver them. To deal with this situation, the available equipment and personnel must be considered.[12,36,39] **Box 5-2** describes one manual technique to quickly deliver an IV fluid bolus. Whatever the intervention, reassessment for its effectiveness and the need for additional measures is necessary. See Chapter 7, "The Child in Need of Stabilization," for more information.

D: Disability

The child's neurologic status is evaluated using the Glasgow Coma Scale (GCS). Consider the child's baseline

BOX 5-2 Push–Pull Technique for Intravenous Fluid Administration

One technique for efficient delivery of controlled fluid boluses is the push–pull method. Commercially manufactured devices are available for administration of such therapies but are not required. A syringe is attached to a port in the IV tubing. A three-way stopcock or kinking of the IV tubing is used to control the direction of the IV fluid. The fluid is pulled from a bag of IV fluids and then manually pushed to the patient using the syringe. **Figure 5-2** shows an example of the equipment setup.

A 20 mL syringe works well for very small children and is a precise way to track the volume. One full 20 mL syringe is needed for each kilogram of weight to administer a 20 mL/kg bolus. For larger children, a larger syringe may be used but can cause hand fatigue and is not necessarily faster.

Regardless of syringe size or device, calculate the number of push–pull sequences necessary and track how many are performed. When using a 60 mL syringe for a 21 kg child, for example, the push–pull process is repeated 7 times to administer 420 mL of fluid for a 20 mL/kg bolus. Using a 20 mL syringe, the push–pull process is repeated 21 times to deliver the same amount. Use care not to contaminate the syringe plunger when using this technique.

Adapted from Cole, E. E., Harvey, G., Burbanski, S., Foster, G., Thabane, L., & Parker, M. J. (2014). Rapid paediatric fluid resuscitation: A randomized controlled trial comparing the efficiency of two provider-endorsed manual paediatric fluid resuscitation techniques in a simulated setting. *BMJ Open, 4,* Article e0005028. https://.doi.org/10.1136/bmjopen-2014-005028; Spangler, H., Piehl, M., Lane, A., & Robertson, G. (2019). Improving aseptic technique during the treatment of pediatric septic shock: A comparison of 2 rapid fluid delivery methods. *Journal of Infusion Nursing, 42*(1), 23–28. https://doi.org/10.1097/NAN.0000000000000307; and Toshniwal, G., Ahmed, Z., & Segnstock, D. (2015). Simulated fluid resuscitation for toddlers and young children: Effect of syringe size and hand fatigue. *Paediatric Anaesthesia, 25*(30), 288–293. https://doi.org/10.1111/pan.12573

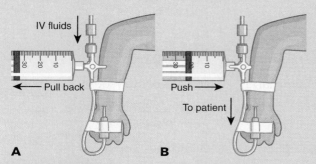

IV fluids

Pull back

Push

To patient

A   **B**

Figure 5-2 *Setup for push–pull technique.*

mentation and developmental stage when calculating the GCS score, as adaptations have been made to the scale. **Table 5-1** explains the GCS assessment parameters based on age. Many versions of the scale score a response "to pain." If the child does not respond to voice or follow commands, use care in the stimulation technique to avoid soft-tissue damage. To minimize injury from overzealous stimulation, "pressure" has replaced "pain" in some adaptations of the scale. Supraorbital or other pressure above the neck is useful in the event of altered sensation due to spinal cord injury.[8]

If the GCS score is less than 8, anticipate the need for intubation to protect the child's airway. A score of less than 8 is also generally considered a state of coma or severe brain injury. While factors other than brain injury, such as hypoglycemia and hypoxia, can alter the score, a score of 13–15 is associated with mild traumatic brain injury and a score of 9–12 is associated with moderate brain injury.[2(Ch6)]

Pupils are assessed for shape, consensual size, and reactivity to light. PERRL indicates the pupils are equal, round, and react to light. PERRLA indicates the pupils

also accommodate by constricting when focusing on an object near the nose after the patient looks at a distant object.[6] Any altered level of consciousness or pupillary changes should prompt consideration of hypoglycemia, hypoxia, brain injury, toxins, or other insults. Obtain a point-of-care blood glucose test for any child with an altered mental status.

E: Exposure and Environmental Control

To ensure no life- or limb-threatening abnormalities have been missed, completely remove the child's clothing, including diapers. This can be done incrementally to reduce the risk of hypothermia to the child. As each area is exposed, inspect for abnormalities such as bleeding, rashes, bruising, deformities, skin discoloration, or wounds. When newly identified life-threatening alterations are identified, intervene as appropriate and reassess.

If the patient arrived on a transport device, it is removed at this time. If there is no suspicion of an unstable spinal or pelvic injury, the patient's back may be quickly assessed.

TABLE 5-1	Glasgow Coma Scale			
Sign	**>5 Years Old**	**2–5 Years Old**	**<2 Years Old**	**Score**
Eye Opening	Spontaneous	Spontaneous	Spontaneous	4
Examples of non-testable situations: eye edema, eye dressings	To sound	To sound	To sound	3
	To pressure	To pressure	To pressure	2
	None	None	None	1
	Non-testable	Non-testable	Non-testable	NT
Verbal Response	Oriented	Oriented	Coos and babbles	5
Examples of non-testable situations: intubation, sedation	Confused	Confused	Irritable/cries	4
	Inappropriate words	Inappropriate words	Cries in response to pressure	3
	Incomprehensible sounds	Incomprehensible sounds	Moans in response to pressure	2
	None	None	None	1
	Non-testable	Non-testable	Non-testable	NT
Motor Response	Obeys command	Obeys commands	Moves spontaneously	6
Examples of non-testable situations: chemical paralysis	Localizes (reaches for swab when inserted into nose)	Localizes	Localizes OR withdraws from pressure	5
	Withdraws from pressure (turns head when swab inserted into nose)	Withdraws from pressure	Withdraws from pressure	4
	Abnormal flexion with stimulus	Abnormal flexion with stimulus	Abnormal flexion with stimulus	3
	Abnormal extension with stimulus	Abnormal extension with stimulus	Abnormal extension with stimulus	2
	None	None	None	1
	Non-testable	Non-testable	Non-testable	NT
Best Total Score				15

Data from American College of Surgeons. (2018). *Advanced trauma life support: Student course manual* (10th ed., p. 110); Jain, S., & Iverson, L. M. (2021, June 20). *Glasgow Coma Scale*. StatPearls Publishing. https://www.ncbi.nlm.nih.gov/books/NBK513298/; Institute of Neurological Sciences NHS Greater Glasgow and Clyde. (2015). *Glasgow Coma Scale: Do it this way.* https://www.glasgowcomascale.org/downloads/GCS-Assessment-Aid-English.pdf?v=3; and Wolters Kluwer. (2022). Glasgow Coma Scale and Pediatric Glasgow Coma Scale. *UpToDate.* https://www.uptodate.com/contents/image/print?imageKey=PEDS%2F59662

For many trauma patients, it is safest to avoid turning the patient until a more thorough exam is completed. Children have an increased risk of morbidity and mortality from hypothermia, so warming measures such as warm blankets, warmed ambient environment, warmed IV fluids, or warmed lights are incorporated into their care. A radiant warmer with a temperature sensing device is useful for small infants.[38]

Data and Considerations to Augment the Primary Survey

The F and G components of the initial assessment identify data and additional considerations that support stabilization beyond the primary survey assessments and interventions. The primary survey can be completed in less than 2 minutes when the patient does not have any life-threatening abnormalities. Many assessments can be completed while talking to the patient. If no immediate interventions are warranted, it is appropriate to move past the primary survey. It may also be appropriate to continue to F and G as long as life-saving interventions have been initiated and are being reevaluated for effectiveness. A fluid bolus is usually delivered within 5–10 minutes. It is not necessary to wait until the fluid bolus is completely infused before continuing the process. It is necessary to ensure that any required primary survey interventions are reevaluated and take priority over routine, noncritical interventions.

F: Full Set of Vital Signs and Family Presence

Many healthcare providers want to obtain vital signs immediately upon arrival of the patient. In reality, vital signs are *not* the priority upon patient arrival. Obtaining vital signs takes valuable time that is best used to quickly identify life-threatening conditions and initiate life-saving interventions such as hemorrhage control, ventilation, and goal-directed therapy for shock. Keep in mind that the primary survey takes minimal time when significant life-saving interventions are not required. Most pediatric patients do not require life-saving interventions during the primary survey. Skipping the stepwise primary survey assessments, however, may lead to missing a life-threatening condition and delaying necessary intervention.

Vital signs include respiratory rate, heart rate, blood pressure, pulse oximetry, temperature, and weight in kilograms. See Chapter 3, "Pediatric Differences," for normal vital signs per age and for more information. To ensure the accuracy of vital signs measurements consider the following:

- Assess the respiratory and heart rates for 60 seconds to detect and account for irregularities.
- Blood pressure can be obtained via palpation, auscultation, or automated noninvasive devices. Several factors can confound the accuracy of pediatric blood pressure measurements, including blood pressure cuff size, equipment calibration, and clinician error. Serial auscultated blood pressure measurements are recommended for the diagnosis of hypertension, and auscultation is often referred to as the "gold standard," though current pediatric-specific data on noninvasive methods are limited.[17,37] Whatever method is used, matching the method to the patient condition is recommended.
- Temperature can be obtained orally, rectally, axillary, or via temporal artery. The route is chosen based on the patient's ability to hold a thermometer under their tongue, available equipment, and patient condition. The rectal method is avoided

in the immunosuppressed child.[18] See Chapter 10, "The Child with a Fever," for more information on each method.

Vital signs provide information on the effectiveness of primary survey interventions and may prompt implementation of additional measures to support the patient's ABCDE. Careful trending and monitoring of the vital signs can identify patient improvement or deterioration. Alterations in perfusion (shock), hypoxia, hypoglycemia, pain, anxiety, ambient temperature, crying, and medications are just a few factors that affect vital signs. Consider abnormal vital signs to be a critical finding until potentially life-threatening conditions are investigated.

The Emergency Nurses Association (ENA) strongly recommends that families be offered the option to be present during the care of their child. Family presence supports collaboration between the caregivers and the healthcare team. Family presence can also reduce pediatric anxiety and pain.[34] A support person whose sole responsibility is to explain to the family what is transpiring and what to anticipate is optimal. Family presence also serves other purposes, such as providing pertinent health history information, identifying alterations from the child's normal condition, interpreting nonverbal behaviors, and noting subtle changes in physiologic status. If a family member poses a threat to the safety or efficacy of the healthcare team, consider placing them in a safe environment away from the resuscitation. Also respect the family's decision to be out of the room during invasive procedures or resuscitation.[14,16] See Chapter 2, "Preparing for Pediatric Emergencies," for more on pediatric patient- and family-centered care.

G: Get Adjuncts and Give Comfort

The LMNOP mnemonic is used to recall adjuncts to the primary survey and pain management. Pain assessment and management are required for all patients. Other adjuncts are considerations and are implemented as ordered by the physician or advanced practice provider. Diagnostic adjuncts to the primary survey such as a radiograph or ultrasound may have been appropriate to evaluate life threats earlier in the assessment. The components of LMNOP follow.

Laboratory Analysis

The need for laboratory analysis is based on the child's illness or injury and may include, but is not limited to, the following:

- Arterial or venous blood gases to evaluate acid–base balance and ventilation
- Blood glucose if interventions for hypoglycemia were implemented in the primary survey or there is a new concern for hypoglycemia

- Blood crossmatch or type and screen for anticipated transfusion
- Coagulation studies
- Complete blood count to assess for infection, anemia, or other dyscrasia
- Cultures (blood, wound, urine) to guide antibiotic therapy
- Lactate levels to gauge end-organ perfusion; lactate is an indicator of the presence and severity of shock
- Metabolic panel to evaluate electrolytes and organ function
- Pregnancy test
- Toxicology screen

Monitor

Attach the patient to a cardiac monitor and set the automatic noninvasive blood pressure cuff to cycle at regular intervals for ongoing evaluation. A 12-lead electrocardiogram may be indicated.

Nasogastric or Orogastric Tube

If the child is intubated, a gastric tube is placed to empty gastric contents. This improves tidal volume and reduces the risk of aspiration. Consider venting preexisting feeding tubes. Nasogastric tubes are contraindicated in patients with evident or suspected facial trauma.

Oxygenation and Capnography

Assess oxygenation and ventilation with pulse oximetry and end-tidal CO_2 monitoring. Pulse oximetry may be inaccurate due to hypothermia, hypotension, vasoconstriction, cold extremities, probe placement, carbon monoxide poisoning, anemia, nail polish, darker skin tone, ambient lighting, ambient temperature, and other factors. Consider the potential for falsely low or high readings when increasing oxygen in response to low oximetry readings or when weaning the patient from oxygen therapy to avoid hyperoxia. Gradually increasing end-tidal CO_2 levels are seen in patients with respiratory depression or insufficiency. The ventilation rate for intubated patients may be increased or decreased based on the end-tidal CO_2 and other respiratory assessments. Generally, the rate of ventilation can be decreased if the end-tidal CO_2 level is low and increased if the end-tidal CO_2 level is high. Significant decreases in end-tidal CO_2 are seen with cardiac arrest and inadvertent displacement of the endotracheal tube.[4(P4),22]

Pain

Pain is assessed using an appropriate scale for the patient's developmental age and physiologic condition. See Chapter 3,

"Pediatric Differences," for a discussion of pain assessment and management. Nonpharmacologic comfort measures include, but are not limited to, the following interventions:

- Distraction (e.g., blowing bubbles, guided imagery, singing)
- Family presence
- Splinting
- Repositioning
- Padding bony prominences
- Verbal reassurance
- Ice (consider hypothermia risk)
- Heat (consider burn risk)

Many nonpharmacologic comfort measures are available but do not replace the need for analgesic medications for moderate to severe pain. Ask the physician or advanced practice provider for a pain medication order if needed. Reevaluate pain management interventions for effectiveness and potential adverse reactions.

Consideration of the Need for Definitive Care

Before, during, or at the conclusion of the primary survey, consideration is given to the need for definitive care. Is intrafacility or interfacility transport indicated? Does the patient need surgery, critical care admission, or transfer to a pediatric-capable facility? These decisions are guided by the patient's condition and available resources. See Chapter 2, "Preparing for Pediatric Emergencies," for more information on pediatric readiness and transfer processes shown to improve patient outcomes.

Secondary Survey

Once life- and limb-threatening conditions have been addressed, the secondary survey begins. For critically ill patients, the cycle of interventions and reassessments may overlap with the secondary survey assessments, but it is important that the primary survey interventions take priority. The purpose of the secondary survey is to correlate a complete history with the physical examination to identify all abnormalities and determine which additional diagnostics or interventions may be necessary. The secondary survey concludes with the reevaluation required while the patient awaits disposition to definitive care. Definitive care may be admission to another department within the facility, transfer to a higher level of care, or discharge to home.

H: History and Head-to-Toe

The secondary survey starts with a patient history and a head-to-toe examination.

History

Information about the patient's illness or injury is obtained from a variety of sources, which may include the following:

- The child, as possible, based on developmental stage and condition
- Caregivers
- Prehospital providers or reports
- Interfacility transport providers
- Report from the sending provider's office or referring healthcare facility
- Bystanders
- Medical records and other documents

The SAMPLE mnemonic is used to recall pertinent questions for the patient history:

- **S**igns and symptoms associated with the illness or injury
- **A**llergies to medications, foods, substances, or environment
- **M**edications, including over-the-counter, supplements, and those routinely administered and given for this illness/injury; ask about the last dose administered
- **P**ast medical and surgical history, including immunizations
- **L**ast meal/output (void and bowel movement)/menstrual period
- **E**vents leading up to the current illness or injury

As the health history is gathered, consideration is given to the age of the pediatric patient and potential risk factors such as immunosuppression or other comorbidities.

Head-to-Toe Examination

The physical assessment of the child is completed in a thorough, organized manner. The nurse uses inspection, palpation, and auscultation to identify any abnormalities while moving from the patient's head downward to the toes. General abnormalities include, but are not limited to, pain or tenderness, bleeding, edema, distention, increased or decreased temperature, adventitious sounds, bony instability (e.g., deformities, crepitus, or a sudden difference in bony contour called a step-off), subcutaneous emphysema, wounds, and skin discoloration. Wounds may include lacerations, abrasions, avulsions, burns, scars, punctures, contusions, and hematomas. Skin discoloration may include redness, ecchymosis, pallor, cyanosis, jaundice, rash, petechiae, and/or purpura. Note that skin discoloration can be difficult to identify on patients with darker skin tones.

General Appearance

The general appearance of the child is assessed initially with the PAT and then reconsidered at this stage. One mnemonic used to guide the general impression is TICLS:

- **T**one: Is the muscle tone demonstrated by the child appropriate? Is the child moving arms and legs, or does the child appear limp or flaccid?
- **I**nteractiveness: Does the child appear to appropriately interact with the environment and/or the caregiver? If age appropriate, does the child play with toys and/or interact with others?
- **C**onsolability: Is the child easily consoled or comforted by the caregiver or a blanket, toy, pacifier, or is there no consoling the child?
- **L**ook/gaze: If the eyes are open, does the child appear to be alert or is the child staring into space? If the child's eyes are closed, do they open to noise or sound, or is the child just sleeping?
- **S**peech/cry: Is the child's speech appropriate or cry loud, strong, and vigorous, or is the speech or cry weak or listless?

Note the child's body position, interactions with caregivers and the healthcare team, cleanliness or dishevelment, smells, incontinence, behaviors, and other observations.

Head, Face, and Neck

While inspecting the head, face, and neck, take note of the following:

- Symmetry of the skull and facial features
- Bleeding or drainage from wounds, ears, eyes, nose, and mouth. If cerebrospinal fluid (CSF) is suspected in drainage, perform a "halo" test. CSF will appear as a faint ring around bloody draining on a sheet, gauze, or pillowcase (**Figure 5-3**).
- Hair distribution
- Loose or missing teeth
- Foreign bodies in the mouth, nose, ears, or wounds
- Piercings
- Use/presence of eyeglasses, contact lenses, hearing aids, or dental devices
- Nasal flaring
- Head bobbing

While inspecting the eyes, take note of the following:

- Presence of ptosis (drooping eyelid), periorbital ecchymosis
- Pupil size, shape, symmetry, and reactivity to light
- Color of sclera and conjunctiva
- Globe shape or disruption
- Hyphema (blood in the anterior chamber)

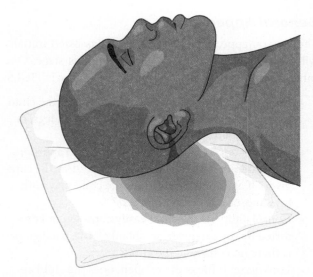

Figure 5-3 *Halo test for cerebrospinal fluid.*

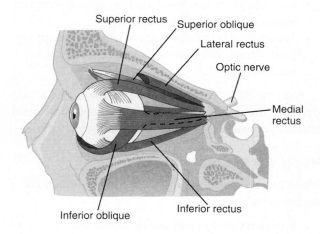

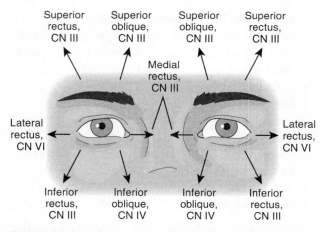

Figure 5-4 *Assessment of extraocular movements.*

- Extraocular movements by tracking the child's gaze through the six cardinal fields (**Figure 5-4**)
- Brief visual acuity by having the child note the number of fingers if developmentally and physically able
- Peripheral visual fields

While palpating the head, face, and neck, take note of the following:

- Fontanelles for bulging or depression (until about 18 months of age)
- Tracheal deviation or jugular venous distention

Chest

While inspecting the chest, take note of the following:

- Rate, quality, and depth of respiration
- Presence of retractions/accessory muscle use
- Presence of symmetrical chest rise or paradoxical chest movement
- Presence of central venous access devices or other medical appliances

While auscultating the chest, take note of the following:

- Heart sounds: S1, S2, extra heart sounds, muffled heart sounds, or friction rub
- Lung sounds: Note presence and location of normal or adventitious lung sounds such as stridor, wheezing, grunting, crackles, rhonchi, or rales

Abdomen and Flanks

While inspecting the abdomen and flanks, take note of the following:

- Medical devices such as a gastrostomy tube, peritoneal dialysis catheter, or diabetic monitoring device
- Pulsations
- Abdominal muscle use with breathing
- Abdominal shape (distended or concave)

While auscultating the abdomen, take note of the following:

- Bowel sounds in all four quadrants

While palpating the abdomen and flanks, take note of the following:

- Rebound tenderness
- Soft, tense, or rigid abdomen

Pelvis and Perineum

While inspecting the pelvis and perineum, take note of the following:

- Priapism
- Bladder or bowel incontinence
- Contraindications to inserting an indwelling urinary catheter, such as blood at the urinary meatus or scrotal/perineal edema/ecchymosis

While palpating the pelvis and perineum, take note of the following:

- Pelvic stability while gently applying downward and medial pressure on the iliac crests; if no pain or instability is noted, apply gentle downward pressure on the pubic symphysis

At this point in the head-to-toe exam, it is logical to consider how to monitor urine output for significantly ill children, depending on the child's developmental stage and physiologic condition. The use of an indwelling catheter is contraindicated with suspected pelvic or perineal trauma or blood at the urinary meatus,[7] and is generally avoided if possible to prevent catheter-associated urinary tract infections.

CLINICAL PEARL

Measuring and Monitoring Urine Output

Monitoring urine output is recommended in critically ill children and certain other conditions to evaluate renal perfusion and function. Methods for measuring urine output include urinals, bedpans, toilet inserts, external catheters, weighing diapers, and indwelling catheters.

Compare the weight of a clean diaper of the same brand and size to the patient's soiled diaper. One gram of weight is equivalent to 1 mL of urine.

Urine output of less than 1 mL/kg/hour can reflect poor end-organ perfusion.

Extremities

When assessing the extremities, it is important to compare the right and left sides. While inspecting the upper and lower extremities, take note of the following:

- Nailbed clubbing
- Shape and color
- Active range of motion

While palpating the upper and lower extremities, take note of the following:

- Quality and equality of bilateral pulses
- Capillary refill time
- Passive range of motion
- Sensation

I: Inspect Posterior Surfaces

While a quick assessment of the back might have been performed in the exposure and environment step, a detailed assessment of the posterior has yet to occur. When spinal or pelvic instability are not a concern, patients can be turned on their side, sit up, or roll themselves over to facilitate inspection and palpation of the posterior surfaces. When spinal or pelvic instability is a concern, turning a patient, even using the log roll maneuver, can cause spinal cord injury from an unstable spine or hemorrhage from an unstable pelvis.

If signs or symptoms of an unstable spine or pelvis were noted in the head-to-toe examination (pain, tenderness, crepitus, neurologic deficit) or are suggested by the history, it is safest to obtain imaging prior to turning the patient due to the potential for harm from the log roll maneuver.[27,30,33,35] If the patient will be transferred, consult with the receiving facility prior to obtaining imaging to reduce unnecessary radiation exposure. If imaging is deferred or confirms the presence of an unstable spine or pelvis, extreme care and consideration of risk and benefit are used with any patient movement. The healthcare team must use the safest technique possible given the available staff and handling devices.

Additional Interventions or Diagnostics

Based on the assessment findings, the nurse anticipates potential interventions or diagnostics. Some interventions are nurse driven, such as mandatory reporting and psychosocial support. The physician or advanced practice provider will determine what is necessary for safe disposition of the patient, but the nurse is responsible for communicating relevant findings and facilitating shared decision making with the family. The decision to admit, transfer, discharge, or continue to evaluate the patient is based on diagnostic results, available resources, patient condition, and family capability. See Chapter 2, "Preparing for Pediatric Emergencies," and Chapter 7, "The Child in Need of Stabilization," for more information on patient transfer to definitive care.

Just Keep Reevaluating

The nurse is responsible for patient reevaluation as long as the patient is in their care. Airway, breathing, circulation, disability, and vital signs assessments should continue. Use the PAT, vital signs trends, and the parents to help monitor for any changes. Notify the healthcare team with concerns. Continue communication with the patient and family so they are aware of and engaged in the plan of care.

The Pediatric Early Warning Score (PEWS) is a validated tool that can detect a decline in the child's status.[9,10,28] A score greater than 2 indicates a likely need for interventions for stabilization.[26,31] Use of the PEWS along with clinical judgment will best enable the nurse to detect subtle changes that can indicate deterioration in the child's status.[10]

CLINICAL PEARL

VIPP Mnemonic for Just Keep Reevaluating

- **V**ital signs
- **I**dentified abnormalities and effectiveness of interventions
- **P**rimary survey
- **P**ain

Emerging Trends

Emergency care of pediatric patients requires awareness of their physiological differences. However, data support that overemphasis of this approach can overly complicate the initial assessment and subsequent treatment.[41] There are many more similarities than differences between children and adults. The A–J mnemonic is utilized for both populations. Taking this approach may reduce the anxiety some nurses have when taking care of children.

Inequities in pediatric health based on race, ethnicity, and socioeconomic status have been documented and acknowledged for some time.[11] Implicit bias that negatively impacts patient care is an international problem. Examples of groups at risk of poor outcomes due to bias include sexual and ethnic minorities, persons with different skin tones, persons with accented speech, persons with limited language proficiency, persons with excess body weight, and persons with disabilities.[19] Rarely do educational materials provide examples of cyanosis, erythema, rashes, or other lesions on persons of color.[29] The U.S. Department of Health and Human Services has created a National Institute on Minority Health and Health Disparities to address the issues related to bias, but much work remains to be done.

Summary

The initial assessment lays the groundwork for pediatric emergency nursing care. The Pediatric Nursing Process represents one way to prioritize care. This systematic approach to the pediatric patient begins with preparation, followed by a general impression based on the Pediatric Assessment Triangle, leading into the A–J assessment

mnemonic. With the primary assessment (A–E), any abnormalities are addressed as found before moving to the next step of the assessment, as these conditions can be life threatening. F and G are adjuncts to the primary assessment and a bridge to the more thorough secondary survey. The secondary assessment includes obtaining a health history and a head-to-toe physical assessment. Appropriate diagnostics and interventions are facilitated. Monitoring and trending of assessment data take place throughout the care of the pediatric patient. This process facilitates use of an organized approach and prompt identification and treatment of conditions that may be subtle in presentation, yet have significant consequences if unrecognized.

References

1. Al-Sarheed, S., Alwatban, J., Alkhaibary, A., Babgi, Y., Al-Mohamadi, W., Mausuadi, E. M., Al Babtain, I., & Azzubi, M. (2020). Cervical spine clearance in unconscious pediatric trauma patients: A Level 1 trauma center experience. *Child's Nervous System, 36,* 811–817. https://doi.org/10.1007/s00381-019-04440-5

2. American College of Surgeons. (2018). *ATLS advanced trauma life support: Student course manual* (10th ed.).

3. American College of Surgeons. (2019). Stop the Bleed® course v. 2.0. https://www.stopthebleed.org/

4. American Heart Association. (2020). *Pediatric advanced life support provider manual.*

5. Balamuth, F., Fitzgerald, J. C., & Weiss, S. L. (2021). Shock. In K. N. Shaw & R. G. Bachur (Eds.), *Fleisher & Ludwig's textbook of pediatric medicine* (8th ed., pp. 72–86). Wolters Kluwer.

6. Baloh, R. W., & Jen, J. C. (2020). Neuro-ophthalmology. In L. Goldman & A. I. Schafer (Eds.), *Goldman-Cecil medicine* (26th ed., pp. 2535–2541). Elsevier.

7. Battaloglu, E., Figuero, M., Moran, C., Lecky, F., & Porter, K. (2019). Urethral injury in major trauma. *Injury, 50*(5), 1053–1057. https://doi.org/10.1016/j.injury.2019.02.016

8. Berger, J. R., & Price, R. (2022). Stupor and coma. In J. Jankovic, J. C. Mazziotta, S. L. Pomeroy, & N. J. Newman (Eds.), *Bradley and Daroff's neurology in clinical practice* (8th ed., pp. 34–51). Elsevier.

9. Branes, H., Solevåg, A., & Solberg, M. (2021). Pediatric early warning score versus a paediatric triage tool in the emergency department: A reliability study. *Nursing Open, 8,* 702–708. https://doi.org/10.1002/nop2.675

10. Chapman, S. M., & Maconochie, I. K. (2018). Early warning scores in paediatrics: An overview. *Archives of Disease in Childhood, 104*(4), 395–399. https://doi.org/10.1136/archdischild-2018-314807

11. Cheng, T. L., Emmanuel, M. A., Levy, D. J., & Jenkins, R. R. (2015). Child health disparities: What can a clinician do? *Pediatrics, 165*(5), 961–968. https://doi.org/10.1542/peds.2014-4126

12. Cole, E. E., Harvey, G., Burbanski, S., Foster, G., Thabane, L., & Parker, M. J. (2014). Rapid paediatric fluid resuscitation: A

randomized controlled trial comparing the efficiency of two provider-endorsed manual paediatric fluid resuscitation techniques in a simulated setting. *BMJ Open, 4,* Article e0005028. https://.doi.org/10.1136/bmjopen-2014-005028

13. Drendel, A. L., Gray, M. P., & Lerner, E. (2019). A systematic review of hospital trauma team activation criteria for children. *Pediatric Emergency Care, 35*(1), 8–15. https://doi.org/10.1097/pec.0000000000001256

14. Dudley, N., Ackerman, A., Brown, K. M., Snow, S. K., American Academy of Pediatrics Committee on Pediatric Emergency Medicine, American College of Emergency Physicians Pediatric Emergency Medicine Committee, & Emergency Nurses Association Pediatric Committee (2015). Patient- and family-centered care of children in the emergency department. *Pediatrics, 135*(1), e255–e272. https://doi.org/10.1542/peds.2014-3424

15. Emergency Medical Services for Children Innovation and Improvement Center. (2021). *National Pediatric Readiness Project.* https://emscimprovement.center/domains/pediatric-readiness-project/

16. Emergency Nurses Association. (2017). *Family presence during invasive procedures and resuscitation* [Clinical practice guideline]. https://enau.ena.org/Users/LearningActivityAssetSingleViewer.aspx?LearningActivityAssetID=SJG9pQGDjT3evvUgo5z1uw%3d%3d

17. Emergency Nurses Association. (2018). *Non-invasive blood pressure measurement* [Clinical practice guideline]. https://enau.ena.org/Users/LearningActivityAssetSingleViewer.aspx?LearningActivityAssetID=In4r4tV8SFlaNVYsTDKuhA%3d%3d

18. Emergency Nurses Association. (2020). *Non-invasive temperature measurement* [Clinical practice guideline]. https://enau.ena.org/Users/LearningActivityAssetSingleViewer.aspx?LearningActivityAssetID=w5BVNLuofjPlgiJwKoEjZg%3d%3d

19. Fitzgerald, C., & Hurst, S. (2017). Implicit bias in healthcare professionals: A systematic review. *BMC Medical Ethics, 18,* Article 19. https://doi.org/10.1186/s12910-017-0179-8

20. Foote, J. M. (2022). Communication and physical assessment of the child and family. In M. J. Hockenberry, C. C. Rodgers, & D. Wilson (Eds.), *Wong's essentials of pediatric nursing* (11th ed., pp. 57–113). Elsevier.

21. Giger, J. N. (2021). Biological variations. In J. N. Giger & L. G. Haddad (Eds.), *Transcultural nursing* (8th ed., pp. 121–158). Elsevier.

22. Heuer, A. J., & Havard, J. (2022). Interpretation of blood gases. In A. J. Heuer (Ed.), *Wilkins' clinical assessment in respiratory care* (9th ed., pp 141–163). Elsevier.

23. Institute of Neurological Sciences NHS Greater Glasgow and Clyde. (2015). *Glasgow Coma Scale: Do it this way.* https://www.glasgowcomascale.org/downloads/GCS-Assessment-Aid-English.pdf?v=3

24. Jain, S., & Iverson, L. M. (2021, June 20). *Glasgow Coma Scale.* StatPearls Publishing. https://www.ncbi.nlm.nih.gov/books/NBK513298/

25. Lewis, C. A. (2022). The pediatric patient. In L. D. Urden, K. M. Stacey, & M. E. Lough (Eds.), *Critical care nursing: Diagnosis and management* (9th ed., pp. 974–996). Elsevier.

26. Ma, X., Liu, Y., Du, M., Ojo, O., Huang, L., Feng, X., Gao, Q., & Wang, X. (2021). The accuracy of the pediatric assessment triangle in assessing triage of critically ill patients in emergency pediatric department. *International Emergency Nursing, 58,* Article 101041. https://doi.org/10.1016/j.ienj.2021.101041

27. Maschmann, C., Jeppesen, E., Rubin, M. A., & Barfod, C. (2019). New clinical guidelines on the spinal stabilisation of adult trauma patients: Consensus and evidence based. *Scandinavian Journal of Trauma, Resuscitation and Emergency Medicine, 27*(1), Article 77. https://doi.org/10.1186/s13049-019-0655-x

28. Miranda, J., Camargo, C. Nascimento Sobrinho, C., Portela, D., & Monoghan, A. (2017). Accuracy of a pediatric early warning score in the recognition of clinical deterioration. *Revista Latino-Americana de Enfermagem, 25*(0). https://doi.org/10.1590/1518-8345.1733.2912

29. Mukwende, M., Tamonyh, P., & Turner, M. (2020). *Mind the gap.* St. George's University of London. https://www.blackandbrownskin.co.uk/mindthegap

30. National Institute for Health and Care Excellence. (2017). *Fractures (complex): Assessment and management* (NICE guideline 37). https://www.nice.org.uk/guidance/ng37

31. Oldroyd, C., & Day, A. (2011). The use of pediatric early warning scores in the emergency department. *Journal of Emergency Nursing, 37*(4), 374–376. https://doi.org/10.1016/j.jen.2011.03.007

32. Recznik, C. T., Simko, L. C., Travers, D., & Devido, J. (2019). Pediatric triage education for the general emergency nurse: A randomized crossover trial comparing simulation with paper-case studies. *Journal of Emergency Nursing, 45*(4), 394–402. https://doi.org/10.1016/j.jen.2019.01.009

33. Rodrigues, I. F. (2017). To log-roll or not to log-roll—that is the question! A review of the use of the log-roll for patients with pelvic fractures. *International Journal of Orthopaedic and Trauma Nursing, 27,* 36–40. https://doi.org/10.1016/j.ijotn.2017.05.001

34. Sağlık, D., & Çağlar, S. (2019). The effect of parental presence on pain and anxiety levels during invasive procedures in the pediatric emergency department. *Journal of Emergency Nursing, 45*(3), 278–285. https://doi.org/10.1016/j.jen.2018.07.003

35. Shodari, A. F., Almaghrabi, M. A., Basindwah, S. A., Alhazmi, B. F., & Fallatah, S. M. (2021). Techniques and tools used in trauma patients transfer: A review. *Saudi Journal of Emergency Medicine, 2*(1), 85–91. https://doi.org/10.24911/SJEMed/72-1598298728

36. Spangler, H., Piehl, M., Lane, A., & Robertson, G. (2019). Improving aseptic technique during the treatment of pediatric septic shock: A comparison of 2 rapid fluid delivery methods. *Journal of Infusion Nursing, 42*(1), 23–28. https://doi.org/10.1097/NAN.0000000000000307

37. Stergiou, G. S., Boubouchairopoulou, N., & Kollias, A. (2017). Accuracy of automated blood pressure measurement in children: Evidence, issues, and perspectives. *Hypertension, 6*(69), 1000–1006. https://doi.org/10.1161/hypertensionaha.116.08553

38. Topjian, A. A., Raymond, T. T., Atkins, D., Chan, M., Duff, J. P., Joyner, B. L., Jr., Lasa, J. J., Lavonas, E. J., Levy, A., Mahgoub, M., Meckler, G. D., Roberts, K. E., Sutton, R. M., & Schexnayder, S. M. (2020). Part 4: Pediatric basic and advanced life

support. *Circulation, 142*, S469–S499. https://doi.org/10.1161/CIR.0000000000000901

39. Toshniwal, G., Ahmed, Z., & Segnstock, D. (2015). Simulated fluid resuscitation for toddlers and young children: Effect of syringe size and hand fatigue. *Paediatric Anaesthesia, 25*(30), 288–93. https://doi.org/10.1111/pan.12573

40. Tran, A., Taljaard, M., Abdulaziz, K. E., Matar, M., Lampron, J., Steyerberg, E. W., & Vaillancourt, C. (2020). Early identification of the need for major intervention in patients with traumatic hemorrhage: Development and internal validation of a simple bleeding score. *Canadian Journal of Surgery*, *63*(5), E422–E430. https://doi.org/10.1503/cjs.010619

41. Walker, A., & Hanna, A. (2020). Kids really are just small adults: Utilizing the pediatric triangle with the classic ABCD approach to assess pediatric patients. *Cureus, 12*(3), Article e7424 https://doi.org/10.7759/cureus.7424

42. Wolters Kluwer. (2021). Glasgow Coma Scale and Pediatric Glasgow Coma Scale. *UpToDate*. https://www.uptodate.com/contents/image/print?imageKey=PEDS%2F59662

43. Wright, K. (2017). Nasopharyngeal and oral airway insertion. In D. L. Weigand (Ed.), *AACN procedure manual for high acuity, progressive, and critical care* (7th ed., pp. 62–68). Elsevier.

The Neonate

Kelly Williams, MSN, RN, CEN, CPN, CPEN, NPD-BC, CNE, TCRN

OBJECTIVES

Upon completion of this chapter, the learner will be able to:

1. Describe the indications for and steps of neonatal resuscitation.
2. Integrate knowledge of anatomic and physiologic characteristics of the neonate into the initial assessment.
3. Identify abnormalities in neonatal assessment.
4. Apply the Pediatric Nursing Process to a neonate.

Introduction

A neonate is a newborn in the first 4 weeks of life. A newborn is considered a neonate 28 days past its due date; therefore, a premature newborn is considered a neonate until 28 days past its due date, even if this stretches beyond 4 weeks after birth. A baby born on April 1 with a due date of May 1 is considered a neonate until May 28, even though the baby is 8 weeks old at that time. Therefore, date of birth and due date are essential components of an infant's history to correctly identify this high-risk population. There are many considerations specific to the neonatal population, which are covered in this chapter.

Fetal Development and Transition to Extrauterine Life

Knowledge of fetal development and the transition to extrauterine life is vital in understanding and applying the steps to neonatal resuscitation. While in utero, the fetal lungs are filled with amniotic fluid and the fetus receives oxygen from the mother's blood via the placenta. The blood traveling to the heart bypasses the lungs through openings in the fetal heart called the foramen ovale and ductus arteriosus. As the neonate takes in deep breaths or cries after birth, the fluid in the lungs is absorbed by the alveoli and air fills the lungs instead. The pulmonary vessels relax, allowing blood to flow through the lungs and absorb the oxygen, which is then transported throughout the body. This transition from the fetal circulation to the neonatal circulation occurs gradually. It may take 10 minutes before the newborn's oxygen saturation reads more than 90%.[52(Ch3)]

Viability refers to the survivability and prognosis of a neonate and is based on the gestation period. An infant born at 26 weeks or later is generally considered to be viable.[34] Viability also references the survivability of a neonate, even with a risk of disability, and after any available medical interventions have been performed.[14]

Neonates are known to be viable at as early as 22 weeks' gestation, but survivability is based on the social and medical conditions in which the neonate was born and the access to and capability of the neonatal care in that region.[46]

Neonatal Resuscitation

A neonate may be born having experienced an interruption in the normal transition to extrauterine life. Interruptions in this transition can stem from birthing difficulties such as placental abruption, nuchal cord (when the umbilical cord is wrapped around the baby's neck), and congenital abnormalities.[37] In such a case, the neonate's organs will not receive an adequate amount of oxygen and the neonate may decompensate. Assessment findings of an abnormal, or interrupted, transition include the following:

- Absent, rapid, or irregular breathing
- Tachycardia or bradycardia
- Decrease in muscle tone
- Pale or blue skin of lips, head, or trunk (central cyanosis)
- Low oxygen saturation
- Low blood pressure

If any of these findings are present, neonatal resuscitation interventions are performed.[52(Ch3)]

> **NOTE**
>
> ## Central Cyanosis Versus Acrocyanosis: Is Cyanosis Normal in a Neonate?
>
> Acrocyanosis is a normal finding in a neonate. Acrocyanosis includes paleness or blueness of the hands, feet, and the skin around the lips. This finding can be present during the neonatal phase when the infant becomes cold, such as after a bath. Warming methods will resolve the cyanosis.
>
> Central cyanosis refers to paleness or blueness of the more central parts of the body, including the lips, the head, and the trunk. It is an abnormal finding in a neonate and indicates a lack of oxygen in the blood. Consider abnormalities of the heart, lungs, or blood. A neonate born presenting with central cyanosis requires resuscitation interventions.[12]

Preparing for Resuscitation

When anticipating a birth in the emergency department (ED), collect the necessary equipment for possible neonatal resuscitation. Ask the following pre-birth questions[52(Ch2)]:

- What is the expected gestational age?
- Is the amniotic fluid clear?
- Are there any additional risk factors?
- What is our umbilical cord management plan?

Steps in Neonatal Resuscitation

Once the neonate is born, an immediate assessment is performed. Three questions are addressed during this assessment:

- Does the baby appear to be term?
- Does the baby have good muscle tone?
- Is the baby breathing or crying?

If the neonate appears to be term, has good muscle tone, and is crying vigorously, the neonate is placed with the mother. If the neonate does not appear to be term, does not have good muscle tone, or is not breathing regularly, then immediate resuscitation is required.

The interventions for neonatal resuscitation are as follows:

- Warm, dry, and stimulate the neonate. Provide warmth by placing the neonate under a radiant warmer. Use a towel or blanket to dry the neonate. Stimulate the neonate while drying or rub the neonate's back, trunk, or extremities.
- Position the neonate's head and neck to open the airway. Use a suction bulb syringe to clear the mouth and then the nose.
- If the neonate is not breathing or is gasping, or if the neonate is breathing but the heart rate is less than 100 beats per minute, initiate positive-pressure ventilation (PPV) at 21% oxygen and 40 to 60 breaths per minute. After the first 15 seconds of PPV, assess the neonate's heart rate and chest rise.
- If the heart rate is not increasing or the chest is not rising with breaths, use the MRSOPA acronym for corrective interventions[52(Ch4)]:
  - **M**ask adjustment
  - **R**eposition head and neck
  - **S**uction the mouth and nose
  - **O**pen the mouth
  - **P**ressure increase using PPV
  - **A**lternative airway
- If there is no improvement after the pressure increase, insert an endotracheal tube or place a laryngeal mask in the neonate and provide 30 more seconds of PPV.[52(Ch5)]

- If the heart rate remains less than 60 beats per minute, increase the oxygen level to 100% and begin compressions.
- Compressions are performed at a rate of 120 compressions per minute. The compression to ventilation ratio is 3:1, yielding 90 compressions and 30 breaths in 1 minute. The rhythm is best counted aloud: "One-and-two-and-three-and-breathe."
- After 60 seconds of compressions, reassess the heart rate. Once the heart rate increases to greater than 60 beats per minute, stop compressions and continue PPV at 40 to 60 breaths per minute. Adjust the oxygen concentration to meet the target pulse oximeter reading.[52(Ch6)]

If fluid volume is required during resuscitation, administer a bolus of 10 mL/kg. Volume expansion is immediately considered for neonates who remain bradycardic despite effective ventilation and for neonates with known blood loss, such as from placental abruption.

CLINICAL PEARL

First-Line Treatment in Neonatal Resuscitation

Ventilating the neonate is the most important and most effective intervention for resuscitation. Effective PPV is the first-line treatment for neonatal resuscitation.[52(Ch7)]

Physiologic Development in the First Month

A neonate may initially lose weight after birth but then regain that weight within the first 10–12 days of extrauterine life. During the first month of life, a neonate grows 1–1.5 inches (2.54–3.81 cm) and gains 4–8 ounces (113.4–226.8 g) in weight each week.[20]

During the neonate phase, the heart is dependent on the beats per minute to increase the cardiac output. A neonate will have a relatively high heart rate and a relatively low blood pressure. By 3 weeks of age, the pulmonary pressure stabilizes below the systemic pressure.[48]

Vital Signs

The expected ranges for vital signs in a neonate are outlined in **Table 6-1**.[8,15,31,35]

Reflexes

An assessment of neonatal reflexes provides information about neurologic function. **Table 6-2** offers guidance on stimulating the primitive neonatal reflexes.[19]

TABLE 6-1	Normal Neonatal Vital Signs
Vital Sign	**Normal Range**
Heart rate (awake)	100–190 beats/min
Heart rate (asleep)	90–160 beats/min
Respiratory rate	30–55 breaths/min
Systolic blood pressure	67–84 mm Hg
Diastolic blood pressure	35–53 mm Hg

Data from American Heart Association. (2020). Part 4: Systematic approach to the seriously ill or injured child. *Pediatric advanced life support provider manual*; Ernst, G. (2020). Pediatric trauma. In J. E. Tintinalli, O. J. Ma, D. M. Yealy, G. D. Meckler, J. S. Stapczynski, D. M. Cline, & S. H. Thomas (Eds.), *Tintinalli's emergency medicine: A comprehensive study guide* (9th ed., pp. 689–697). McGraw Hill; Lucia, D., & Glenn, J. (2017). Pediatric emergencies. In C. K. Stone & R. L. Humphries (Eds.), *Current diagnosis and treatment: Emergency medicine* (8th ed., pp. 964–1016). McGraw Hill; and Mersch, J. (2020). *Pediatric vital signs ranges and charts*. https://www.emedicinehealth.com/pediatric_vital_signs/article_em.htm

TABLE 6-2	Neonate Reflexes	
Neonatal Reflex	**Stimulus to Elicit Reflex Response**	**Response**
Palmar grasp	Finger in neonate's palm	Grasping of the finger
Tonic neck	Supine position with head to one side	Fencing position
Moro	Sudden vertical drop	Open hands, extend and abduct arms
Plantar grasp	Touch ball of foot with thumb	Toes curl
Rooting	Stroke the cheek near mouth	Head turns toward stimulus
Sucking/swallowing	Touch lips with finger	Begins to suck and swallow

Data from Hawes, J., Bernardo, S., & Wilson, D. (2020). The neonatal neurological examination: Improving understanding and performance. *Neonatal Network, 39*(3), 116–128. https://connect.springerpub.com/content/sgrnn/39/3/116

Safe Haven Laws

Safe Haven laws allow an unharmed, newborn infant to be surrendered to a healthcare facility for medical treatment and placement without repercussions to the parent. Laws vary depending on locality. It is important for ED nurses to review the stipulations of their local Safe Haven law. Healthcare facilities are deemed safe havens in all 50 states of the United States, the District of Columbia, and Puerto Rico. Some local ordinances also allow a newborn to be surrendered at other emergency facilities, such as a fire station. While not all other countries have laws similar to the U.S. Safe Haven laws, an emerging trend is the availability of "baby boxes," which can be found in many places around the globe. These boxes are temperature-controlled hatches that send an alarm if a baby is left in one.[11] Even in areas without Safe Haven laws, such as South Africa, baby boxes have been put in use to mitigate infant abandonment.[18] It is important to be familiar with your healthcare organization's protocol upon receiving a surrendered infant.[44]

Selected Conditions, Assessment Findings, and Interventions

There are many conditions to consider when presented with a sick neonate. This section considers the most common neonatal conditions, assessment findings that lead to diagnosis, and proper interventions.

THEMISFITS, NEO SECRETS, and TORCH

Various mnemonics outline the most common etiologies for abnormal assessment findings when a neonate presents to the ED with a complaint. This section briefly outlines three of these mnemonics.

THEMISFITS

THEMISFITS is a mnemonic used to remember potential etiologies of abnormal neonatal assessment findings.[36]

- **T**rauma: Injury is not a normal finding in a neonate. Therefore, any suspicious assessment findings should be investigated as a sign of child maltreatment. External findings include bruising or a frenulum tear. Signs of neurologic damage include fixed and dilated pupils, seizure, bulging fontanel, or posturing.
- **H**eart disease: Poor feeding, vomiting, or cyanosis can signal congenital heart disease (CHD). See

the section "Congenital Heart Disease" for more information.
- **E**ndocrine: Adrenal insufficiency due to congenital adrenal hyperplasia is the most common endocrine disease found in the neonate. Assessment findings include hyperpigmentation of the skin or enlarged genitalia. This is treated with circulatory support and the administration of hydrocortisone.
- **M**etabolic: Hypoglycemia is the primary metabolic disorder found in neonates. The neonate may present with altered mental status, seizures, tachycardia, and diaphoresis. A bedside glucose reading is obtained immediately.
- **I**nborn errors of metabolism: See the section "Inborn Errors of Metabolism."
- **S**eizures: Neonates are at a high risk of seizures related to central nervous system abnormalities such as hydrocephalus or metabolic disease.
- **F**ormula: Incorrect formula constitution can result in altered mental status or seizure. If the formula is mixed with too much water, hyponatremia can occur; if the formula is mixed with too small an amount of water, hypernatremia can occur.
- **I**ntestinal: Abdominal emergencies can occur in neonates. These include malrotation with volvulus, necrotizing enterocolitis, and Hirschsprung's disease. Assessment findings may include vomiting, abdominal distention, and bloody stools. Immediate surgery may be required.
- **T**oxins: Toxins are considered as a possible cause of altered mental status.
- **S**epsis: Sepsis is the leading cause of critical illness in the neonate. Assessment findings may include fever or hypothermia, altered mental status, respiratory distress, and signs of inadequate perfusion.

NEO SECRETS

Another mnemonic to consider potential etiologies of abnormal neonatal assessment findings is NEO SECRETS[43]:

- **In**born errors of metabolism
- **E**lectrolyte abnormalities
- **O**verdose
- **S**eizures
- **E**nteric emergencies
- **C**ardiac abnormalities
- **R**ecipe (formula, additives)
- **E**ndocrine crisis
- **T**rauma
- **S**epsis

CLINICAL PEARL

Hypoglycemia in Neonates

Hypoglycemia is the most common metabolic disturbance in neonates. When a neonate presents as unwell in the ED, a blood glucose level is checked immediately. A prolonged period of low blood glucose in a neonate results in an interruption in neurodevelopment or brain damage.

Neonates experience a period of transient hypoglycemia as they transition to extrauterine life, but their blood glucose returns to normal levels within a few hours after birth. Premature neonates are at a higher risk of prolonged hypoglycemia due to decreased glycogen stores and increased metabolic demands.

Signs of hypoglycemia in a neonate include:

- Sweating
- Poor feeding
- Weak or high-pitched cry
- Tremors
- Hypothermia
- Irritability
- Lethargy
- Hypotonia
- Seizures
- Coma
- Trouble breathing
- Cyanosis

Assessment findings of hypoglycemia in a neonate can vary. Sometimes a neonate with hypoglycemia may present as asymptomatic. When a neonate presents to the ED, a blood glucose level is the priority.[1]

TORCH

TORCH syndrome refers to an infection in a fetus or newborn that is transmitted from the mother through the placenta.[24] TORCH is a mnemonic for the agents that cause infection:

- **T**oxoplasmosis
- **O**ther agents (syphilis)
- **R**ubella (German measles)
- **C**ytomegalovirus
- **H**erpes simplex

Assessment findings include lethargy, fever, difficulty eating, liver or spleen enlargement, and anemia. Neonates may also present with petechiae or purpura or jaundice of the skin. Treatment is specific to the causative agent.[24]

Congenital Heart Disease

CHD is the most common birth defect and the most common type of cardiac disease encountered in the first year of life.[4,22] It is the leading cause of death among children with congenital malformations.[39] CHD is defined as a structural abnormality of the heart that occurs during fetal development.[22,39] The most common defect is a ventricular septal defect (VSD). Respiratory distress is the complaint that most commonly brings the infant into the ED for evaluation. CHD has been associated with malnutrition and failure to thrive, as the infant has increased energy requirements but demonstrates a decrease in oral intake, malabsorption, and a decrease in growth factors.[4,49] CHD is diagnosed through an echocardiogram and requires rapid recognition and aggressive treatment.[22]

The fetal heart begins developing as early as 3 weeks post conception.[48] Factors that place a fetus at risk for developing a congenital heart defect include genetic disposition and environmental exposure. Maternal risk factors include malnutrition, alcohol intake, high altitude (hypoxia), specific medication intake, and underlying health disease.[26]

Many times, symptoms arise soon after birth, so that CHD is diagnosed prior to the neonate going home. However, some neonates are discharged home prior to any diagnosis. This delay in diagnosis leads to higher morbidity and mortality rates. Therefore, when an infant presents to the ED with signs and symptoms of CHD, immediate intervention is critical.[3]

Signs and symptoms of CHD in an infant manifest as signs of shock or pulmonary edema.[3] Parents may report irritability, decreased activity, crying during feedings, decrease in appetite, and poor weight gain. Assessment findings include fast or irregular breathing, a blue or purple discoloration of the skin and mucus membranes,

NOTE

Blue Baby Syndrome

"Blue baby syndrome" is another name for infant methemoglobinemia. An infant with this condition will have a bluish discoloration, notably on the lips and hands, and especially when crying. This is a sign that the abnormal hemoglobin is not able to transport oxygen to the tissues. Methemoglobinemia can be genetic, or it can be caused by food and drink high in nitrate, or certain medications such as benzocaine and dapsone. Mild cases may not require treatment. Methylene blue, ascorbic acid, blood transfusion, exchange transfusion, and hyperbaric oxygen therapy may be used when treatment is necessary.[32]

cyanosis, tachypnea, tachycardia, auscultation of a heart murmur, and hepatomegaly.[39] Echocardiography has largely replaced the historically standard hyperoxia test and can definitively diagnose CHD.[16] If echocardiography is not available, a cardiac anomaly is more likely than a respiratory issue if the infant does not respond to hyper-oxygenation treatment administered for 10 minutes.[16,42]

Cyanotic Congenital Heart Disease

CHD can be classified as cyanotic or acyanotic. Cyanotic CHD, also known as critical CHD (CCHD), can be caused by either ductal-dependent lesions or non-ductal-dependent lesions. Differential cyanosis, which is characterized by normal color in the upper body and cyanosis in the lower body, may be seen with CCHD. Preductal and postductal oxygen saturation measurements can detect differential cyanosis when it might not be visibly obvious.[3] This section covers some of the most common forms of CCHD.

> **CLINICAL PEARL**
>
> ### Heart Disease?
>
> Neonates with respiratory or shock symptoms and no fever or exposure to ill respiratory contacts may be exhibiting signs of CHD. A quick screening tool that can help identify patients with this condition is preductal and postductal saturation measurements. Measuring pulse oximetry on the right hand and comparing it to a measurement taken on either foot can indicate an issue with the heart when the difference between the measurements at the two sites is more than 3% or the oxygen saturation level is less than 90% when measured at either.[13,40]

Ductal-Dependent Lesions

In an unborn fetus, the ductus arteriosus (DA) is an opening that connects the aorta to the pulmonary artery (**Figure 6-1**), detouring blood away from the lungs. The fetus receives oxygenated blood from the maternal placenta. At birth, the neonate begins to breathe and use the lungs, so the DA is no longer needed. The opening closes within a couple of days after birth.

In a neonate with a ductal-dependent lesion, the closure of the DA can cause cyanosis.[3] If this occurs, the DA must remain open and patent. Prostaglandin is administered as a life-saving intervention to keep the DA open; it promotes pulmonary and systemic blood flow. Prostaglandin can also be used as an interim measure to improve circulation prior to surgical intervention.[2]

> **CLINICAL PEARL**
>
> ### Apnea During Prostaglandin Administration
>
> An infant receiving prostaglandin is at risk for apnea. Prior to administration of prostaglandin, airway supplies should be gathered in preparation for possible endotracheal intubation.
>
> An emerging trend is the promotion of caffeine administration in infants receiving prostaglandin as an antagonist to an apneic spell. This practice has been tested in rats but has not yet been approved for human use; however, caffeine is already utilized in neonatal intensive care units to treat apnea of immaturity.[50]

Tetralogy of Fallot

Tetralogy of Fallot is the most common CCHD.[39] This condition comprises four congenital defects: VSD, right

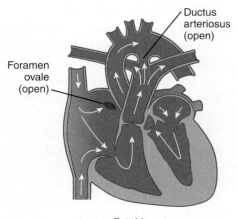

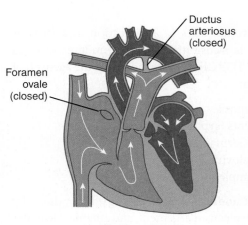

Fetal heart

Newborn heart

Figure 6-1 *Fetal heart versus newborn heart.*

ventricular outflow tract obstruction, an overriding aorta, and right ventricular hypertrophy.[53]

Ventricular Septal Defect. VSD is a hole that connects the two ventricles, allowing oxygen-rich blood to mix with oxygen-poor blood. Because the blood from the left ventricle can travel to the right ventricle, a larger amount of blood is being pumped into the lungs. This causes the heart and the lungs to work harder and the lungs to become congested.[7]

Right Ventricle Outflow Tract Obstruction (Pulmonary Stenosis). A right ventricle outflow tract obstruction, or pulmonary stenosis, is a narrowing of the pulmonary valve. The pulmonary valve is located between the right ventricle and the pulmonary artery. When this valve cannot open fully, the heart must work harder to pump blood and the lungs receive less blood to oxygenate. This results in cyanosis.[6,33]

Overriding Aorta. In an overriding aorta, the aorta is attached between the right and left ventricles rather than to just the left ventricle. As a result, oxygen-poor blood enters the aorta rather than being sent to the lungs via the pulmonary artery. As blood flow to the lung decreases, cyanosis occurs.[33]

Right Ventricular Hypertrophy. Right ventricle hypertrophy occurs with VSD. The VSD allows more blood to be received through the right ventricle, and this extra stress causes thickening of the muscles of the ventricle wall.[33]

Transposition of the Great Arteries

Transposition of the great arteries is the second most common CCHD. It is usually diagnosed within a week after birth.[39] Transposition of the great arteries occurs when the aorta is connected to the right ventricle and the pulmonary trunk is connected to the left ventricle (**Figure 6-2**). A septal defect can also be present, allowing some oxygen-rich blood to leak into the blood flow that is delivered to the body, providing a temporary fix until surgery can be performed. Without mixing of the blood or surgical intervention, this defect is incompatible with life.[47]

Assessment findings include cyanosis within the first 30 days of life, tachypnea, and a murmur if a VSD is present. Neonates may be breathing faster than 60 breaths per minute but not have any accompanying signs of distress such as retractions, grunting, or flaring.[47]

Diagnosis is made by echocardiogram. Treatment includes immediate oxygenation. Prostaglandin is administered to keep the ductus arteriosus patent. Corrective treatment involves surgical repair.[47]

Complaints Related to Formula

Human milk is considered the gold standard around the world for the nourishment of infants. However, if an infant is formula-fed, the best formula is an iron-fortified product that contains protein-based cow's milk.[30]

Formula Intolerance

Not all infants are able to tolerate protein-based cow's milk. Assessment findings of formula intolerance include

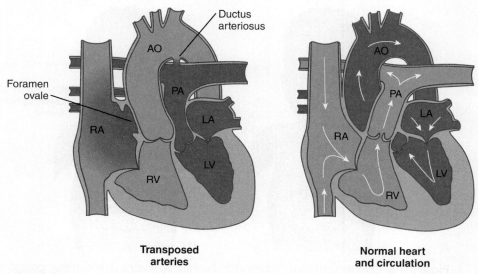

Transposed
arteries

Normal heart
and circulation

Figure 6-2 *Transposition of the great arteries.*

spitting up, fussiness, gas pains, crying, and watery or hard stool. Spitting up is the primary complaint worldwide attributed to formula intolerance. Treatment includes switching to an alternative type of formula. Soy formula is the most common alternative and its use resolves most signs and symptoms.[30]

Hyponatremic Seizure

In infants younger than 6 months of age with an otherwise normal exam, hyponatremia is the leading cause of new-onset nonfebrile seizures. The most common contributing factor is over-dilution of infant formula. Over-dilution of formula is associated with status epilepticus, intubation, and hypothermia.[21]

Assessment findings include altered mental status, edema, hypothermia, and seizure. Seizures in neonates most commonly present with subtle findings such as oral–buccal–lingual movements, ocular movements, or bicycling of the lower extremities.[27] Clinicians also consider etiologies such as hypoglycemia, maltreatment, sepsis, and ingestion.[21] Parents report over-dilution of the formula in response to symptoms of formula intolerance or the need to make the formula last longer because of financial restrictions.[21,38]

Hyponatremic seizures are treated with 3% hypertonic solution to address the underlying cause. Infants experiencing a hyponatremic seizure are less likely to respond to an anticonvulsant medication. Discharge teaching includes the dangers of over-dilution and the proper dilution measurements for infant formula.[21]

Intestinal Emergencies

Neonates may present with signs and symptoms of a variety of intestinal disorders. These include volvulus, intussusception (see Chapter 11, "The Child with Vomiting"),

necrotizing enterocolitis (NEC), and congenital diaphragmatic hernia.

Necrotizing Enterocolitis

NEC is most common in premature neonates and is the primary cause of short bowel syndrome in the pediatric population.[27] It is characterized by ischemic necrosis of the intestinal mucosa, which results in inflammation and invasion of gas into the intestinal wall.[28] Assessment findings include vomiting, abdominal distention and tenderness, bloody stools, apnea, bradycardia, and temperature instability.[27] NEC is associated with hypovolemia and impaired cardiac contractility. Volume replacement is the first-line treatment to mitigate hypovolemic shock.[45] Other emergent treatment includes intubation, infusion of vasopressors, bowel rest and decompression, antibiotics, and surgical intervention.[27,28]

Congenital Diaphragmatic Hernia

In congenital diaphragmatic hernia (CDH), the intra-abdominal contents herniate into the thoracic cavity.[27] The diaphragm does not form normally during fetal development, and the intestines, stomach, and liver are found within the chest (**Figure 6-3**). This results in improper development of the lungs.[52(Ch10)] CDH can lead to pulmonary hypoplasia or pulmonary hypertension.

Signs and symptoms can present within the first 24 hours after birth. Assessment findings include respiratory distress, unilateral absence of breath sounds, and a scaphoid-shaped abdomen.

Diagnosis is confirmed with radiograph. CDH can easily be mistaken for a pneumothorax, so accurate diagnosis is critical for proper treatment. Treatment includes a gastric tube for decompression and surgical intervention.[27]

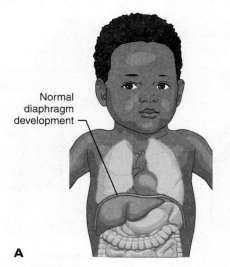
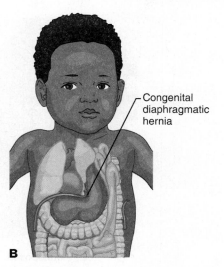

Figure 6-3 *Congenital diaphragmatic hernia.* **A.** *Infant without congenital diaphragmatic hernia.* **B.** *Infant with congenital diaphragmatic hernia.*

Neonate Born with CDH

Resuscitation of a neonate with known CDH does not include the administration of PPV. In patients with CDH, gas enters the stomach and intestines if PPV is administered with a face mask. These organs expand within the chest and decrease the ability of the lungs to inflate. If positive pressure is increased in an attempt to improve ventilation, a pneumothorax can develop.

When resuscitating a neonate with known CDH, immediately intubate the trachea. Insert a large orogastric tube and place it on suction to prevent distention. Do not administer PPV with a face mask for any neonate with known CDH.[52(10)]

Jaundice

Neonatal jaundice is a condition caused by altered metabolism of bilirubin, resulting in hyperbilirubinemia. This is a common finding in neonates, and its severity is determined by history, exam, and blood work.

Assessment findings include a yellow discoloration of the skin, conjunctiva, and sclera. Jaundice will usually start in the face and then progress downward and outward to the trunk and extremities. Treatment for severe jaundice includes phototherapy or exchange transfusion[9,25,41] Left untreated, jaundice can become neurotoxic, resulting in acute bilirubin encephalopathy or kernicterus, an irreversible condition leading to sensory and intellectual disabilities.[25]

Neonatal Abstinence Syndrome

Neonatal abstinence syndrome is also referred to as neonatal opioid withdrawal syndrome. This condition occurs in neonates born to mothers who used opioids during pregnancy and is considered a disorder of neurobehavioral dysregulation.[23,51]

Assessment findings include irritability, crying, disturbed alertness, hypertonicity, tremors and jitters, skin breakdown, vomiting, diarrhea, hypersensitivity or hyposensitivity to stimuli, and failure to thrive. Disturbances are found in autonomic control, motor and tone control, alertness and attention control, and sensory processing.[23]

The Finnegan Neonatal Abstinence Scoring System is a tool used to assess a withdrawing neonate every 3 to 4 hours. The score determines whether nonpharmacologic or pharmacologic interventions are appropriate.[17] If pharmacologic intervention is necessary, opioids may be administered and the neonate gradually weaned.[51]

Discharge instructions include that the infant may demonstrate residual symptoms that can last for months and should have frequent follow-up visits with the pediatrician.[23]

Inborn Errors of Metabolism

More than 5,000 types of inborn errors of metabolism have been identified. An inborn error of metabolism is an inherited disorder that prevents the natural breakdown of food into energy.[27] The most common variant is phenylketonuria, for which the neonate is tested soon after birth. In phenylketonuria, the enzyme that breaks down and processes amino acids is lacking, so normal growth and development are repressed.[10]

Assessment findings for inborn errors of metabolism include poor feeding, vomiting, diarrhea, and lethargy eventually leading to coma. Other assessment findings include hepatomegaly, jaundice, liver dysfunction, hypoglycemia, or hyperammonemia. Diagnosis is clinical, through blood work including ammonia level and culture studies. Treatment involves keeping the neonate on nothing by mouth (NPO) status, providing maintenance fluids, assisting elimination of ammonia, and treating metabolic acidosis.[27]

Summary

Children of all ages are considered vulnerable and high-risk patients. The neonate, an infant within the first 28 days of life (or 28 days after the due date), is the highest-risk pediatric patient. Be prepared to resuscitate any neonate born in the ED. Nursing knowledge of neonatal-specific conditions will facilitate early recognition of symptoms and preparation for urgent intervention. Other conditions, such as sepsis, intussusception, and volvulus, can be found in the neonate but also occur in older children; these topics are covered in other chapters of this provider manual. See Chapter 7, "The Child in Need of Stabilization," and Chapter 11, "The Child with Vomiting," for more information on these topics.

References

1. Abramowski, A., Ward, R., & Hamdan, A. H. (2020, September 9). *Neonatal hypoglycemia*. StatPearls Publishing. https://www.ncbi.nlm.nih.gov/books/NBK537105/

2. Akkinapally, S., Hundalani, S. G., Kulkarni, M., Fernandes, C. J., Cabrera, A. G., Shivanna, B., & Pammi, M. (2018). Prostaglandin E$_1$ for maintaining ductal patency in neonates with ductal-dependent cardiac lesions. *Cochrane Database of Systematic Reviews, 2*, Article CD011417. https://doi.org/10.1002/14651858.CD011417.pub2

3. Altman, C. (2020). Identifying newborns with critical congenital heart disease. *UpToDate*. Retrieved August 12, 2021, from https://www.uptodate.com/contents/identifying-newborns -with-critical-congenital-heart-disease

4. Amelia, P., Adriansyah, R., Lubis, B., & Akil, M. (2020). The association between cyanotic and acyanotic congenital heart disease with nutritional status. *Open Access Macedonian Journal of Medical Sciences, 8*(B), 245–248. https://doi.org/10.3889 /oamjms.2020.3978

5. American Heart Association. (n.d.). *Patent ductus arteriosus (PDA)*. https://www.heart.org/en/health-topics/congenital -heart-defects/about-congenital-heart-defects/patent-ductus -arteriosus-pda

6. American Heart Association. (n.d.). *Pulmonary valve stenosis*. https://www.heart.org/en/health-topics/congenital -heart-defects/about-congenital-heart-defects/pulmonary -valve-stenosis

7. American Heart Association. (n.d.). *Ventricular septal defect (VSD)*. https://www.heart.org/en/health-topics/congenital-heart -defects/about-congenital-heart-defects/ventricular-septal -defect-vsd

8. American Heart Association. (2020). *Pediatric advanced life support provider manual*.

9. Ansong-Assoku, B., Shah, S. D., Adnan, M., & Ankola, P. A. (2022, February 19). *Neonatal jaundice*. StatPearls Publishing. https://www.ncbi.nlm.nih.gov/books/NBK532930/

10. Atwal, P. S. (2019). *Phenylketonuria*. National Organization for Rare Disorders. https://rarediseases.org/rare-diseases /phenylketonuria/

11. Baker, V. (2019). Drop-off baby boxes: Can they help save lives in the US? https://www.bbc.com/news/world-us-canada-46801838

12. Bretz, M. (2021, September). *Cyanosis in infants and children*. Cincinnati Children's. https://www.cincinnatichildrens.org /health/c/cyanosis

13. Cleveland, L. M. (2022). Health promotion of the newborn and family. In M. J. Hockenberry, C. C. Rogers, & D. Wilson (Eds.), *Wong's essentials of pediatric nursing* (11th ed., pp. 175–212). Elsevier.

14. DiStefano, L. M., Wood, K., Mactier, H., Bates, S. E., & Wilkinson, D. (2021). Viability and thresholds for treatment of extremely preterm infants: Survey of UK neonatal professionals. *Archives of Disease in Childhood—Fetal and Neonatal Edition*. https://doi .org/10.1136/archdischild-2020-321273

15. Ernst, G. (2020). Pediatric trauma. In J. E. Tintinalli, O. J. Ma, D. M. Yealy, G. D. Meckler, J. S. Stapczynski, D. M. Cline, & S. H. Thomas (Eds.), *Tintinalli's emergency medicine: A comprehensive study guide* (9th ed., pp. 689–697). McGraw Hill.

16. Geggel, R. L. (2021). Diagnosis and initial management of cyanotic heart disease in the newborn. *UpToDate*. Retrieved January 16, 2022, from https://www.uptodate.com/contents /diagnosis-and-initial-management-of-cyanotic-heart-disease -in-the-newborn

17. Gomez-Pomar, E., & Finnegan, L. P. (2018). The epidemic of neonatal abstinence syndrome, historical references of its origins, assessment, and management. *Frontiers in Pediatrics, 6*, Article 33. https://doi.org/10.3389/fped.2018.00033

18. Goulden, A. (2019). *Baby boxes allow mothers to drop-off unwanted children*. https://apolitical.co/solution-articles/en /baby-boxes-allow-mothers-to-drop-off-unwanted-children

19. Hawes, J., Bernardo, S., & Wilson, D. (2020). The neonatal neurological examination: Improving understanding and performance. *Neonatal Network, 39*(3), 116–128. https://connect .springerpub.com/content/sgrnn/39/3/116

20. Healthwise. (2020, May 27). *Growth and development, newborn*. University of Michigan Health. https://www.uofmhealth .org/health-library/hw42229

21. Houck, J., Ganti, L., & Vera, A. E. (2019). A case of hyponatremia-induced seizures in an infant secondary to water intoxication from the use of almond milk. *Cureus, 11*(10), Article e5899. https://doi.org/10.7759/cureus.5899

22. Jamali, A. A., Kanhar, I. A., Jamali, A. A., Jamali, G. M., Shaikh, B., & Tanwani, B. (2018). Congenital heart diseases: Frequency of different acyanotic and cyanotic lesions in children. *International Research Journal of Pharmacy and Medical Sciences, 1*(3), 41–45. http://irjpms.com/wp-content/uploads/2018/04 /IRJPMS-PP1651-18.pdf

23. Jansson, L. M., & Patrick, S. W. (2019). Neonatal abstinence syndrome. *Pediatric Clinics of North America, 66*(2), 353–367. https://doi.org/10.1016/j.pcl.2018.12.006

24. Johnson, K. E. (2019). Overview of TORCH infections. *UpToDate*. Retrieved August 12, 2921, from https://www.uptodate .com/contents/overview-of-torch-infections

25. Kapadia, V. S., & Brion, L. P. (2017). Neonatal jaundice. In T. K. McInerny, H. M. Adam, D. E. Campbell, T. G. DeWitt, J. M. Foy, & D. M. Kamat (Eds.), *Textbook of pediatric care* (2nd ed.). American Academy of Pediatrics. https://pediatriccare .solutions.aap.org/chapter.aspx?sectionid=139979288&boo kid=1626

26. Kalisch-Smith, J., Ved, N., & Sparrow, D. (2020). Environmental risk factors for congenital heart disease. *Cold Spring Harbor Perspectives in Biology, 12*, Article a037234. https://doi .org/10.1101/cshperspect.a037234

27. Kennedy, T. M., & Sharieff, G. Q. (2020). The crashing neonate. In E. Rose (Ed.), *Pediatric emergencies: A practical, clinical guide* (pp. 15–30). Oxford University Press.

28. Kim, J. H. (2020). Neonatal necrotizing enterocolitis: Management. *UpToDate*. Retrieved August 12, 2021, from https://www.uptodate.com/contents/neonatal-necrotizing -enterocolitis-management

29. Lantin-Hermoso, M. R., Berger, S., Bhatt, A. B., Richerson, J. E., Morrow, R., Freed, M. D., & Beekman, R. H. (2017). The care of children with congenital heart disease in their primary medical home. *Pediatrics, 140*(5), Article e20172607. https:// doi.org/10.1542/peds.2017-2607

30. Lasekan, J., & Baggs, G. (2021). Efficacy of soy-based formulas in alleviating gastrointestinal symptoms in infants with milk-based formula intolerance: A randomized clinical trial. *Clinical Pediatrics, 60*(3), 184–192. https://doi.org /10.1177%2F0009922820973017

31. Lucia, D., & Glenn, J. (2017). Pediatric emergencies. In C. K. Stone & R. L. Humphries (Eds.), *Current diagnosis and treatment: Emergency medicine* (8th ed., pp. 964–1016). McGraw Hill.

32. Ludlow, J. T., Wilkerson, R. G., & Nappe, T. M. (2020). *Methemoglobinemia*. StatPearls Publishing. https://www.ncbi.nlm.nih.gov/books/NBK537317/

33. Mancini, M. (2021). *Tetralogy of Fallot*. National Organization for Rare Disorders. https://rarediseases.org/rare-diseases/tetralogy-of-fallot/

34. Mercucio, M. R., & Drago, M. (2021). Periviable birth (limit of viability). *UpToDate*. Retrieved August 12, 2021, from https://www.uptodate.com/contents/periviable-birth-limit-of-viability

35. Mersch, J. (2020). *Pediatric vital signs ranges and charts*. eMedicineHealth. https://www.emedicinehealth.com/pediatric_vital_signs/article_em.htm

36. Mojica, M. (2019, April 15). *The critically ill infant*. Core EM. https://coreem.net/core/the-critically-ill-infant/

37. NeoResus. (2017, December). Disorders of transition. https://www.neoresus.org.au/learning-resources/key-concepts/disorders-of-transition/

38. O'Brien Pharmacy. (2021). *Diluting baby formula: When frugality can be fatal*. https://obrienpharmacy.com/2015/09/diluting-baby-formula-when-frugality-can-be-fatal/

39. Ossa Galvis, M. M., Bhakta, R., Tarmahomed, A., & Mendez, M. (2021). *Cyanotic heart disease*. StatPearls Publishing. https://www.ncbi.nlm.nih.gov/books/NBK500001/

40. Oster, M. (2019). Newborn screening for critical congenital heart disease using pulse oximetry. *UpToDate*. Retrieved August 19, 2021, from https://www.uptodate.com/contents/newborn-screening-for-critical-congenital-heart-disease-using-pulse-oximetry

41. Pan, D. H., & Rivas, Y. (2017). Jaundice: Newborn to age 2 months. *Pediatrics in Review, 38*(11), 499–510. https://doi.org/10.1542/pir.2015-0132

42. Puri, K., Allen, H. D., & Qureshi, A. M. (2017). Congenital heart disease. *Pediatrics in Review, 38*(10), 471–486. https://doi.org/10.1542/pir.2017-0032

43. Radwine, Z. (2014, August 12). *The sick neonate*. emDocs. http://www.emdocs.net/sick-neonate/

44. Rousseau, J. B., & Friedrichs, J. B. (2021). Providing a safe haven: Staff response to a simulated infant relinquishment in the emergency department. *Journal of Emergency Nursing, 47*(2), 352–358. https://doi.org/10.1016/j.jen.2020.12.005

45. Schwarz, C. E., & Dempsey, E. M. (2020). Management of neonatal hypotension and shock. *Seminars in Fetal and Neonatal Medicine, 25*(5), Article 101121. https://doi.org/10.1016/j.siny.2020.101121

46. Stanojevic, M. (2021, May). Limits of viability: Should we play God? *Psychitria Danubina, 33*(3). https://pubmed.ncbi.nlm.nih.gov/34010253/

47. Szymanski, M. W., Moore, S. M., Kritzmire, S. M., & Goyal, A. (2021). *Transposition of the great arteries*. StatPearls Publishing. https://www.ncbi.nlm.nih.gov/books/NBK538434/

48. Tan, C. M. J., & Lewandowski, A. J. (2020). The transitional heart: From early embryonic and fetal development to neonatal life. *Fetal Diagnosis and Therapy, 47*(5), 373–386. https://doi.org/10.1159/000501906

49. Ulfah, D. A., Lestari, E. D., Salimo, H., Widjaya, S. L., & Artiko, B. (2017). The effect of cyanotic and acyanotic congenital heart disease on children's growth velocity. *Paediatrica Indonesiana, 57*(3), 159–162. https://doi.org/10.14238/pi57.3.2017.160-3

50. University Hospitals Cleveland Medical Center. (2019, April 29). Caffeine prevents PGE1-induced disturbances in respiratory neural control: Therapeutic implications for infants treated for congenital heart disease. *ScienceDaily*. https://www.sciencedaily.com/releases/2019/04/190429125358.htm

51. Wachman, E. M., Schiff, D. M., & Silverstein, M. (2018). Neonatal abstinence syndrome: Advances in diagnosis and treatment. *Journal of the American Medical Association, 319*(13), 1362–1374. https://doi.org/10.1001/jama.2018.2640

52. Weiner, G., Zaichkin, J., & Kattwinkel, J. (Eds.). (2021). *Textbook of neonatal resuscitation* (8th ed.). American Academy of Pediatrics.

53. Wilson, R., Ross, O., & Griksaitis, M. J. (2019). Tetralogy of Fallot. *BJA Education, 19*(11), 362–369. https://doi.org/10.1016/j.bjae.2019.07.003

The Child in Need of Stabilization

Diona Giordano, DNP, RN, FNP-BC

OBJECTIVES

Upon completion of this chapter, the learner will be able to:

1. Describe characteristics and selected causes of pediatric decompensation.
2. Differentiate etiologies and management of pediatric shock.
3. Apply the Pediatric Nursing Process to the critically ill child

Introduction

A distressed pediatric patient presenting to the emergency department (ED) can be unnerving, even for the most experienced emergency nurse. Children may become critically ill from common childhood infections, traumatic injuries, immune responses, respiratory compromise, and more. Most cardiopulmonary arrests in children arise from respiratory failure, shock, or the deadly combination of both.[4(Pa7),30] Astute assessment, knowledge of normal infant and child parameters, and a solid understanding of pediatric pathophysiology are important components of the nurse's clinical practice. Early identification and intervention can mean the difference between management and resuscitation. Although there are many reasons why a child may present in respiratory failure or shock, the purpose of this chapter is to review shock pathophysiology, assessment, and interventions to support the nurse's clinical decision making to improve pediatric outcomes.

Respiratory Failure

Respiratory failure, a common cause of pediatric morbidity and mortality, occurs when cellular oxygen demand exceeds the rate at which oxygen is supplied via blood-gas exchange. Prolonged hypoxia leads to cellular death and organ dysfunction. Respiratory failure is characterized by altered responsiveness, skin color changes, and weakening respiratory effort.[4(Pa7)] Respiratory distress, evidenced by increased work of breathing, requires prompt intervention to prevent its progression to respiratory failure.

Respiratory compromise may arise from upper airway conditions, lower airway conditions, disordered breathing, and lung tissue disease. Upper airway concerns include foreign body aspiration, secretions, swelling, masses, and anatomic anomalies such as stenosis (narrowing) or tracheomalacia (tracheal cartilage collapse). Lower airway issues include asthma and bronchiolitis. Disordered breathing may be associated with neurologic, metabolic, or toxicologic causes and presents with altered respiratory effort and ineffective breathing patterns. Lung tissue disease includes pneumonia, trauma, edema, and inflammatory responses.[4(Pa7)]

Other than genetic or underlying cardiac conditions, respiratory distress progressing to failure is the leading cause of pediatric cardiac arrest.[4(Pa3)] See Chapter 8, "The Child with a Cough," for more information on the differentiation between respiratory distress and respiratory failure, potential causes, and condition-specific interventions.

Shock

Respiratory distress is also a sign of the body's attempts to compensate in case of shock. Shock is simply defined as inadequate tissue perfusion, but has many causes. This condition results from the body's inability to compensate for disruptions due to injury or illness, leading to impaired oxygen/nutrient flow to the vital organs. Astute assessment of a child's condition is essential to identify the presence and cause of shock and thereby facilitate goal-directed interventions. Failing to intervene results in shock progression. Untreated shock leads to an irreversible state of cell death and organ dysfunction.[25]

CLINICAL PEARL

The Pediatric Nursing Process

Every step of the primary survey is designed to identify and manage respiratory distress and shock. When interventions are undertaken during the primary survey, the goal is to support or restore tissue perfusion so as to prevent decompensation and the need for resuscitation.

1. Assess and support the airway (oxygen intake).
2. Assess and support breathing and ventilation (alveolar gas exchange).
3. Assess and support circulation (blood flow to the tissues).
4. Assess and support disability (inability to protect the airway, hypoglycemia).
5. Look for other life-threatening conditions; keep the patient warm to decrease metabolic demand and prevent worsening acidosis and coagulopathy.[11]

Pathophysiology

Adequate ventilation and perfusion require inhaled oxygen, alveolar transfer of oxygen to the blood, delivery of oxygenated blood to the tissues, and exhalation of carbon dioxide. Blood flow to the tissues depends on cardiac output, defined as the amount of blood pumped from the heart per minute. Cardiac output is the product of stroke volume and heart rate, where stroke volume is the amount of blood pumped with each ventricular contraction. Cardiac output (CO) = stroke volume (SV) × heart rate (HR).

An increased heart rate will not increase cardiac output if the rate is too fast and unable to adequately fill the ventricles. Stroke volume is affected by preload, afterload, and contractility. Shock results from inadequately oxygenated blood or conditions that affect a child's circulating blood volume (preload), vascular resistance (afterload), contractility, or obstruction of blood flow.[4(Pa9),31] **Figure 7-1** illustrates the factors affecting cardiac output.

Aerobic (with oxygen) metabolism is the normal state of cellular perfusion and is supported with adequate oxygenated blood flow to the tissues. When there is inadequate oxygenated blood flow (decreased tissue perfusion), anaerobic (without air) metabolism takes place. This process is much less efficient and creates lactate, an acid, as a by-product. In prolonged states of anaerobic metabolism, inadequate nutrients to maintain cellular integrity create an acidic environment, leading to cell death.[4(Pa9),6,25,26]

Management of the child with inadequate ventilation or perfusion involves supporting the airway, breathing, and circulation to provide an adequate amount of oxygenated blood to the tissues. Determining why perfusion is inadequate will facilitate goal-directed therapy. Recognition of shock is the first step in providing such care.

Stages of Shock

Shock can be described as proceeding in three stages: compensated, decompensated/hypotensive, and irreversible. In compensated shock, the body recognizes perfusion has decreased and initiates compensatory mechanisms. If perfusion is not restored, these compensatory mechanisms will eventually lose the energy to continue and become ineffective. Decompensation is evidenced by hypotension. In irreversible shock, widespread cellular death leads to multisystem organ dysfunction. Outcomes are generally poor for patients in irreversible shock. However, progression through these stages is not inevitable.

Recognition of early signs of compensation and early intervention can often restore tissue perfusion and stop the progression.[4(Pa9),6,8,25,26,31] Mental status, capillary refill time, skin color, pulse quality and rate, vital sign trends, and other clinical assessment findings are key to early identification of shock. **Table 7-1** briefly describes the pathophysiologic basis for the assessment findings associated with each stage of shock, and **Box 7-1** presents more information on pulse pressure and mean arterial pressure.

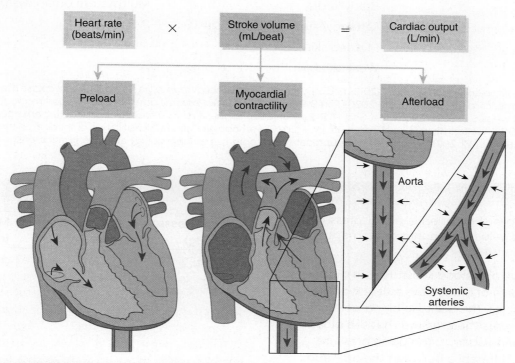

Figure 7-1 *Factors affecting cardiac output.*

TABLE 7-1	Stages of Shock and Pathophysiologic Basis for Assessment Findings	
Stage of Shock	**Assessment Findings**	**Pathophysiologic Basis**
Compensated	Capillary refill 2–3 seconds Cool extremities Decreased urine output Elevated lactate level Increased diastolic blood pressure Mild irritability or sleepiness Mild pallor Orthostatic vital sign changes Tachycardia Tachypnea Weak peripheral pulses	Vasoconstriction shunts blood to vital organs (heart, lungs, brain) Renal hypoperfusion, retention of sodium and water Lactate is a by-product of anaerobic metabolism Reduced cerebral glucose and oxygen supply alter brain function Increased heart and respiratory rate to increase cardiac output and oxygen supply
Decompensated/hypotensive	Altered mental status Hypotension Increased work of breathing Pallor Weak to absent peripheral pulses	Compensatory mechanisms are inadequate and begin to fail

(continues)

TABLE 7-1   Stages of Shock and Pathophysiologic Basis for Assessment Findings (*continued*)

Stage of Shock	Assessment Findings	Pathophysiologic Basis
Irreversible	Bradycardia	Multisystem organ dysfunction
	Lethargy/stupor/unresponsive	
	Mottled skin	
	Weak to absent peripheral pulses	

Data from American College of Surgeons. (2018). Pediatric trauma. In *Advanced trauma life support student course manual* (10th ed., Chapter 10); American Heart Association. (2020). Part 9: Recognizing shock. *Pediatric advanced life support manual*; Balamuth, F., Fitzgerald, J., & Weiss, S. L. (2021). Shock. In K. Shaw & R. Bachur (Eds.), *Fleisher & Ludwig's textbook of pediatric emergency medicine* (7th ed., pp. 55–78). Wolters Kluwer; and Pomerantz, W. J. (2020). Pathophysiology and classification of shock in children. *UpToDate*. Retrieved September 22, 2021, from https://www.uptodate.com/contents/pathophysiology-and-classification-of-shock-in-children

---

BOX 7-1 Pulse Pressure and Mean Arterial Pressure

Derived from the patient's blood pressure, these calculated values are noninvasive measurements of tissue perfusion.

- The systolic blood pressure (SBP) represents the force of blood flow as it leaves the ventricles. The diastolic blood pressure (DBP) represents the pressure that the blood is flowing against. The pulse pressure is the difference between the SBP and the DBP.
- Vasoconstriction, a compensatory mechanism for shock, will increase the DBP and cause a "narrowed" pulse pressure. Vasodilation, a pathophysiologic response seen in distributive shock, will decrease the DBP and cause a "widened" pulse pressure.
- The mean arterial pressure (MAP) reflects arterial perfusion to the organs. This calculation accounts for time spent in systole and diastole.
- Blood pressure, pulse pressure, and MAP trends are much more meaningful than one set of vital signs.

Blood Pressure (mm Hg)	Pulse Pressure (mm Hg)	MAP* (mm Hg)
120/80	40, normal	93
110/90	20, narrowed	97
110/50	60, widened	70
80/40	40, normal	53

* Consider that normal blood pressures are lower in children and that MAP targets are adjusted accordingly when administering vasopressors.

Data from Lough, M. E., Berger, S. J., Larsen, A., & Sandoval, C. P. (2022). Cardiovascular diagnostic procedures. In L. D. Urden, K. M. Stacy, & M. E. Lough (Eds.), *Critical care nursing: Diagnosis and management* (9th ed., pp. 206–297). Elsevier; Lough, M. E. (2022). Cardiovascular anatomy and physiology. In L. D. Urden, K. M. Stacy, & M. E. Lough (Eds.), *Critical care nursing: Diagnosis and management* (9th ed., pp. 167–189). Elsevier; and Lough, M. E. (2022). Cardiovascular clinical assessment. In L. D. Urden, K. M. Stacy, & M. E. Lough (Eds.), *Critical care nursing: Diagnosis and management* (9th ed., pp. 190–205). Elsevier.

Pediatric Considerations

Normal vital signs vary by age. Generally, children's heart and respiratory rates are higher and their blood pressures are lower than those of adults. Normal pediatric vital signs reference ranges, which are available as printed resources or may be embedded in the electronic health record, can help the nurse recognize subtle abnormalities that are early warning signs of shock. Vital signs trends are also useful to detect subtle physiologic signs of compensation. While hypotension is a late sign of shock, rising diastolic blood pressure is an early indicator of vasoconstriction and the body's attempt to shunt blood to the vital organs in response to decreased perfusion. **Table 7-2** presents normal vital signs by age and **Box 7-2** covers pediatric hypotension guidelines. Always consider patient activity and clinical condition when interpreting vital signs data: Lower heart and respiratory rates may be normal for a healthy sleeping child but inadequate for an awake or ill child.

TABLE 7-2 Normal Vital Signs for Pediatric Patients

Age	Heart Rate (beats/min)	Respiratory Rate (breaths/min)	Systolic Blood Pressure (mm Hg)
Term neonate, < 1 month	90–190	35–60	67–84
Infant, 1–12 months	90–180	30–55	72–104
Toddler, 1–3 years	80–140	22–40	86–104
Preschooler, 3–5 years	65–120	18–35	89–112
School-age, 5–12 years	70–120	16–30	90–115
Adolescent, 12–18 years	60–100	12–20	100–130

Data from American Heart Association. (2020). Part 4: Systematic approach to the seriously ill or injured child. *Pediatric advanced life support provider manual*; Ernst, G. (2020). Pediatric trauma. In J. E. Tintinalli, O. J. Ma, D. M. Yealy, G. D. Meckler, J. S. Stapczynski, D. M. Cline, & S. H. Thomas (Eds.), *Tintinalli's emergency medicine: A comprehensive study guide* (9th ed., pp. 689–697). McGraw Hill; and Lucia, D., & Glenn, J. (2017). Pediatric emergencies. In C. K. Stone & R. L. Humphries (Eds.), *Current diagnosis and treatment: Emergency medicine* (8th ed., pp. 964–1016). McGraw Hill.

BOX 7-2 Pediatric Advanced Life Support (PALS) Guidelines for Hypotension

PALS defines hypotension based on systolic blood pressure (SBP) as follows:

- Neonate (0 to 28 days old): SPB < 60 mm Hg
- Infants (1 to 12 months): SBP < 70 mm Hg
- Children (1 to 10 years): SBP < 70 + (2 × age in years) mm Hg
- Children (older than 10 years): SBP < 90 mm Hg

These blood pressures defining hypotension commonly overlap with the lower normal SBP value spectrum.

Data from American Heart Association. (2020). Part 4: Systematic approach to the seriously ill or injured child. *Pediatric advanced life support provider manual*.

CLINICAL PEARL

Rapid Physical Assessment

Taking 10 seconds to inspect and palpate can provide crucial information even prior to obtaining a full set of vital signs. Consider the significant information gained by the following assessments:

- Are there signs of increased work of breathing?
- Palpate a pulse. Is it fast or slow? Irregular? Weak or bounding?
- Are the peripheral pulses weaker than the central pulses?
- What is the capillary refill time?
- Is the skin normal, warm, and dry, or pale, cool, and diaphoretic?
- How is the child responding to the parents or healthcare team?

Tachycardia is an early indicator of shock but is not considered specific or reliable as a diagnostic tool. Fever, pain, and fear may also cause tachycardia. Patients with cardiotoxic drug ingestions, spinal cord injuries, or bradycardic dysrhythmias may be in shock without tachycardia.[26]

A common medical axiom is "Treat the patient, not the numbers." This understanding is particularly important when evaluating pediatric vital signs. If the child appears ill, immediate intervention is required. It is safest to assume that abnormal vital signs are an indicator of shock until proven otherwise and to correlate normal vital signs with the patient's physical presentation.

The body's response to shock is complex and involves multiple interrelated body systems. In times of inadequate perfusion, the body preferentially perfuses the vital organs (heart, lungs, and brain). Most children have strong compensatory mechanisms but limited reserves. Shock progresses, leading to pediatric decompensation, as the compensatory mechanisms fail. This can happen quickly because the compensatory mechanisms work very well until, quite suddenly, they cannot. **Table 7-3** describes the clinical significance of pediatric anatomic and physiologic differences relevant to the shock response.

TABLE 7-3 Pediatric Differences Relevant to Shock	
Characteristics	**Clinical Significance**
› Stroke volume depends on the amount of blood returning to the heart (preload), myocardial contractility, and resistance against blood flow into the peripheral vasculature (afterload). › Given the pediatric heart's smaller contractile mass and shorter myocardial fibers, stroke volume cannot be increased. › Tachycardia is the primary mechanism to maintain cardiac output.	› Heart rate, rather than stroke volume, increases to maintain cardiac output. › Tachycardia is considered a sign of inadequate tissue perfusion until proven otherwise. › Very fast heart rates reduce preload because of inadequate ventricular filling time. › Vasoconstriction, with resultant increased systemic vascular resistance, can increase afterload and further impair stroke volume and cardiac output.
› Infants have a cardiac output twice that of adults.	› Cardiac output provides for increased oxygen needs but leaves little cardiac output in reserve.
› The higher metabolic rate in pediatric patients results in a higher oxygen demand. › Oxygen consumption in infants is twice that of adults. › Infants have little to no myocardial contractility in reserve to increase stroke volume.	› Additional stressors (e.g., hypothermia/hyperthermia, tachypnea, pain, injury, anxiety) result in additional metabolic demands. › A slow or irregular respiratory rate in an acutely ill infant or child is an ominous clinical sign. › Infants rely on heart rate to increase cardiac output and meet increased metabolic demand.

› The greater percentage of total body water weight in pediatric patients requires increased circulating blood volume to meet tissue perfusion needs.
 › Circulating blood volume:
   • Infant: 90 mL/kg
   • Child: 80 mL/kg
   • Adult: 70 mL/kg
	› Increased potential for dehydration.
	 › Increased insensible water losses cause circulatory compromise.
	 › Hypotension occurs after approximately 30% loss of volume. In a 10-kg patient, 30% is < 300 mL.

› Systemic vascular resistance (vasoconstriction) usually increases as a compensatory mechanism to maintain perfusion to vital organs and blood pressure. › Systolic blood pressure will remain normal or even increase in early shock. › Increased diastolic blood pressure is reflective of increased systemic vascular resistance. › Vasodilation occurs in distributive shock, decreasing systemic vascular resistance. › Abnormal systemic vascular resistance results in disruption of blood flow to nonvital tissues and organs.	› Weak peripheral pulses and prolonged capillary refill may indicate abnormal vasoconstriction, while flushed skin and bounding pulses may indicate abnormal vasodilation. › Assess systemic vascular resistance by timing capillary refill and comparing the strength of central pulses to the strength of peripheral pulses. › Narrowed pulse pressure (the difference between the systolic and diastolic readings) is a sign of compensation. › Hypotension is a sign of circulatory decompensation. The combination of decreased heart and/or respiratory rate with poor perfusion is an ominous sign.

Characteristics	Clinical Significance
› Even in compensated shock, automated blood pressure readings may be difficult to obtain. › Automated blood pressure devices are accurate only when distal perfusion is adequate. › Increased peripheral vascular resistance may give falsely high or low readings. › Obtain a manual blood pressure reading and compare it with the automated blood pressure reading.	› Treat the patient based on the clinical exam. › Assess capillary refill as an indicator of peripheral perfusion (normal capillary refill time is less than 2 seconds in a warm ambient environment), along with radial/brachial or femoral pulses. › Preferable sites for assessment of capillary refill are those located at the level of the heart. In the smaller pediatric patient, a finger or toe is often not the most appropriate site.

Data from American College of Surgeons. (2018). Pediatric trauma. In *Advanced trauma life support student course manual* (10th ed., Chapter 10); Balamuth, F., Fitzgerald, J., & Weiss, S. L. (2021). Shock. In K. Shaw & R. Bachur (Eds.), *Fleisher & Ludwig's textbook of pediatric emergency medicine* (8th ed., pp. 55–78); Waltzman, M. (2021). Initial evaluation of shock in children. *UpToDate*. https://www.uptodate.com/contents/initial-evaluation-of-shock-in-children#!; Davis, A. L., Carcillo, J. A., Aneja, R. K., Deymann, A. J., Lin, J. C., Nguyen, T. C., Okhuysen-Cawley, R. S., Relvas, M. S., Rozenfeld, R. A., Skippen, P. W., Stojadinovic, B. J., Williams, E. A., Yeh, T. S., Balamuth, F., Brierley, J., de Caen, A. R., Cheifetz, I. M., Choong, K., Conway, E., Jr., . . . Zuckerberg, A. L. (2017). American College of Critical Care Medicine clinical practice parameters for hemodynamic support of pediatric and neonatal septic shock. *Critical Care Medicine, 45*(6), 1061–1093. https://doi.org/10.1097/CCM.0000000000002425; Pasman, E. A., & Watson, C. M. (2019). Shock in pediatrics. *Medscape*. Retrieved September 21, 2021, from https://emedicine.medscape.com/article/1833578-overview; and Pomerantz, W. J. (2020). Pathophysiology and classification of shock in children. *UpToDate*. Retrieved September 22, 2021, from https://www.uptodate.com/contents/pathophysiology-and-classification-of-shock-in-children

Types and Causes of Shock

When assessing a child or infant who may be exhibiting signs of shock, thoughtful consideration should be given to the type and cause of shock. Implementing effective goal-directed therapy for shock requires determination of the cause. Shock is an imbalance between energy and oxygen consumption due to a physiologic disruption. What is the physiologic disruption? Is the shock due to a "pump" (heart), "pipe" (vascular structures), or "tank" (fluid volume) problem, or a combination of these? Which factor impacting cardiac output is altered—heart rate or stroke volume? Is the stroke volume compromised due to changes in preload, afterload, or contractility? The answers to these questions will help determine the cause and categorize the shock as one of four types: hypovolemic, obstructive, cardiogenic, or distributive.

Hypovolemic Shock

Hypovolemic shock is a "tank" (fluid volume) problem. Considered the most common form of shock, hypovolemic shock is a result of intravascular volume depletion.[4(Pa9),31] This volume deficit will affect preload. Preload is a component of stroke volume; therefore, if fluid loss (intravascular or hemorrhage) occurs, preload will decrease, resulting in decreased cardiac output. Contractility will be unaffected or slightly increased, but the afterload (vascular resistance) may increase due to the body's attempt to compensate by constricting the vessels to maintain or increase blood pressure. Causative factors for intravascular loss include vomiting and diarrhea from gastroenteritis, urinary diuresis from diabetes insipidus, shifting of interstitial fluids or third spacing from burns, and heat stroke. Another cause of body fluid deficit is hemorrhage, where causes of blood loss may include traumatic injury, surgery, gastrointestinal bleeding, and epistaxis.[25,31]

Interventions for impending or actual hypovolemic shock focus on finding the source of the fluid loss and ensuring fluid replenishment. With hemorrhagic sources of hypovolemic shock, the initial goal-directed therapy is bleeding control. This may require direct pressure, tourniquets, interventional radiology, or surgical intervention. For all forms of hypovolemic shock, the "tank" must be filled (preload) to deliver an adequate supply of oxygenated blood to the rest of the body. "Filling the tank" may be accomplished in a variety of ways, including

NOTE

Shock Associated with Trauma

Trauma is associated with hypovolemic (hemorrhagic) and obstructive (cardiac tamponade, tension pneumothorax) shock. See Chapter 9, "The Child with an Injury," for more information on traumatic injuries and resuscitation.

providing small, frequent, amounts of oral fluids, administering intravenous (IV) fluid boluses, and administering blood products.[4(Pa10),25,31]

Obstructive Shock

Obstructive shock is a "pump" (heart) or "pipe" (vasculature) problem resulting from a physical obstruction. The obstruction compresses the heart and/or the vasculature. This can occur due to either congenital or acquired conditions such as cardiac tamponade, tension pneumothorax, pulmonary embolism, ductal-dependent lesions, pulmonary hypertension, and hypertrophic cardiomyopathy. In obstructive shock, intravascular volume is unaffected. Although heart contractility is considered normal, an obstruction limits the pumping mechanism of the heart. The preload and afterload may be decreased due to an obstruction limiting ventricular filling or the afterload may be increased due to an obstruction preventing normal vascular flow. Interventions focus on the relief of the obstruction and may include pericardiocentesis, thoracostomy, prostaglandin administration, and surgery.[4(Pa9,10),6,27]

CLINICAL PEARL

Pulsus Paradoxus in Obstructive Shock

A drop in blood pressure with inspiration, called pulsus paradoxus, results from increased intrathoracic pressure that exacerbates the vascular obstruction. Invasive blood pressure monitoring or taking a blood pressure during inspiration is not necessary to identify this important clinical finding associated with obstructive shock. Pay attention to the palpated pulse and pulse oximetry waveform as the patient inhales. When pulsus paradoxus is present, the pulse will be weaker and/or the pulse oximetry waveform will dampen.[4(Pa9),7]

Cardiac Tamponade

Cardiac tamponade is a condition caused by an accumulation of fluid in the pericardial sac. This fluid compresses the heart, progressively limiting its ability to pump effectively. The heart is unable to adequately fill. Cardiac tamponade is commonly associated with hypotension, muffled heart sounds, and jugular vein distention (Beck's triad). If the patient has hypovolemia, however, jugular vein distention may not be prominent. Pericardiocentesis and/or surgery may be required to treat shock associated with a cardiac tamponade.[4(Pa9),31]

Pulmonary Embolism

Pulmonary embolism is a blockage within one or more of the pulmonary arteries. It is most often caused by blood clots but can also be caused by fat, air, fluid, or bacteria. Risk factors for pulmonary embolism include obesity, hormone use (e.g., oral contraceptives), hypercoagulable status, prolonged immobility, surgery, and trauma.[4(Pa7),23,34] Pulmonary embolism is suspected in a child or infant presenting as cyanotic and/or hypotensive with respiratory distress. Guidelines for intervention rely heavily on adult recommendations and include anticoagulation, thrombolysis, and thrombectomy.[23,34]

Tension Pneumothorax

A pneumothorax occurs when the protective lining of the lung, called the pleura, becomes compromised. Air entering the pleural space causes alveolar collapse, limiting gas exchange. A pneumothorax may be caused by trauma or due to underlying lung disease such as cystic fibrosis, asthma, and pneumonia. Some spontaneous pneumothoraces are not associated with lung disease.[14,22] In recent years, an increased incidence of pediatric pneumothoraces has been associated with the growing popularity of vaping.[22,33]

A tension pneumothorax develops when enough air enters the pleural space to put pressure on the heart and great vessels. This pressure then obstructs cardiac function, leading to obstructive shock. Tachycardia, respiratory distress, and hypotension are common findings. Jugular vein distention and tracheal deviation are considered late signs.

NOTE

Congenital Heart Disease

Congenital heart disease may cause obstructive or cardiogenic shock, depending on the pathophysiology. Congenital heart defects affect the structure of the heart, valves, or blood vessels.[27] An infant or child may present with cyanosis to the extremities, nails, or lips; changes in breathing patterns; and fatigue, especially with feeding.[10] Shock, cyanosis, and respiratory symptoms are hallmark presentations of critical congenital heart disease.[1] Interventions may include prostaglandin administration, interventional radiology, and surgery.[15] See Chapter 6, "The Neonate," for more information.

Jugular vein distention will not occur in patients with significant hypovolemia, and tracheal deviation is often not appreciated in children. Treatment of a tension pneumothorax involves release of the trapped air via thoracostomy, finger thoracostomy (needle decompression, chest tube), or surgical intervention.[4(P10),14,22]

Cardiogenic Shock

Cardiogenic shock results from problems with the "pump" (heart) and may be idiopathic. Pump failure due to cardiomyopathy can originate from infection (myocarditis), inherited disease, surgical intervention, trauma, or toxins.[25,26] Pump failure due to dysrhythmias may result from toxins, heart disease, hypoxia, or hypothermia.[26] Cardiac contractility and rate are affected. Interventions focus on supporting the heart function by strengthening contractility or correcting the heart rate.[4(Pa10)]

Both atrial and ventricular dysrhythmias may result in cardiogenic shock. Rhythms that are too fast decrease ventricular filling time. This leads to decreased stroke volume and potentially inadequate cardiac output. Rhythms that are too slow can also decrease cardiac output, as younger pediatric patients have a limited capability to increase stroke volume. When the heart rate is not sufficient to maintain perfusion, cardiogenic shock occurs.[4(Pa9),26] **Table 7-4** provides more information on pediatric rhythm disturbances.

Distributive Shock

Distributive shock is a "pipe" (vasculature) problem caused by systemic vasodilation. While the fluid volume may be adequate, a relative hypovolemia occurs. Normal body fluid volume is not enough to fill the much larger "tank" resulting from extensive vasodilation. Vasoconstriction causes the cool, pale skin and weak pulses noted in other forms of shock. Because distributive shock is caused by vasodilation, these signs are not typically seen. Distributive shock is discussed in terms of three main types: anaphylactic, neurogenic, and septic. As with all forms of shock, the goal-directed therapy is driven by the pathophysiology.[4(Pa9),6,31]

Anaphylactic

Anaphylaxis is an overwhelming allergic reaction. Systemic vasodilation results from a release of inflammatory mediators such as histamine, prostaglandins, kinins, and serotonins. Patients present with hives, flushing, facial and airway swelling, stridor, vomiting and diarrhea, and/or wheezing. The priority intervention is administration of intramuscular epinephrine. Airway management including intubation, inhaled albuterol, and IV fluids may be required. Adjunctive treatments include antihistamines and steroids but are *not* considered life-saving interventions.[4(Pa10),9]

Neurogenic

Neurogenic shock is usually a result of high thoracic or cervical spinal cord injuries, which interrupt the sympathetic nervous system response. Sympathetic stimulation results in tachycardia and vasoconstriction. The interrupted sympathetic response increases the influence of the parasympathetic nervous system. This parasympathetic stimulation then results in bradycardia and vasodilation. Spinal precautions and careful monitoring of respiratory status are recommended. Goal-directed therapy includes careful management of IV fluids to "fill the tank." Bradycardia predisposes the patient to fluid volume overload and pulmonary edema if large, rapid fluid boluses are administered. Medications to increase heart rate and vascular tone may be required to maintain perfusion.[4(Pa10),25,31]

Septic

Overwhelming infection triggers a systemic inflammatory response syndrome that can result in septic shock. This is considered the most common form of distributive shock in the pediatric population.[25] Vasoactive mediators are released, resulting in systemic vasodilatation. IV fluids should be administered based on the patient's condition and require careful monitoring to avoid volume overload. For hypotension, administer 10–20 mL/kg per bolus, up to a total of 40–60 mL/kg over the first hour. Epinephrine or norepinephrine infusions are used if the patients shows signs of abnormal perfusion after fluid administration. Ideally, antibiotics will be administered within 1 hour of the patient's arrival at the ED. Obtain blood cultures prior to IV antibiotic administration if this does not cause a significant delay.[4(Pa10),32] See Chapter 10, "The Child with a Fever," for more information on sepsis.

CLINICAL PEARL

Distributive Shock Presents Differently

- Be alert for bradycardia and vasodilation with warm, dry skin with neurogenic shock.
- Be alert for "flash" capillary refill (< 1 second) and bounding pulses with septic or anaphylactic shock.[4(Pa9),6]

TABLE 7-4 Pediatric Rhythm Disturbances: Causes, Characteristics, Symptoms, and Interventions

Rhythm Disturbance	History and Causes	ECG Characteristics	Signs and Symptoms	Interventions
Sinus bradycardia (too slow)	Hypothermia, hypoxia Increased intracranial pressure Suspected overdose or ingestion Head or chest trauma Increased vagal tone from suctioning, intubation attempts, coughing, or other stimulation Calcium-channel blockers, beta blockers, or digoxin Inadequate oral intake	Heart rate less than normal for age or less than 60 beats/min P wave present QRS narrow, rhythm regular	Signs of poor perfusion Increased work of breathing Change in level of consciousness, fussy, irritable, listless Can be asymptomatic ECG shows atrial and ventricular rates are slow	Identify and treat reversible causes; ensure adequate oxygenation and ventilation. If bradycardia is the result of vagal stimulation or atrioventricular (AV) block, consider IV/IO atropine: › Dosing: 0.02 mg/kg › Minimum dose: 0.1 mg › Maximum dose: 0.5 mg If the heart rate remains less than 60 beats/min, initiate cardiopulmonary resuscitation (CPR) and administer IV/IO epinephrine: › Dosing: 0.01 mg/kg › May repeat every 3 to 5 minutes › Maximum single dose: 1 mg Consider cardiac pacing.
Sinus tachycardia (too fast)	Hypoxia Medications (albuterol, amphetamines) Sepsis Crying Agitation Anxiety Fever Pain	Heart rate greater than normal for age P wave present, QRS narrow, rhythm regular Heart rate fluctuates with activity Beat-to-beat variability	Rapid, thready peripheral pulses Increased work of breathing Flash (less than 1 second) or delayed (more than 2 seconds) capillary refill Dry mucous membranes	Treat the underlying cause.

Rhythm Disturbance	History and Causes	ECG Characteristics	Signs and Symptoms	Interventions
	Congenital heart disease (CHD) Hyperthyroidism Heart failure Hypovolemia (trauma or illness) Consumption of a stimulant (e.g., energy drink, synthetic drug, nicotine, caffeine, cocaine) Alcohol withdrawal Drug withdrawal Pulmonary embolism	Rate normally less than 220 beats/min in infants and less than 180 beats/min in children; if it exceeds these values, consider supraventricular tachycardia	Decreased number of wet diapers Increased stool, diarrhea, or vomiting	
Supraventricular tachycardia (SVT) (too fast)	Poor feeding Irritable, fussy, or inconsolable Sweating when feeding Palpitations Chest pain Exercise intolerance Respiratory distress Cough or cold medications History of previous episodes of SVT or Wolff-Parkinson-White (WPW) syndrome CHD	Heart rate greater than 220 beats/min in infants and greater than 180 beats/min in children P wave difficult to distinguish due to rate; may be buried in QRS; QRS narrow and regular No beat-to-beat variability or change with activity	Pale, mottled, or cyanotic Signs of poor perfusion Weak or absent peripheral pulses Altered level of consciousness, listless Heart rate too fast to count Signs of heart failure, including crackles Hypotension	Treatment is based on the patient's clinical status and stability. If the child is **stable**: 12-lead ECG and IV/IO access. Vagal maneuvers to slow conduction.[a] If vagal maneuvers are ineffective, consider IV/IO adenosine: › With continuous ECG monitoring, administer adenosine rapidly through the IV closest to the central circulation and flush immediately › Initial dose: 0.1 mg/kg (maximum dose 6 mg) › Second dose if needed: 0.2 mg/kg (maximum dose 12 mg) Determine risk factors for hypovolemia, sepsis, fever, cardiac disease, electrolyte abnormality or overdose; treat underlying cause.

(continues)

TABLE 7-4 Pediatric Rhythm Disturbances: Causes, Characteristics, Symptoms, and Interventions *(continued)*

Rhythm Disturbance	History and Causes	ECG Characteristics	Signs and Symptoms	Interventions
				If the child is *unstable*: Adenosine if IV/IO access is present. Do not delay cardioversion for IV/IO access. Synchronized cardioversion with 0.5-1 J/kg, may increase to 2 J/kg if initial dose is ineffective. Consider sedation if IV access is present. Consider IV/IO amiodarone 5 mg/kg over 20 to 60 minutes (maximum dose 150 mg)
Ventricular tachycardia (VT) with a pulse (too fast)	Dizziness. Loss of consciousness. Suspected overdose (cyclic antidepressants, stimulants, cocaine). Structural heart disease or CHD. Myocarditis or cardiomyopathy. Long QT syndrome. Electrolyte imbalance (hypokalemia, hypomagnesemia, or hypocalcemia). Drugs that cause long QT syndrome	Three or more consecutive beats originating from the ventricles. QRS is wide (0.09 seconds). Rate can vary from 120 to 200 beats/min. P waves are not identifiable; T waves are typically opposite in polarity from the wide QRS. Torsades de pointes (TdP): a form of polymorphic VT; has a rapid rate and wide QRS, as well as variations in the QRS axis	Signs of poor perfusion. Decreased level of consciousness. May lose pulses—reassess frequently. Increased work of breathing. Palpitations. Hypotension. Sustained VT can deteriorate into ventricular fibrillation. Additional history for TdP: Patient may have history of long QT syndrome or take drugs known to lengthen the QT interval. Hypokalemia and hypomagnesemia	If the child is *stable*: Identify and treat reversible causes. Consider adenosine if regular with monomorphic QRS (suggestive for SVT with aberrancy). Consider IV/IO amiodarone 5 mg/kg over 20 to 60 minutes (maximum dose 150 mg). If the child is *unstable*: Synchronized cardioversion at 0.5-1 J/kg. May increase to 2 J/kg if initial dose is ineffective. Consider sedation. Polymorphic VT/TdP. Consider magnesium. Synchronized cardioversion may be difficult. Attempt to increase the size of the R wave or change leads. May give an unsynchronized shock to unstable patients.

a Vagal maneuvers include applying a bag of ice to the face without occluding the airway and bending the knees to the chest. Older children can be instructed to bear down, blow through an occluded straw, or try to blow the plunger out of a syringe. Eyeball pressure and carotid massage are to be avoided.

Data from American Heart Association. (2020). Part 11 and Part 12. *Pediatric advanced life support provider manual.*

Management of the Child in Septic Shock

The 2020 Surviving Sepsis Campaign guidelines[32] include the following interventions, which are to be implemented within 1 hour of initial recognition of septic shock:

- IV/IO access
- IV fluid bolus, 10–20 mL/kg per bolus up to 40–60 mL/kg
  - Monitor closely for signs of volume overload
- Blood culture collection: Attempt to obtain prior to antibiotic administration but do not delay antibiotics if unable to obtain
- IV antibiotics

Note that fluid boluses are not recommended for normotensive children being treated in healthcare systems without pediatric intensive care access.

Clinical markers of improving perfusion include heart rate, blood pressure, capillary refill time, level of consciousness, lactate level, and urine output. Epinephrine and norepinephrine are preferable to dopamine for children with abnormal perfusion after 40–60 mL/kg of IV fluids.[32]

Goal-Directed Therapy for Shock

Causes of hypovolemic shock include hemorrhage, gastrointestinal losses, poor intake, diuresis, or third-spacing of fluids. Causes of obstructive shock include cardiac tamponade, tension pneumothorax, pulmonary embolism, and congenital heart disease. Causes of cardiogenic shock include cardiomyopathy, heart failure, and rhythm disturbances. Causes of distributive shock include anaphylaxis, spinal cord injury, and sepsis. **Figure 7-2** illustrates each type of shock. **Table 7-5** summarizes shock presentations and goal-directed therapies.

Cardiopulmonary Resuscitation

The International Liaison Committee on Resuscitation (ILCOR) develops periodic consensus statements on resuscitation science with treatment recommendations. These guidelines represent a scientific collaboration with the American Heart Association, the Australian and New Zealand Committee on Resuscitation, the European Resuscitation Council, the Heart and Stroke Foundation of Canada, the InterAmerican Heart Foundation, the Resuscitation Council of Asia, and the Resuscitation Council of Southern Africa. Refer to ilcor.org for more information about the collaborative process and consensus statements.[24] The American Heart Association uses these consensus statements as a basis for its Basic Life Support (BLS), Pediatric Advanced Life Support (PALS), and Adult Cardiovascular Life Support (ACLS) courses. This section is a summary of the PALS and ACLS skill steps.

Resuscitation Skill Steps for Adults, Children, and Infants

For resuscitation purposes, an adult patient is defined as any patient with signs of puberty such as chest hair, underarm hair, or any breast development. Patients are infants from 28 days past their due date to 1 year of age. Neonates (less than 28 days past their due date) are treated according to the Neonatal Resuscitation Program

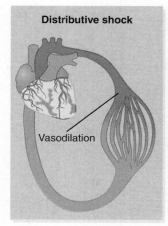
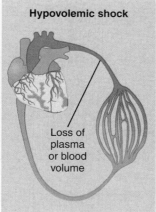
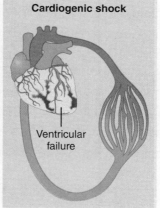
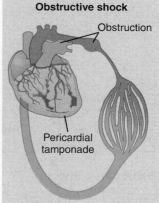

Figure 7-2 *Types of shock.*

TABLE 7-5	Summary of Shock Presentation and Goal-Directed Therapy
Hypovolemic Shock	
Assessment findings	Early signs:
	› Tachycardia and tachypnea
	› Slight alteration in mental status
	› Slightly prolonged capillary refill time (2–3 seconds)
	› Slightly increased diastolic pressure
	Late signs:
	› Prolonged capillary refill time
	› Weak pulses and hypotension
	› Cool, pale, mottled skin
	› Altered mental status
	› Hemorrhage, external or internal (can be occult)
	Signs of dehydration:
	› Dry mucous membranes
	› Sunken eyes
	› Sunken fontanelle
	› Absence of tears
History findings	› Fever, vomiting, diarrhea
	› Decreased appetite and poor oral intake
	› Decreased urine output
	› Burn injury
	› Trauma (focus on mechanism of injury)
Diagnostics	› Focused assessment with sonography for trauma (FAST) examination
	› Computed tomography (CT)
	› Urinalysis/specific gravity
	› Complete blood count (CBC)
	› Electrolytes (including glucose)
	› Chest radiographs
	› Blood gas (arterial, venous, or capillary) to include base deficit
	› Lactate level
Interventions	› Prevent fluid loss; stop uncontrolled bleeding
	› Administer antiemetics as ordered
	› Oral rehydration therapy as appropriate for clinical condition (i.e., alert, no potential for airway compromise)
	› Administer an isotonic crystalloid fluid bolus, 20 mL/kg, and reassess
	› Anticipate blood product administration for hemorrhagic shock
	› Administer balanced component therapy; prevent coagulopathy[11]
	› Consider initiating massive transfusion protocol
Cardiogenic Shock	
Assessment findings	› Abnormal breath sounds (crackles, rales, diminished)
	› Abnormal heart sounds (gallop, heart murmur)
	› Edema

Cardiogenic Shock

	› Evidence of acute or previous chest trauma, surgical scar
	› Extremely high or low heart rate
	› Hepatomegaly
	› Jugular venous distention
	› Orthopnea (difficulty breathing when lying flat)
History findings	› Hypotension and syncope
	› Possible ingestion
	› Previous cardiac surgery or congenital heart defect (CHD)
	› Supraventricular tachycardia: History of decreased feeding, tires easily, sweating when feeding or crying, decreased crying, and acrocyanosis (bluish discoloration of hands and feet due to hypoxemia)
	› Viral illness followed by decreased activity
Diagnostics	› Ultrasound
	› Electrocardiogram and echocardiogram
	› Chest radiograph to rule out cardiomegaly
	› Medication levels for suspected ingestion
Interventions	› Cardiology consult
	› Decrease oxygen and metabolic demands
	› IV/IO fluids, 5–10 mL/kg isotonic crystalloid administered over 10–30 minutes; re-assess for improvement of perfusion status and monitor closely for signs of fluid overload
	› Vagal maneuvers, antidysrhythmics, and cardioversion
	› Vasopressors and/or inotropes

Obstructive Shock

Assessment findings	› Anxiety, feeling of impending doom
	› Evidence of thoracic trauma
	› Pulsus paradoxus (decrease in systolic blood pressure during inspiration)
	› Jugular venous distention (may not be visible in younger patients or in the presence of hypovolemia)
	› Muffled heart sounds
	› Elevated diastolic blood pressure
	› Asymmetrical chest rise and fall
	› Unilateral decreased or absent breath sounds (hyperresonant pediatric breath sounds may mask this assessment finding)
History findings	› Blunt-force trauma to chest, neck, or trunk
	› Recent long bone fracture
	› Neonate with little or no prenatal care, home birth
	› Pulmonary embolism risks: Sickle cell disease, central venous catheter, coagulation disorder, birth control use

(continues)

TABLE 7-5	Summary of Shock Presentation and Goal-Directed Therapy (*continued*)		
Obstructive Shock			
Diagnostics	› Chest radiograph or CT › FAST exam › Echocardiogram › Pericardiocentesis › Fluoroscopy		
Interventions	› Treat ductal-dependent lesions with prostaglandin E₁ infusion › Pericardiocentesis for cardiac tamponade › Finger thoracostomy, needle decompresssion, chest tube for tension pneumothorax › Possible anticoagulants or surgical intervention for pulmonary embolism		
Distributive Shock			
Assessment findings	Anaphylactic	› Respiratory distress, airway spasm, difficulty swallowing › Stridor, hoarseness, respiratory distress, wheezing › Tachycardia › Hives, flushing, urticaria; swelling of lips, tongue, or throat › Hypotension with widened pulse pressure › Syncope › Vomiting, diarrhea	
	Neurogenic	› Bradycardia › Hypotension with widened pulse pressure › Warm, dry extremities	
	Septic	› Tachycardia › Altered mental status › Hypotension with widened pulse pressure › Flash capillary refill (< 1 second) in early shock › Hyperthermia, normothermia, or hypothermia	
History findings	Anaphylactic	› Exposure to known or unknown allergen › Sudden onset of symptoms	
	Neurogenic	› History of trauma with neurologic deficit or access to neuromuscular-blocking agents or dissociative agents	
	Septic	› History of fever, exposure to communicable disease, or other symptoms of infectious disease › History of immunosuppression	
Diagnostics	Anaphylactic	› Blood gas › Monitoring, including pulse oximetry and capnography	
	Neurogenic	› CT/magnetic resonance imaging (MRI), chest radiograph	

	Septic	› Laboratory studies
		  · CBC
		  · Cultures of blood, urine, cerebral spinal fluid, wounds, and indwelling devices	

Distributive Shock

		· Lactate
		· Procalcitonin
		› Blood gas (to include base deficit)
		› Radiographic studies as indicated for cough or joint pain
Interventions	Anaphylactic	› Intramuscular epinephrine, administered in the thigh
		› Nebulized albuterol for bronchospasm/wheezing
		› Consider second-line treatment with diphenhydramine, famotidine, ranitidine, and steroids
		› Prepare to support airway and breathing
		› 20 mL/kg isotonic crystalloid bolus
	Neurogenic	› Spinal motion restriction if appropriate
		› Prepare to support airway and breathing
		› 20 mL/kg of isotonic crystalloid bolus, to exclude hypovolemia as the cause of hypotension, followed by maintenance fluids
		› Vasopressor or inotrope therapy as needed for fluid-refractory hypotension
		› Provide warming measures such as blankets or warmed fluids to prevent hypothermia
	Septic	› 20 mL/kg isotonic crystalloid bolus, prepare to repeat up to 60 mL/kg in first hour
		› Antibiotic administration in first hour
		› Vasopressor therapy as needed for fluid refractory hypotension

Data from American Heart Association. (2020). Part 9 and Part 10. *Pediatric advanced life support provider manual*; Balamuth, F., Fitzgerald, J., & Weiss, S. L. (2021). Shock. In K. Shaw & R. Bachur (Eds.), *Fleisher & Ludwig's textbook of pediatric emergency medicine* (8th ed., pp. 55–78). Wolters Kluwer; and Waltzman, M. (2021). Initial evaluation of shock in children. *UpToDate*. Retrieved September 22, 2021, from https://www.uptodate.com/contents/initial-evaluation-of-shock-in-children

guidelines developed in collaboration with the American Academy of Pediatrics, but these protocols are generally reserved for the newly born as they transition from intrauterine to extrauterine life.[4(Pa2)] See Chapter 6, "The Neonate," for more information on neonatal resuscitation.

When any patient is noted to be unresponsive or apneic, first consider scene safety. Look for normal breathing while palpating for a pulse for no less than 5 seconds but no more than 10 seconds. If no pulse is palpable, a lone rescuer with no immediate mechanism to summon help (e.g., alarm button in the room, people in hearing range) considers whether the arrest is sudden or the result of hypoxia. Sudden witnessed arrests are more likely to benefit from immediate defibrillation. Unwitnessed arrests or those likely to have resulted from hypoxia are more likely to benefit from immediate chest compressions and ventilations. The lone rescuer might leave the patient to call for help and bring a defibrillator prior to initiating compressions for sudden witnessed arrests. Otherwise, call for help and a defibrillator while beginning high-quality

RED FLAG

Pulselessness is not the only indication for pediatric chest compressions. A heart rate of less than 60 beats/min with signs of poor perfusion (e.g., altered mental status, delayed capillary refill, cool skin, mottling, pallor, diaphoresis, hypotension) is ominous in a child. This child needs airway and breathing support with positive-pressure ventilation. If the heart rate does not increase after adequate oxygenation and ventilation, begin CPR.[4(Pa11)]

cardiopulmonary resuscitation (CPR) starting with chest compressions. Provide chest compressions with minimal interruptions (less than 10 seconds).[3(Pa3),4(Pa5)]

The compression and ventilation technique varies slightly depending on age. For patients with signs of puberty (e.g., chest hair, underarm hair, pubic hair, any breast development), use two hands to compress the chest at a depth of at least 2 inches (5 cm) and a rate of 100 to 120 compressions per minute. In the absence of an advanced airway, provide cycles of 30 compressions with a pause for 2 breaths. When an advanced airway is placed, provide continuous compressions. One breath is delivered every 6 seconds with no pauses in compressions.[3(Pa3)]

For infants and children without any signs of puberty, compress the chest at a depth of at least one-third the diameter of the chest and a rate of 100 to 120 compressions per minute. One or two hands may be used for children, while two fingers or two thumbs may be used for infants. Use of two thumbs with the hands encircling the infant's chest is preferred for infants, but this technique requires two rescuers so as to minimize the pauses in compressions to deliver ventilations. In the absence of an advanced airway, two rescuers will provide cycles of 15 compressions with a pause for 2 breaths. When an advanced airway is placed, provide continuous compressions. One breath is delivered every 2 to 3 seconds with no pauses in compressions.[4(Pa5)]

Ventricular Fibrillation/Pulseless Ventricular Tachycardia

Ventricular fibrillation and pulseless ventricular tachycardia are considered "shockable" rhythms, which means that defibrillation may convert them to a perfusing rhythm. Lone rescuers may prioritize attaching a defibrillator in cases of sudden, witnessed cardiac arrest. Otherwise, apply a defibrillator as soon as possible while chest compressions are being performed. Pause only to determine the rhythm. When the rhythm is identified as ventricular fibrillation or pulseless ventricular tachycardia, the intervention sequence is as follows[3(Pa3),4(Pa5)]:

- Resume compressions and charge the defibrillator.
- Follow the device manufacturer's guidelines, but generally the initial defibrillation energy dose is 120–200 J for adults and 2 J/kg for children.
- Pause compressions to deliver a shock; resume compressions immediately after the shock is delivered.
- Perform 2 minutes of CPR, pausing for less than 10 seconds to switch compressors and reevaluate the patient's rhythm.
- Obtain IV or IO access for fluid and medication administration.
- If the rhythm is still shockable (ventricular fibrillation/pulseless ventricular tachycardia), resume compressions while charging the defibrillator. The energy dose is up to 360 J for adults and 4 J/kg for children.

- Pause compressions to deliver a shock; resume compressions immediately after the shock is delivered.
- Administer IV epinephrine every 3 to 5 minutes. The dose is 1 mg for adults and 0.01 mg/kg, to a maximum of 1 mg, for children.
- Consider placement of an advanced airway and use of capnography.
- Continue 2-minute cycles of CPR with pauses only to switch compressors and reevaluate the patient's rhythm.
- If the rhythm is still shockable (ventricular fibrillation/pulseless ventricular tachycardia), resume compressions while charging the defibrillator. Subsequent energy doses are up to 360 J for adults and 10 J/kg for children, per the device manufacturer's recommendations.
- Administer amiodarone intravenously (300 mg for adults and 5 mg/kg for children) or lidocaine intravenously, 1 mg/kg.
- Continue 2-minute cycles of CPR with pauses only to switch compressors and reevaluate the patient's rhythm.

Potential underlying causes of cardiac arrest are listed in **Table 7-6**. Consider and treat underlying causes, prioritizing hypoxia and hypovolemia.

Pulseless Electrical Activity or Asystole

When the rhythm is identified as pulseless electrical activity or asystole, the intervention sequence is as follows[3(Pa3),4(Pa5)]:

- Resume CPR, starting with chest compressions.
- Obtain IV or IO access to administer epinephrine as soon as possible.

TABLE 7-6 Causes of Cardiac Arrest	
The Hs	**The Ts**
Hypovolemia (trauma, illness)	Tension pneumothorax
	Tamponade (cardiac)
Hypoxia	Toxins/tablets
Hydrogen ion (acid-base balance)	Thrombosis (pulmonary embolism)
Hypokalemia/hyperkalemia (other electrolytes and glucose)	Thrombosis (coronary, acute myocardial infarction)
Hypothermia	

Data from American Heart Association. (2020). Part 5. *Advanced cardiovascular life support*; American Heart Association. (2020). Part 5. *Pediatric advanced life support provider manual.*

- Administer IV epinephrine every 3 to 5 minutes. The dose is 1 mg for adults and 0.01 mg/kg, to a maximum of 1 mg, for children.
- Continue 2-minute cycles of CPR with pauses only to switch compressors and reevaluate the patient.

  - In pulseless electrical activity, the only change in the patient may be a palpable pulse.
  - A team member can palpate the pulse during compressions. This evaluates the quality of the compressions and will help quickly identify the return of a spontaneous pulse when the compressors are switched.
  - Consider placement of an advanced airway and use of capnography.
  - Consider and treat underlying causes (refer to Table 7-6), prioritizing hypoxia and hypovolemia.

Post-Resuscitation Care for Children

Immediate post-resuscitation care priorities are to optimize the airway, breathing and ventilation, and circulation while continuing goal-directed therapy for persistent shock. Maintenance fluids with or without dextrose and electrolytes are administered based on the patient's age, weight, hydration status, electrolyte balance, and glucose level. Be alert for and treat hypoxia, hypotension, and hypoglycemia. Avoid hyperoxia and hyperthermia. Targeted temperature management is considered for pediatric patients who are unresponsive after return of spontaneous circulation. Other neurologic support includes avoiding hyperthermia and aggressive seizure management. Closely monitor vital signs, capnography, capillary refill, level of consciousness, glucose, pain, and urinary output.[4(Pa13)]

Pediatric patients with simple and complex medical needs may present to EDs with varying pediatric resources and expertise. Acknowledge the facility's capabilities and consider regional resources early to support early expert consultation and management. Well-developed processes and guidelines will ensure the best possible patient outcomes. See Chapter 2, "Preparing for Pediatric Emergencies," for more information on pediatric transfers.

Often, transfer of a pediatric patient to a higher level of care is necessary and lifesaving. However, each transfer should be reviewed to diminish the risk of preventable harm to patients and families. Consider and mitigate the following transport risks[16,29]:

- Delay in accessing pediatric expertise and services
- Extended transport time
- Helicopter, airplane, or motor vehicle crashes
- Inadequate transport team availability or expertise

- Inadvertent extubation or loss of venous access
- Physiologic deterioration
- Hemodynamic instability, hypercarbia, hypoxia, and increased intracranial pressure
- Radiation exposure from duplicate or unnecessary imaging studies
- Uncontrolled agitation or pain

Shared decision making can mitigate much preventable harm. Lack of communication or information heightens stress, increases burdens, and damages patient/family, facility, and transport team trust.[16] Identifying stopgaps with transferring EDs, transport providers, and receiving facilities is crucial to promote safe patient transport and transfer of care. Incorporating a formal handoff procedure and documentation tool may provide for a seamless transition for the critical pediatric patient, enabling all parties involved with the transfer to be on the same page, with all questions answered and with less opportunity for assumptions. Utilizing a formal written form or even incorporating telemedicine platforms for report handoff have been suggested to improve transport processes.[16]

Emerging Trends

The COVID-19 pandemic led a plethora of publications to provide healthcare workers and the public with information and guidance on care. This information was desperately sought to help healthcare workers save patients' lives while protecting themselves and their families from the virus. Public health officials were challenged to develop guidance based on this rapidly growing body of literature given its varying levels of scientific rigor. A second consensus statement with interim guidance for healthcare worker protection during resuscitation was released in January 2022. The authors acknowledged that it "is not a guidelines statement which is based on formal evidence review" and that "these revisions should always be adapted to changing public health recommendations and local protocols and resources."[5(p3)] The need to critically evaluate evolving research and use appropriate PPE has never been more vital or publicly apparent.

In the adult trauma patient with hypovolemia due to blood loss, administration of whole blood has reemerged as a viable alternative to component therapy. For pediatric trauma patients, administration of whole blood has the potential to be beneficial. However, utilization of un-crossmatched blood could cause hemolytic reactions in children due to their physiologically small blood volume. With further research, these concerns may be addressed with low-titer products and theoretically allow for greater usage of this therapy in pediatric trauma patients.[21]

Summary

The Pediatric Nursing Process provides the nurse with an excellent framework to identify children at risk of or experiencing decompensation and to prioritize life-saving interventions. Upon forming a general impression of the patient using the Pediatric Assessment Triangle, the nurse can identify hemorrhage, unresponsiveness, or apnea. If the hemorrhage is uncontrolled or further investigation of the unresponsive or apneic patient confirms that there is no pulse, reprioritize ABC to C-ABC. Priority interventions are to control hemorrhage or begin chest compressions.

Hypoxia resulting from respiratory compromise is a common cause of pediatric decompensation. Shock is defined as inadequate tissue perfusion. Every step of the primary survey is designed to identify and provide life-saving interventions for shock. See Chapter 5, "Initial Assessment: The Pediatric Nursing Process," for more information. Early identification of shock facilitates goal-directed therapy. Familiarity with the causes of shock and strategies to reverse hypovolemic, obstructive, cardiogenic, or distributive shock will help the nurse anticipate stabilizing interventions. After resuscitation, safely transport the patient to the most appropriate level of care based on the child's condition and need for specialty expertise. The clinical goals for pediatric patients in need of stabilization are immediate recognition, aggressive intervention to restore and maintain tissue perfusion, and timely transfer to definitive care.

References

1. Altman, C. A. (2021). Identifying newborns with critical congenital heart disease. *UpToDate.* Retrieved September 22, 2021, from https://www.uptodate.com/contents/identifying-newborns-with-critical-congenital-heart-disease
2. American College of Surgeons. (2018). *Advanced trauma life support student course manual* (10th ed.).
3. American Heart Association. (2020). *Advanced cardiovascular life support provider manual.*
4. American Heart Association. (2020). *Pediatric advanced life support provider manual.*
5. Atkins, D. L., Sasson, C., Hsu, A., Aziz, K., Becker, L. B., Berb, R. A., Bhanji, F., Bradley, S. M., Brooks, S. C., Chan, M., Chan, P. S., Cheng, A., Clemency, B. M., deCaen, A., Duff, J. P., Edelson, D. P., Flores, G. E., Fuchs, S., Girotra, S., … Morgan, R. W. (In press). 2022 guidance for BLS/ACLS in COVID-19 patients. *Circulation: Cardiovascular Quality and Outcomes.* https://doi.org/10.1161/CIRCOUTCOMES.122.008900
6. Balamuth, F., Fitzgerald, J., & Weiss, S. L. (2021). Shock. In K. Shaw & R. Bachur (Eds.), *Fleisher & Ludwig's textbook of pediatric emergency medicine* (7th ed., pp. 55–78). Wolters Kluwer.
7. Borlaug, B. A. (2021). Pulsus paradoxus in pericardial disease. *UpToDate.* Retrieved February 22, 2022, from https://www.uptodate.com/contents/pulsus-paradoxus-in-pericardial-disease
8. Brown, K. M., & Riley, M. S. (2021). Shock. In S. Fuchs & M. McEvoy (Eds.), *Pediatric education for prehospital providers* (4th ed., pp. 75–91). Jones & Bartlett Learning.
9. Campbell, R. L. (2021). Anaphylaxis: Emergency treatment. *UpToDate.* Retrieved February 22, 2022, from https://www.uptodate.com/contents/anaphylaxis-emergency-treatment
10. Centers for Disease Control and Prevention. (n.d.). *Congenital heart defects.* https://www.cdc.gov/ncbddd/heartdefects/facts.html
11. Christiaans, S. C., Duhachek-Stapelman, A. L., Russell, R. T., Lisco, S. J., Kerby, J. D., & Pittet, J. (2014). Coagulopathy after severe pediatric trauma: A review. *Shock, 41*(6), 476–490. https://doi.org/10.1097/SHK.0000000000000151
12. Davis, A. L., Carcillo, J. A., Aneja, R. K., Deymann, A. J., Lin, J. C., Nguyen, T. C., Okhuysen-Cawley, R. S., Relvas, M. S., Rozenfeld, R. A., Skippen, P. W., Stojadinovic, B. J., Williams, E. A., Yeh, T. S., Balamuth, F., Brierley, J., de Caen, A. R., Cheifetz, I. M., Choong, K., Conway, E., Jr., Cornell, T., . . . Zuckerberg, A. L. (2017). American College of Critical Care Medicine clinical practice parameters for hemodynamic support of pediatric and neonatal septic shock. *Critical Care Medicine, 45*(6), 1061–1093. https://doi.org/10.1097/CCM.0000000000002425
13. Ernst, G. (2020). Pediatric trauma. In J. E. Tintinalli, O. J. Ma, D. M. Yealy, G. D. Meckler, J. S. Stapczynski, D. M. Cline, & S. H. Thomas (Eds.), *Tintinalli's emergency medicine: A comprehensive study guide* (9th ed., 689–697). McGraw Hill.
14. Foster, D. (2020). Primary spontaneous pneumothorax. *Critical Decisions in Emergency Medicine, 35*(3), 10–11.
15. Geggel, R. L. (2021). Diagnosis and initial management of cyanotic heart disease in the newborn. *UpToDate.* Retrieved February 12, 2022, from https://www.uptodate.com/contents/diagnosis-and-initial-management-of-cyanotic-heart-disease-in-the-newborn
16. Hamline, M. Y., & Rosenthal, J. L. (2020). Interfacility transfers: A process ridden with improvement opportunities. *Hospital Pediatrics, 10*(2), 195–197. https//doi.org/10.1542/hpeds.2019-0305
17. Lough, M. E. (2022). Cardiovascular anatomy and physiology. In L. D. Urden, K. M. Stacy, & M. E. Lough (Eds.), *Critical care nursing: Diagnosis and management* (9th ed., pp. 167–189). Elsevier.
18. Lough, M. E. (2022). Cardiovascular clinical assessment. In L. D. Urden, K. M. Stacy, & M. E. Lough (Eds.), *Critical care nursing: Diagnosis and management* (9th ed., pp. 190–205). Elsevier.
19. Lough, M. E., Berger, S. J., Larsen, A., & Sandoval. C. P. (2022). Cardiovascular diagnostic procedures. In L. D. Urden, K. M.

Stacy, & M. E. Lough (Eds.), *Critical care nursing: Diagnosis and management* (9th ed., pp. 206–297). Elsevier.

20. Lucia, D., & Glenn, J. (2017). Pediatric emergencies. In C. K. Stone & R. L. Humphries (Eds.), *Current diagnosis and treatment: Emergency medicine* (8th ed., pp. 964–1016). McGraw Hill.

21. Mar, P., & Edwards, M. J. (2021). Whole blood resuscitation for pediatric trauma: Why we must move forward. *Current Surgery Reports, 9*(9). https://doi.org/10.1007/s40137-021-00287-5

22. Miscia, M. E., Lauriti, G., Lisi, G., Riddio, A., & Chiesa, P. L. (2020). Management of spontaneous pneumothorax in children: A systematic review and meta-analysis. *European Journal of Pediatric Surgery, 30*(1), 2–12. https://doi.org/10.1055/s-0039-3402522

23. Navandan, N., Stein, J., & Mistry, R. (2019). Pulmonary embolism in children. *Pediatric Emergency Care, 35*(2), 143–151. https://doi.org/10.1097/PEC.0000000000001730

24. Nolan, J. P., Maconochie, I., Soar, J., Olasveengen, T. M., Greif, R., Wyckoff, M. H., Singletary, E. M., Aickin, R., Berg, K. M., Mancini, M. E., Bhanji, F., Wyllie, J., Zideman, D., Neumar, R. W., Perkins, G. D., Castren, M., Morley, P. T., Montgomery, W. H., Nadkarni, V. M., … Hazinski, M. F. (2020). Executive summary: 2020 international consensus on cardiopulmonary resuscitation and emergency cardiovascular care science with treatment recommendations. *Circulation, 142.* S2–S27. https://doi.org/10.1161/CIR.0000000000000890

25. Pasman, E. A., & Watson, C. M. (2019). Shock in pediatrics: Pathophysiology. *Medscape.* Retrieved September 22, 2021, from https://emedicine.medscape.com/article/1833578-overview#a5

26. Pomerantz, W. J. (2020). Pathophysiology and classification of shock in children. *UpToDate.* Retrieved September 22, 2021, from https://www.uptodate.com/contents/pathophysiology-and-classification-of-shock-in-children

27. Rao, P. S. (2021). Principles of management of the neonate with congenital heart disease. In P. S. Rao & D. Vidyasagar (Eds.), *A multidisciplinary approach to perinatal cardiology* (Vol. 1, pp. 426–446). Cambridge Scholars Publishing.

28. Selbst, S. M., & Rogers, B. D. (2020). Septic-appearing infant. In K. N. Shaw & R. G. Bachur (Eds.), *Fleisher and Ludwig's textbook of emergency medicine* (8th ed., pp. 500–507). Wolters Kluwer.

29. Semkiw, K., Anderson, D., & Natale, J. (2020). Mitigating the risk of intrahospital transport for pediatric patients at risk of physiologic instability. *Patient Safety Network: Web M&M Case Studies.* Retrieved February 13, 2022, from https://psnet.ahrq.gov/web-mm/mitigating-risk-intrahospital-transport-pediatric-patients-risk-physiologic-instability

30. Vega, R. M., Kaur, H., & Edemekong, P. F. (2021, October 9). Cardiopulmonary arrest in children. *StatPearls.* https://www.ncbi.nlm.nih.gov/books/NBK436018/

31. Waltzman, M. (2021). Initial evaluation of shock in children. *UpToDate.* Retrieved September 22, 2021, from https://www.uptodate.com/contents/initial-evaluation-of-shock-in-children

32. Weiss, S. L., Peters, M. J., Alhazzani, W., Agus, M. S. D., Flori, H., Inwald, D. P., Nadel, S., Schlapbach, L. J., Tasker, R. C., Argent, A. C., Brierly, J., Carcillo, J., Carrol, E. D., Carroll, C. L., Cheifterz, I. M., Choong, K., Cies, J. J., Cruz, A. T., De Luca, D., … Tissieres, P. (2020). Surviving Sepsis Campaign international guidelines for the management of septic shock and sepsis-associated organ dysfunction in children. *Pediatric Critical Care Medicine, 21*(2), e52–e106. https://doi.org/10.1097/pcc.0000000000002198

33. Wieckowska, J., Assaad, U., & Aboudan, M. (2021). Pneumothorax secondary to vaping. *Respiratory Medicine Case Reports, 33,* 101421. https://doi.org/10.1016/j.rmcr.2021.101421

34. Winant, A. J., & Lee, E. Y. (2020). Pediatric pulmonary embolism. In R. Cleveland & E. Lee (Eds.), *Imaging in pediatric pulmonology* (2nd ed., pp. 325–336). Springer. https://doi.org/10.1007/978-3-030-23979-4_16

The Child with a Cough

Anne-Marie Sweeney, DNP, RN(EC), CNCC(C), CNN(C)

OBJECTIVES

Upon completion of this chapter, the learner will be able to:

1. Describe characteristics of pediatric respiratory distress and failure.
2. Identify various causes of pediatric respiratory distress and failure.
3. Apply the Pediatric Nursing Process to a child with a respiratory concern.

Introduction

Because respiratory emergencies are a leading cause of pediatric death, early identification and intervention is key to preventing decompensation of the child with such an emergency. Any condition that increases oxygen demand, impairs oxygen intake, or compromises tissue perfusion can lead to respiratory distress. While in respiratory distress, the child is able to do the work of breathing but worsening respiratory distress exhausts the patient's reserves and may rapidly turn into respiratory failure. Progression to respiratory failure indicates the child's breathing is inadequate to supply the tissues with needed oxygen. Without intervention, severe hypoxia, organ failure, and cardiac arrest are likely. Respiratory distress and respiratory failure can be the result of acute upper and lower respiratory conditions. Respiratory compromise may also result from or be exacerbated by neuromuscular disorders, skeletal abnormalities, central nervous system disorders, and congenital anomalies. The selected conditions discussed in this chapter may present with respiratory distress and deteriorate to respiratory failure without prompt recognition and intervention.

Initial Assessment

While forming a general impression of the patient using the Pediatric Assessment Triangle, it may become apparent that the child is in respiratory distress. Assess the patient for abnormal sounds (stridor, grunting), abnormal positioning (tripoding to maximize airway expansion), retractions, nasal flaring, and rapid or slow respirations. The child in respiratory distress may look anxious or focused on their respiratory effort. The child in respiratory failure will have markedly decreased alertness. Pallor, cyanosis, or mottling may be evident. **Table 8-1** identifies the primary survey assessments and interventions in airway and breathing. **Table 8-2** describes the progression from respiratory distress to respiratory failure and impending arrest.[1,16]

TABLE 8-1	Pediatric Nursing Process: Airway and Breathing	
	Assessment	**Potential Interventions***
Airway	Difficulty keeping airway open (tongue obstruction, snoring, flexed neck)	Head tilt–chin lift or jaw-thrust maneuver Oropharyngeal or nasopharyngeal airway Positioning: towel under shoulders/torso, allow position of comfort (sitting upright, tripod position)
	Secretions/foreign bodies	Nasal suctioning, oropharyngeal suctioning Manual removal of foreign bodies
	Facial/airway edema, anaphylaxis	Intramuscular epinephrine Surgical airway
Breathing	Increased respiratory rate	Administer oxygen
	Decreased respiratory rate	Assist ventilation with a bag-mask device
	Stridor, wheezing	Inhaled epinephrine, albuterol
	Unilateral absent breath sounds, unilateral hyperinflated chest, resistance felt with manual ventilation	Finger thoracostomy, needle decompression, chest tube
	Open sucking chest wound	Apply three-sided dressing, prepare for chest tube

*Not an all-inclusive list. Support inadequate breathing with bag-mask ventilation and prepare for noninvasive positive-pressure ventilation, intubation, or a rescue airway for children in significant respiratory distress or respiratory failure.

TABLE 8-2	Respiratory Distress Versus Respiratory Failure	
Respiratory Distress	**Severe Respiratory Distress**	**Respiratory Failure/Impending Arrest**
Alert, mildly anxious	Anxious, irritable, focused on breathing, not interacting normally with environment, becoming tired	Lethargic, not interacting, or unresponsive
Mild tachypnea	Marked tachypnea	Extreme tachypnea or bradypnea, apnea, gasping, agonal respirations
Mild nasal flaring, retractions	Severe nasal flaring, retractions Abdominal breathing (also called seesaw breathing)	Extremely increased work of breathing OR Minimal respiratory effort
Mild stridor, grunting (glottic stop at end of inhalation) Wheezing or other adventitious sounds with good air exchange	Pronounced stridor, grunting Wheezing or other adventitious sounds with diminished air exchange	Minimal air movement
Mild tachycardia	Marked tachycardia	Extreme tachycardia or bradycardia

Respiratory Distress	Severe Respiratory Distress	Respiratory Failure/Impending Arrest
Normal pulse oximetry level	Normal to decreased pulse oximetry level	Low oxygen saturation despite high-flow oxygen administration
Pale	Pale, cool	Cyanosis, mottling
Normal capillary refill	Capillary refill > 2 seconds	Very delayed capillary refill

Data from American Heart Association. (2020). Part 7. *Pediatric advanced life support provider manual*; and Lewis, C. A. (2022). The pediatric patient. In L. D. Urden, K. M. Stacy, & M. E. Lough (Eds.), *Critical care nursing* (9th ed., pp. 974–996). Elsevier.

RED FLAGS

Signs of increased work of breathing include the following:

· Abnormal positioning
· Grunting
· Head bobbing
· Nasal flaring
· Retractions
· Accessory muscle use
· Tachypnea

Red flags include the following:

· Altered mental status
· Anxiety
· Central cyanosis
· Decreased and/or absent air entry on auscultation
· Oxygen saturation less than 92%
· Prolonged capillary refill
· Respiratory rate greater than 60 breaths/min
· Suprasternal retractions (sometimes called tracheal tug)

Selected Conditions

The conditions discussed in this section include bronchiolitis, pneumonia, foreign body aspiration, asthma, epiglottitis, croup, and pertussis.

Bronchiolitis

Bronchiolitis is a lower respiratory tract infection resulting in increased mucus production and inflammation of the bronchioles, causing small airway obstruction, air trapping, and atelectasis.[8,14,18,22,23] Bronchiolitis is most often caused by respiratory syncytial virus (RSV).

Assessment Findings

Assessment findings associated with bronchiolitis include the following[8,14,18,23]:

· Child younger than 2 years of age
· One- to 3-day history of fever and runny nose
· Respiratory distress and cough that worsens with crying
· Tachypnea and retractions
· Wheezing, crackles
· Skin color change/pallor
· Low pulse oximetry reading

Children at risk of severe illness or succumbing to bronchiolitis include those who were born at less than 36 weeks' gestation, had a low birth weight, are younger than 12 weeks of age, or have comorbidities such as lung, heart, immunodeficiency, or neurologic conditions. Environmental factors that increase the risk of bronchiolitis include exposure to smoke, crowded households, older/other siblings in the home, and daycare attendance.[8,14,18,23]

Interventions

Interventions for bronchiolitis are mainly supportive. Nasal suctioning helps to keep the nasal passages free of obstruction. Ensuring the nasal passages are clear is important, especially in younger children who are obligate nose breathers. Oxygen saturation should be at least 92%. Oxygen therapy with a heated, humidified, high-flow nasal cannula (HFNC) or non-invasive positive-pressure ventilation may prevent progression to respiratory failure and the need for endotracheal intubation in high-risk patients. Hydration is maintained with oral or intravenous fluids.[8,14,18,22]

The severity of bronchiolitis is determined by assessing and monitoring respiratory distress. Over-the-counter medications are to be avoided with the exception of an antipyretic medication, if needed for comfort. No known treatment has been shown to shorten illness or hospital stay. Treatments such as bronchodilators, epinephrine, corticosteroids, and nebulized hypertonic saline are not routinely recommended but may be considered for patients with severe bronchiolitis.[8,14,18,22]

Pneumonia

Pneumonia—an acute infection of the pulmonary parenchyma[2,8,14,18]—remains a leading cause of pediatric death worldwide.[4] This infection may be caused by bacteria, viruses, or fungi (**Table 8-3**).[4,29] Pneumonia can occur throughout the year. Risk factors for pneumonia include being from lower socioeconomic groups, environmental crowding, contact with school-age children, and exposure to cigarette smoke. Children with comorbidities may be more susceptible to both pneumonia and the development of serious sequelae. Vaccinations for influenza and pneumonia have been shown to protect children from disease.[4,8,14,18]

Assessment Findings

Pediatric pneumonia presentations vary and are often nonspecific; suspect pneumonia in an ill child even without respiratory symptoms. Assessment findings may include fever, cough, tachypnea, hypoxemia, and increased work of breathing. During the lung exam, auscultation may reveal wheezes; crackles; and decreased, abnormal, or absent breath sounds. Infants might not have abnormal breath sounds or a cough, but instead present with fussiness or difficulty feeding. Children old enough to speak or indicate may complain of chest and/or abdominal pain.[2,8,14,18]

Interventions

Monitor the patient's respiratory effort closely; prepare for advanced airway management if deterioration is noted. Interventions for pneumonia include supportive care and early antibiotic treatment. Fever and pain can be managed with acetaminophen or ibuprofen. Assess for dehydration and manage this condition with oral or intravenous rehydration as required and tolerated. Suctioning may be required to ensure nasal passages and airways are kept clear. A child with an oxygen saturation of less than 92% is treated with oxygen therapy titrated to a target saturation of 92–98%.[3,8,14,18]

Diagnostic tests for pneumonia may not be necessary if assessment supports the proposed diagnosis and treatment. Radiography of the chest can be considered if assessment findings are inconclusive or the child does not respond to treatment for the respiratory illness.[2,8,14,18] Computed tomography or lung ultrasound may be considered if more extensive imaging is required or clarification of radiography is needed. Lung ultrasound has been shown to be a safe and reliable diagnostic alternative to chest radiography.[15,21,35]

Laboratory investigations depend on the severity of illness and whether the child is to be hospitalized. Laboratory tests could include a complete blood count, C-reactive protein, and electrolytes to assess for the degree of dehydration. Microbiologic testing (cultures) of blood, sputum, or pleural fluid may be required if the patient develops complications of pneumonia or with pneumonia treatment. Assessment of oxygenation with blood gases is considered on an individual basis but is likely to be needed if signs of respiratory failure are noted or advanced airway interventions are required.[3,8,14,18]

Treatment for pneumonia includes early antibiotic therapy. Hospitalization is considered for children presenting with more severe symptoms, not responding to initial treatment, or with other significant comorbidities. Additional medications such as bronchodilators and corticosteroid therapy are considered based on the child's individual assessment and needs.[3,8,14,18] Pneumonia, like any other infection, can lead to sepsis and distributive shock. See Chapter 7, "The Child in Need of Stabilization," and Chapter 10, "The Child with a Fever," for more information.

Foreign Body Aspiration

Foreign body aspiration (FBA) into the respiratory system is potentially life threatening, as obstruction of the

TABLE 8-3	Predominant Causes of Pneumonia by Age
Age	**Cause**
Neonate: early (< 7 days old)	› Aspiration of infected amniotic fluid › Transplacental transmission
Neonate: late (> 7 days old)	› Parental transmission › Anomaly of the airway › Prolonged hospital stay
Infant/child < 5 years of age	› Viral
Child > 5 years of age	› Bacterial

Data from Barson, W. J. (2022). Pneumonia in children: Epidemiology, pathogenesis, and etiology. *UpToDate*. Retrieved March 31, 2022, from https://www.uptodate.com/contents /pneumonia-in-children-epidemiology-pathogenesis-and -etiology; and Speer, M. E. (2021). Neonatal pneumonia. *UpToDate*. Retrieved March 31, 2022, from https://www .uptodate.com/contents/neonatal-pneumonia

airway impairs oxygenation and ventilation, leading to hypoxia and potentially cardiac arrest.[10,14,24] FBA is suspected with any reports of choking. FBA is also suspected with a clinical presentation of impaired oxygenation and ventilation with no obvious cause, especially in children younger than 2 years of age.[10,14,24]

Assessment Findings

Assessment findings with FBA depend on the degree of blockage, the location of the object, and the amount of time elapsed since aspiration. The most commonly noted symptom is cough, followed by tachypnea and stridor. On inspection, the child may appear to be in respiratory distress, have cyanosis, and/or have an altered mental status. Auscultation may reveal wheezing or absent air entry in a specific region of lung field. Because the patient presentation may be delayed, FBA needs to be considered for respiratory issues that are not improved with expected treatment—for example, abnormal chest radiography and lack of improvement after antibiotic treatment.[10,14,24]

Interventions

Interventions and treatment for FBA include supportive care and identification of the foreign body. Supportive care includes keeping the child calm and ensuring the pharynx and mouth are kept clear. Oxygen therapy is provided to maintain an oxygen saturation greater than 92%. A chest radiograph may identify radiopaque foreign bodies; areas of hyperinflation, atelectasis, or pneumonia distal to the object; or a mediastinal shift away from the foreign body. Abscesses or bronchiectasis may appear if the foreign body has been trapped in the airway for some time. A neck radiograph is indicated for children with stridor, hoarseness, or other findings suspicious for a laryngotracheal foreign body. Low-dose computed tomography (CT) may be warranted to identify FBA and may prevent bronchoscopy, as CT can detect radiolucent foreign bodies.[12] Bronchoscopy is considered when there is a high likelihood or strong suspicion of FBA to facilitate removal of the foreign body.[10,14,24]

Asthma

Asthma is a significant problem worldwide and one of the most common chronic childhood illnesses.[6,7,10,11,14,18,25] A reactive disease of the lungs, asthma is characterized by airway inflammation, bronchial smooth-muscle constriction, mucus plugging, and airway remodeling in some patients.[17] Symptoms can range from mild to severe. Asthma can be controlled, though not cured, and can have an unpredictable course with increasing exacerbations and hospitalizations.

The most commonly noted symptoms of asthma are cough and wheezing. Airway inflammation and hyper-responsiveness occur in response to certain triggers, such as respiratory tract infection (viral or bacterial), exercise, weather, tobacco smoke, allergens, irritant exposure (aerosolizing products), and stress. A comprehensive assessment includes allergies, asthma triggers, family history, environment, past medical history, medications, healthcare utilization, school attendance, physical activity, and psychosocial profile.[6,7,10,11,14,18,25]

Assessment Findings

The child may present to the hospital only during asthma exacerbations. Assessment findings for the child with an exacerbation of asthma include tachypnea, hypoxia, wheezing, accessory muscle use, retractions, and a prolonged expiratory phase.[28] While initiating immediate interventions for respiratory distress, obtain a history to determine the level of asthma symptom control and asthma severity to help determine the patient's risk of deterioration. A variety of measures—including clinical findings, symptom frequency, response to rescue medications, and numeric tools—are used to evaluate asthma control and exacerbation severity. When emergent intervention is not required, measure the patient's peak expiratory flow rate before and after medical management to gauge improvement and for comparison with the patient's baseline.[13] **Table 8-4** correlates signs and symptoms of mild, moderate, and severe asthma exacerbations with score ranges for two numeric assessment tools.[13,28] Be familiar with facility-specific clinical assessment tools.

> **RED FLAG**
>
> A silent chest implies that the child's air flow is so poor that wheezes cannot be produced and immediate medical treatment is required.[6,7,10,11,14,18,25]

A child also may present to the hospital for other reason(s) and have asthma, suboptimal asthma control, or associated atopic conditions. The child in this case may present with decreased air entry, wheezes, prolonged expiratory phase, dry cough, rhinitis, signs of sinusitis, conjunctivitis, signs of acute respiratory illness, transverse nasal crease (due to repeated upward rubbing of the nose), halitosis from rhinitis, nasal polyps, and eczema or atopic dermatitis. Such a patient may require treatment for asthma or asthma-related findings in addition to the reason for presentation to the emergency department.[6,7,10,11,14,18,25]

TABLE 8-4   Asthma Exacerbation Severity

	Mild	Moderate	Severe
Assessment			
Respirations	Slight tachypnea	Tachypnea	Extreme tachypnea
Lung sounds	Good air exchange Expiratory wheezing	Wheezing throughout expiration Possible inspiratory wheezing	Inspiratory and expiratory wheezing Minimal air exchange (silent chest)
Inspiratory to expiratory ratio	1:1	1:2	> 1:2
Accessory muscle use	None to minimal	Common	Significant
Oxygen saturation	> 95%	90–95%	< 90%
Peak expiratory flow	≥ 70%	51–69%	≤ 50 %
Speech	Sentences	Phrases	Words
Position	Comfortable lying flat	Prefers sitting upright	Tripoding, cannot recline
Pulmonary Index Score	1–6	7–11	≥ 12
Pediatric Respiratory Assessment Measure	0–4	5–8	9–12

Data from Global Initiative for Asthma. (2021). *Global strategy for asthma management and prevention, 2021 update.* https://ginasthma.org/wp-content/uploads/2021/05/GINA-Main-Report-2021-V2-WMS.pdf; and Scarfone, R. J. (2020). Acute asthma exacerbations in children younger than 12 years: Emergency department management. *UpToDate.* Retrieved April 6, 2022, from https://www.uptodate.com/contents/acute-asthma-exacerbations-in-children-younger-than-12-years-emergency-department-management

Interventions

Emergency department management may be guided by numeric assessment tools or regional protocols according to the child's age and clinical condition. A child who has taken multiple recent doses of a short-acting beta agonist is less likely to improve quickly. Treatment options are added as warranted based on the child's response to treatment and include the following[13,14,28]:

- Oxygen
- Inhaled short-acting beta agonists to dilate the bronchioles
  - Includes albuterol (also known as salbutamol) and levalbuterol.
  - Via metered-dose inhaler with a spacer (**Figure 8-1**), air-driven nebulizer, or oxygen-driven nebulizer; also can be delivered with a mask (**Figure 8-2**).
  - Nebulizers may be administered continuously.
  - All administration options may be repeated.
  - If possible, measure the patient's peak expiratory flow rate before and after administration.
- Oral or intravenous corticosteroids

- Nebulized ipratropium (anticholinergic)
- Nebulized or intravenous magnesium sulfate (relaxes smooth muscles in the airway)
- Intravenous terbutaline (short-acting beta agonist)
- Heliox—may decrease air flow resistance but its administration should not delay intubation
- Trial of noninvasive positive-pressure ventilation if tolerated
  - Sedation is not recommended to facilitate noninvasive positive-pressure ventilation.
- Endotracheal intubation
  - Ketamine is also a bronchodilator and is therefore recommended for sedation prior to intubation.

Diagnostic tests for asthma presentations in the emergency department may not be required, as assessment findings may indicate the need for treatment. Chest radiography is not routinely recommended but may be used to identify underlying conditions such as a pneumothorax, FBA, or pneumonia in patients with atypical presentations, localized lung sound abnormalities, or failure to improve.[6,7,10,11,14,18,25]

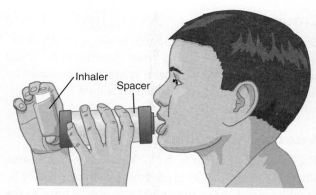

Figure 8-1 *Spacer with mouthpiece for metered-dose inhaler.*

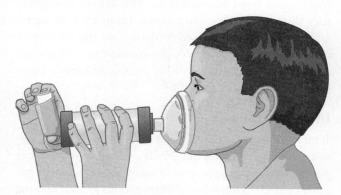

Figure 8-2 *Spacer with mask for metered-dose inhaler.*

The goals of outpatient asthma management are to maintain normal activity levels with good control of symptoms while minimizing lung remodeling and medication side effects. Management requires close follow-up with an action plan based on symptoms and peak expiratory flow monitoring. Medications are prescribed in a stepwise approach based on symptom control, patient/parental preference and adherence, and practical considerations such as cost and inhaler technique.

Pharmacologic therapies for asthma include short-acting beta agonists for immediate symptom relief, with long-acting beta agonists and corticosteroids being used for symptom control. These medications are usually inhaled and given via metered-dose inhalers using a spacer device with a mouthpiece or appropriately sized face mask, via breath-activated inhaler for older children who can sustain an inhalation with sufficient force, or via nebulizer for those patients who cannot manage the inhaler and/or require oxygen therapy. Inhaler technique and medication adherence are evaluated before moving to the next steps, which may include leukotriene receptor antagonists, increased doses of inhaled controller medications, referral to a specialist, and oral corticosteroids.[6,7,9–12,14,18,26]

For children with allergy-triggered asthma, immunotherapy is considered.[6,7,9–11,14,18,26,28]

In addition to pharmacologic management, provision of appropriate education to the child and the family is crucial.[19] Such education not only includes medication administration, but also emphasizes prevention of exacerbations by avoiding irritants or allergens. Children who have exacerbations with activity or exercise are instructed to use medications prior to engaging in such activity.

The monitoring of pulmonary function is an important component of asthma education and management for children with persistent disease. Children older than 6 years of age are provided with a peak flow meter and instructed in how to use the device correctly. Peak flow measurements can reveal subtle changes in respiratory function that may not cause symptoms for several days. To use a peak flow meter, patients must establish a "personal best," which represents the best reading they can obtain when they are as asymptomatic as possible. Peak flows between 50% and 80% of an individual's personal best are cause for concern. Even if symptoms are mild, treatment should be provided as agreed upon with the child's primary care provider. If peak flows do not improve or there is a severe decrease in peak flow to less than 50% of the patient's personal best, immediate medical attention is required.[6,7,10,11,14,18,27]

Epiglottitis

Epiglottitis is an inflammation of the epiglottis and adjacent supraglottic structures. Without interventions, it may progress to a life-threatening airway obstruction. Epiglottitis in children is most often caused by *Hemophilus influenzae* type b. With routine immunization for this infection, the incidence of epiglottitis has decreased.[18,32]

Assessment Findings

Assessment findings for epiglottitis include the three Ds—dysphagia, drooling, and distress—along with a high fever that begins abruptly and progresses rapidly, usually over a course of hours (frequently less than 12 hours). The child may experience respiratory distress or stridor; have a choking sensation during inspiration; or be anxious, restless, and irritable. Speech will be muffled and is often described as "hot potato voice." The child may assume a tripod position to maximize chest wall expansion (**Figure 8-3**).[18,32]

Interventions

Interventions for epiglottitis include airway management, supplemental oxygen, and early antibiotic treatment. Immediate management of the child's airway and oxygenation is a priority. Consulting an airway specialist and/or otolaryngologist early is ideal to ensure

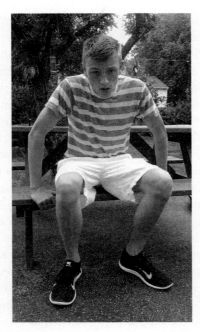

Figure 8-3 *Tripod position.*

provision of appropriate care. Humidified oxygen therapy is indicated for patients with oxygen saturations less than 92%.[18,33] Assisted ventilation with a bag-mask device may be necessary for patients with inadequate respirations.

If assisted ventilation is required for a prolonged period or is not helping, endotracheal intubation becomes the priority. Endotracheal intubation ideally takes place using laryngoscopy in the operating room, with the equipment available for performing an emergent surgical airway procedure. Supraglottic airway devices such as a laryngeal mask airway are not recommended or effective for epiglottitis. Diagnostic tests (blood and epiglottic cultures) and antimicrobial therapy are initiated once the child's airway has been secured. The administration of glucocorticoids is not routinely recommended, as evidence of its benefits is lacking. Fever and pain are managed with appropriate medications.[18,33]

NOTE

Avoid Agitation, Manage the Airway

Children presenting with concerning signs and symptoms of epiglottitis should not have diagnostics completed that interfere with or delay treatment. Crying may lead to abrupt airway obstruction. Every effort should be made to avoid unnecessary stress and agitation until after the airway is secured.[18,33]

Croup

Croup, also known as laryngotracheitis, is an upper respiratory disorder resulting from inflammation of the larynx and subglottic airway. It is most often caused by respiratory viruses. Croup is usually a mild illness, typically resolving in 3 days.[8,14,18,31]

Assessment Findings

The hallmark of croup is the barking cough that is usually worse at night. A viral prodrome characterized by irritability, nasal congestion, and fever occurs prior to the onset of the cough. Symptoms such as hoarseness and stridor are dependent on the amount of upper airway obstruction from inflammation. The degree of respiratory distress—stridor, retractions, diminished air entry, and cyanosis—are assessed to determine the severity of croup. Signs of lower airway involvement such as wheezing or other alterations in lung sounds indicate a more serious underlying condition.[8,14,18,31,34,37]

Interventions

Interventions for croup depend on the severity of symptoms. **Table 8-5** shows the Westley Croup Severity Score parameters and recommended medical management per severity level.[34] Home-based interventions include altering the air environment (night air, cool mist humidifiers, or sitting in a steamy bathroom), administering antipyretics for fever and discomfort, keeping the nasal passages clear, and encouraging intake of fluids. For more severe symptoms, place the child in a position of comfort, decrease agitation, and consider oxygen therapy and medications.[8,14,18,31,32]

Corticosteroids and nebulized epinephrine are administered for moderate to severe croup. Oxygen therapy is initiated for patients with oxygen saturations less than 92% or those who are experiencing respiratory distress. Administration of heliox to improve airflow may be considered for patients with severe respiratory distress. If the croup severity progresses or presents as respiratory failure, intubation is considered.[8,14,18,31,34]

Diagnostic tests are not usually required for croup. However, if assessment findings are atypical of croup, a chest or soft-tissue radiograph of the neck may be ordered. The steeple sign (**Figure 8-4**) indicates upper airway narrowing and supports the diagnosis of croup.[8,14,18,31,32]

Pertussis

Pertussis, also known as whooping cough, is a contagious acute respiratory infection caused by *Bordetella pertussis*, a bacterium that is spread by airborne droplets.[5,8,14,18,30,36,37] Whooping cough usually occurs in children younger than the age of 4 years who are not

TABLE 8-5   Westley Croup Severity Score

Clinical Features	Assigned Score		
Level of consciousness	Normal, including sleep = 0 Disoriented = 5		
Cyanosis	None = 0 With agitation = 4 At rest = 5		
Stridor	None = 0 With agitation = 1 At rest = 2		
Air entry	Normal = 0 Decreased = 1 Markedly decreased = 2		
Retractions	None = 0 Mild = 1 Moderate = 2 Severe = 3		
Score	**Severity**	**Description**	**Management**
≤ 2	Mild	Occasional barky cough, no stridor at rest, mild or no retractions	Symptomatic care, antipyretics, mist, oral fluids Single dose of oral corticosteroid
3–7	Moderate	Frequent barky cough, stridor at rest, mild to moderate retractions but minimal distress or agitation	Single dose of oral corticosteroid Consider nebulized epinephrine Consider hospitalization if patient's condition does not improve with treatment
8–11	Severe	Frequent barky cough, stridor at rest, marked retractions/distress/agitation	Single dose of oral, intramuscular, or intravenous corticosteroid Consider repeat doses of nebulized epinephrine Probable hospitalization unless patient's condition is much improved with treatment
≥ 12	Impending respiratory failure	Decreased level of consciousness, stridor at rest, severe retractions, poor air entry, cyanosis/pallor	Single dose of intramuscular or intravenous corticosteroid Repeated doses of nebulized epinephrine as indicated Consider intensive care unit admission Consult otolaryngology or anesthesia for intubation in a controlled environment

Data from Woods, C. R. (2021). Epiglottitis (supraglottitis): Management. *UpToDate*. Retrieved April 8, 2022, from https://www.uptodate.com/contents/epiglottitis-supraglottitis-management

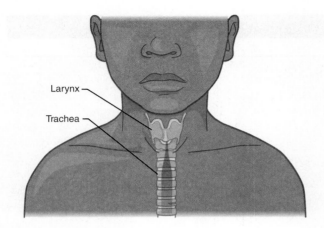

Figure 8-4 *Steeple sign.*

immunized. Immunizations have decreased the number of cases, but the disease can occur in people of all ages if they are not immunized.

Assessment Findings

Pertussis is a clinical diagnosis of paroxysms of coughing, with an inspiratory whoop and possible post-tussive vomiting. Classic pertussis is divided into three stages: catarrhal, paroxysmal, and convalescent[5,8,14,18,20,30,37]:

- **Catarrhal stage:** One to 2 weeks of a mild cold.
- **Paroxysmal stage:** Coughing spells increase and whooping becomes more distinct. The child may gag, develop cyanosis, and appear to struggle to breathe. Paroxysms of cough may occur spontaneously or may be the result of external stimuli. Post-tussive vomiting may also occur and is more common in infants. This stage may last for up to 8 weeks.
- **Convalescent stage:** The cough subsides over several weeks to months, but may worsen with recurrence of respiratory infection.

Interventions

Interventions for pertussis include supportive care, isolation, and early antibiotic treatment. They include having the child remain calm (excitement and crying may worsen the cough) and allowing the child to assume a position of comfort. The child and caregivers should be placed in isolation with droplet precautions. Other interventions include antipyretics for fever and discomfort, keeping the nasal passages clear with gentle suctioning, and encouraging intake of fluids.[5,8,14,18,30]

Diagnostic tests may be done but should not delay the early administration of antibiotics. Such tests may include cultures from the patient's nasal passages or serology to detect antibodies. A chest radiograph is unlikely to be of benefit.[5,8,14,18,30,37]

Treatments for pertussis include humidified oxygen therapy for patients with oxygen saturations less than 92% and early administration of antibiotics. The patient should avoid known triggers such as exercise or cold temperatures. Administration of antitussives, corticosteroids, and aerosolized bronchodilators has not shown benefit in the treatment of pertussis.[5,8,14,18,30,36]

Summary

The child presenting to the hospital with a cough or other respiratory symptoms requires assessment to evaluate the degree of respiratory distress or identify respiratory failure. Assessment findings can often aid the provider in identifying the specific etiology. The early identification of worsening respiratory distress or of respiratory failure with initiation of treatments and therapies can prevent more serious hypoxia and cardiac arrest from occurring. Every respiratory concern requires individual assessment and tailored interventions. Hospital admission or referral to a specialist is based on the severity of respiratory illness on presentation and response to treatment.

References

1. American Heart Association. (2020). Part 7. In *Pediatric advanced life support provider manual*. First American Heart Association Printing.

2. Barson, W. J. (2021). Community-acquired pneumonia in children: Clinical features and diagnosis. Retrieved March 31, 2022, from https://www.uptodate.com/contents/community-acquired-pneumonia-in-children-clinical-features-and-diagnosis

3. Barson, W. J. (2021). Pneumonia in children: Inpatient treatment. *UpToDate*. Retrieved March 31, 2022, from https://www.uptodate.com/contents/pneumonia-in-children-inpatient-treatment

4. Barson, W. J. (2022). Pneumonia in children: Epidemiology, pathogenesis, and etiology. *UpToDate*. Retrieved March 31, 2022, from https://www.uptodate.com/contents/pneumonia-in-children-epidemiology-pathogenesis-and-etiology

5. Boslett, B. A., & Schwartz, B. S. (2021). *Bordetella pertussis* infection (whooping cough). In M. A. Papadakis, S. J. McPhee, & M. W. Rabow (Eds.), *Current medical diagnosis & treatment 2021* (60th ed., Part 33-10). McGraw-Hill.

6. Chesnutt, A. N., Chesnutt, M. S., Prendergast, N. T., & Prendergast, T. J. (2021). Approach to management asthma. In M. A. Papadakis, S. J. McPhee, & M. W. Rabow (Eds.), *Current medical diagnosis & treatment 2021* (60th ed., Part 9-05). McGraw-Hill.

7. Dabelić, A. (2020). Respiratory problems. In J. E. South-Paul, S. C. Matheny, & E. L. Lewis (Eds.), *Current diagnosis & treatment: Family medicine* (5th ed., pp. 285–299). McGraw-Hill Lange.

8. Dewar, S. B., & Bernard H. M. (2020). Common acute infections in children. In J. E. South-Paul, S. C. Matheny, & E. L. Lewis (Eds.), *Current diagnosis & treatment: Family medicine* (5th ed., pp. 36–55). McGraw-Hill Lange.

9. El Hussein, M. T., & Pitts, M. (2021). Asthma management: An update. *NP Current, 7,* 14–19. https://npcurrent.ca/pdfs/NPCurrent_Issue7-2021_Hussein_WEB.pdf

10. Foley, A., & Sweet, V. (2020). Respiratory emergencies. In V. Sweet & A. Foley (Eds.), *Sheehy's emergency nursing; Principles and practice* (7th ed., pp. 216–226). Elsevier.

11. Freire, G., Shefrin, A., & Zemek, R. (2020). Wheezing in infants and children. In J. E. Tintinalli, O. Ma, D. M. Yealy, G. D. Meckler, J. Stapczynski, D. M. Cline, & S. H. Thomas (Eds.), *Tintinalli's emergency medicine: A comprehensive study guide* (9th ed., pp. 798–810). McGraw-Hill.

12. Gibbons, A. T., Casar Berazaluce, A. M., Hanke, R. E., McNich, N. L., Person, A., Mehlam, T., Ribin, M., & Ponsky, T. A. (2020). Avoiding unnecessary bronchoscopy in children with suspected foreign body aspiration using computed tomography. *Journal of Pediatric Surgery, 55,* 176–181. https://doi.org/10.1016/j.jpedsurg.2019.09.045

13. Global Initiative for Asthma. (2021). Global strategy for asthma management and prevention, 2021 update. https://ginasthma.org/wp-content/uploads/2021/05/GINA-Main-Report-2021-V2-WMS.pdf

14. Health Canada, First Nations and Inuit Health Branch. (2020). Respiratory system. *Clinical practice guidelines for nurses in primary care: Pediatric and adolescent care (Chapter 10).* Government of Canada. https://www.canada.ca/en/indigenous-services-canada/services/first-nations-inuit-health/health-care-services/nursing/clinical-practice-guidelines-nurses-primary-care/pediatric-adolescent-care/chapter-10-respiratory-system.html

15. Heuvelings, C. C., Belard, S., Familusi, M. A., Spijker, R., Grobusch, M. P., & Zar, H. J. (2019). Chest ultrasound for the diagnosis of pediatric pulmonary disease: A systematic review and meta-analysis of diagnostic test accuracy. *British Medical Bulletin, 129,* 35–51. https://doi.org/10.1093/bmb/ldy041

16. Lewis, C. A. (2022). The pediatric patient. In L. D. Urden, K. M. Stacy, & M. E. Lough (Eds.), *Critical care nursing* (9th ed., pp. 974–996). Elsevier.

17. Liu, M. (2022). Pathogenesis of asthma. *UpToDate.* Retrieved April 4, 2022, from https://www.uptodate.com/contents/pathogenesis-of-asthma

18. Logee, K. (2020). Pediatric emergencies. In V. Sweet & A. Foley (Eds.), *Sheehy's emergency nursing: Principles and practice* (7th ed, pp. 556–575). Elsevier.

19. Martinez-Gonzalez, C. L., Camargo-Fajardo, M. C. C., Segura-Medina, P., & Quezada-Bolarios, P. (2019). Therapeutic patient education in learning objectives improves asthma control in Mexican children. *Journal of Medical Systems, 44*(4), Article 79. https://doi.org/10.1007/s10916-020-1539-3

20. Moore, A., Harnden, A., Grant, C. C., Patel, S., & Irwin, R. S. (2019). Clinically diagnosing pertussis-associated cough in adults and children: CHEST Guideline and Expert Panel Report. *Chest, 155*(1), 147–154. https://doi.org/10.1016/j.chest.2018.09.027

21. Orso, D., Ban, A., & Guglielmo, N. (2018). Lung ultrasound in diagnosing pneumonia in childhood: A systematic review and meta-analysis. *Journal of Ultrasound, 21*(3), 183–195. https://doi.org/10.1007/s40477-018-0306-5

22. Piedra, P. A., & Stark, A. R. (2020). Bronchiolitis in infant and children: Treatment, outcome, and prevention. *UpToDate.* Retrieved September 3, 2021, from https://www.uptodate.com/contents/bronchiolitis-in-infants-and-children-treatment-outcome-and-prevention?topicRef=6018&source=see_link

23. Piedra, P. A., & Stark, A. R. (2022). Bronchiolitis in infant and children: Clinical features and diagnosis. *UpToDate.* Retrieved September 3, 2021, from https://www.uptodate.com/contents/bronchiolitis-in-infants-and-children-clinical-features-and-diagnosis?topicRef=6020&source=see_link

24. Ruiz, F. E. (2021). Airway foreign bodies in children. *UpToDate.* Retrieved June 7, 2021, from https://www.uptodate.com/contents/airway-foreign-bodies-in-children

25. Sawicki, G., & Haver, K. (2021a). Asthma in children younger than 12 years: Initial evaluation and diagnosis. *UpToDate.* Retrieved June 9, 2021, from https://www.uptodate.com/contents/asthma-in-children-younger-than-12-years-initial-evaluation-and-diagnosis

26. Sawicki, G., & Haver, K. (2021b). Asthma in children younger than 12 years: Overview of initiating therapy and monitoring control. *UpToDate.* Retrieved June 9, 2021, from https://www.uptodate.com/contents/asthma-in-children-younger-than-12-years-overview-of-initiating-therapy-and-monitoring-control

27. Sawicki, G., & Haver, K. (2021c). Asthma in children younger than 12 years: Quick relief (rescue) treatment for acute symptoms. *UpToDate.* Retrieved June 9, 2021, from https://www.uptodate.com/contents/asthma-in-children-younger-than-12-years-quick-relief-rescue-treatment-for-acute-symptoms

28. Scarfone, R. J. (2020). Acute asthma exacerbation in children younger than 12 years: Emergency department management. *UpToDate.* Retrieved April 6, 2022, from https://www.uptodate.com/contents/acute-asthma-exacerbations-in-children-younger-than-12-years-emergency-department-management

29. Speer, M. E. (2021). Neonatal pneumonia. *UpToDate.* Retrieved March 31, 2022, from https://www.uptodate.com/contents/neonatal-pneumonia

30. Top, K. A., & Halperin, S. A. (2018). Pertussis and other *Bordetella* infections. J. L. Jameson, A. S. Fauci., D. L. Kasper, S. L. Hauser, D. L. Longo, & J. Loscalzo (Eds.), *Harrison's principles of internal medicine* (20th ed., Chapter 155). McGraw-Hill.

31. Woods, C. R. (2021). Croup: Clinical features, evaluation and diagnosis. *UpToDate.* Retrieved September 5, 2021, from https://www.uptodate.com/contents/croup-clinical-features-evaluation-and-diagnosis

32. Woods, C. R. (2021). Epiglottitis (supraglottitis): Clinical features and diagnosis. *UpToDate.* Retrieved April 8, 2022, from https://www.uptodate.com/contents/epiglottitis-supraglottitis-clinical-features-and-diagnosis

33. Woods, C. R. (2021). Epiglottitis (supraglottitis): Management. *UpToDate.* Retrieved September 5, 2021, from https://www.uptodate.com/contents/epiglottitis-supraglottitis-management

34. Woods, C. R. (2021). Management of croup. *UpToDate*. Retrieved April 8, 2022, from https://www.uptodate.com /contents/management-of-croup

35. Yan, J., Yu, N., Wang, Y., Gao, Y., & Pan, L. (2020). Lung ultrasound vs chest radiography in the diagnosis of children pneumonia: Systematic evidence. *Journal of Ultrasound, 21*(3), 183–195. https://doi.org/10.1097/md.0000000000023671

36. Yeh, S. (2021). Pertussis infection in infants and children: Treatment and prevention. *UpToDate*. Retrieved April 8, 2022, from https://www.uptodate.com/contents/pertussis-infection-in -infants-and-children-treatment-and-prevention

37. Yeh, S., & Mink, C. M. (2020). Pertussis infection in infants and children: Clinical features and diagnosis. *UpToDate*. Retrieved June 6, 2021, from https://www.uptodate.com /contents/pertussis-infection-in-infants-and-children-clinical -features-and-diagnosis

The Child with an Injury

Shannon Miller, SANE-P, TNS, CPNP-PC, DNP

OBJECTIVES

Upon completion of this chapter, the learner will be able to:

1. Recognize the anatomic, physiologic, and developmental characteristics of the pediatric patient with trauma that contribute to the signs and symptoms associated with injury.
2. Identify mechanisms of injury seen in the pediatric patient with trauma.
3. Discuss interventions for the effective management of the pediatric patient with trauma.

Introduction and Epidemiology

Traumatic injury remains the number one cause of mortality in children between 1 and 18 years of age, with unintentional injuries resulting in more than 10,000 deaths annually in the United States.[9] Unintentional trauma has a greater impact on morbidity and mortality than any other disease in the pediatric population. In 2020, motor vehicle crashes accounted for 40% of traumatic deaths, while falls accounted for 30.5% of nonfatal injuries.[9] From an international perspective, injury in childhood remains one of the most immediate health threats, resulting in the death of 869,000 children ages 5 to 14 in 2020.[39] Sub-Saharan Africa and Southeast Asia have the highest regional mortality rates for children in this age group.[39]

Despite significant advances in prevention and clinical management, there continues to be an unequal distribution of resources with competency in caring for seriously injured children. Urban centers often have adequate pediatric injury resources, but the ability to provide timely trauma care in rural areas is strained. The American College of Surgeons (ACS) has established trauma quality programs and develops standards to verify trauma centers, but has also clearly stated that "The designation of trauma centers is a regulatory process performed by authorized regional governmental or other agencies."[3(p.3)] Regional authorities and healthcare facilities are tasked with assessing the geographic need to help establish trauma care systems that make the best use of available resources. See Chapter 2, "Preparing for Pediatric Emergencies," for more information on pediatric preparedness and transferring pediatric patients to definitive care.

Anatomic, Physiologic, and Developmental Characteristics

Chapter 7, "The Child in Need of Stabilization," describes pediatric differences relevant to resuscitation. Other trauma-relevant anatomic and physiologic characteristics of children include the following[2(Ch10),14]:

- Hypotension with hemorrhagic shock indicates the child has lost more than 45% of their circulating blood volume.[2(Ch10)]
- Compared to adults, children's bones are thinner and pliable, offering less protection to underlying organs. Significant underlying organ injury can be present without any bony disruption.
- A child's head is disproportionately large and heavy, and the neck muscles are weak, predisposing the child to head and neck trauma.
- A large occiput will flex the supine neck in children younger than 8 years.
- The tongue is larger in proportion to the mouth, while the trachea is smaller in diameter and shorter; inhalation injuries or other trauma that leads to oropharyngeal edema poses a greater risk to the airway.
- The cranium is thinner and more pliable in young children. While skull fractures are unusual, intracranial tissue is more susceptible to injury since the skull does not effectively dissipate energy.
- Cranial sutures are not fused until after infancy; increased intracranial pressure may present with a bulging fontanelle.
- A flexible rib cage and a soft, thin chest wall are more compliant and offer less effective protection for the lungs and upper abdomen.
- The protuberant abdomen, immature abdominal muscles, rib cage sitting higher in the abdominal cavity, and small pelvis offer little protection to the underlying solid and hollow abdominal organs.
- The solid organs and kidneys are relatively larger and more prone to injury.
- The sigmoid and ascending colon are not fully attached in the peritoneal cavity and, therefore, are more prone to injury from acceleration and deceleration forces.
- Bones are pliable and fracture differently. Growth plate (physeal), greenstick, and buckle fractures are typical.
- Children are at increased risk of cancer due to radiation exposure; imaging decision trees and techniques to minimize radiation exposure are utilized to keep radiation doses as low as possible.

The cervical spine of a child is less protected than the cervical spine of an adult and prone to injury for a variety of reasons. Differences include the following[14,22]:

- Large head compared to the body
- Weak musculature supporting the spine
- Increased laxity of ligaments supporting the spinal cord
- Unossified vertebra/growth plates present
- Immature vertebral joints with more horizontally inclined facets

Developmental considerations that heighten the potential for injury include the following:

- Infants are mobile from birth and can fall off raised surfaces.
- Coordination evolves as children learn to crawl, walk, climb, jump, and play.
- Children are easily distracted, have a limited grasp of cause and effect, and lack experience with situations that can cause traumatic injury.
- Children have difficulty judging the speed and distance of oncoming vehicles.
- Young children may have trouble localizing sound and recognizing sounds of danger.
- The visual field is primarily at a much lower eye level.
- Toddlers and school-age children are egocentric and believe that if they see the car, the driver sees them.
- Adolescents may be easily distracted by mobile phones while walking near traffic.
- Risk-taking behavior is common.

Mechanisms of Injury

Traumatic injuries occur when the body is subjected to greater force than it can withstand. Acceleration and deceleration forces are generated via increases or decreases in the body's velocity. An example is being thrown from a horse. Acceleration forces propel the body away from the horse, and deceleration forces stop the body when it lands on the ground. Structures within the body may move at different speeds when the velocity changes, causing tearing or shearing where these structures are connected. Force can also be broadly categorized as blunt or penetrating. Other mechanisms of injury include burns and submersions. Moreover, mechanisms can overlap, such as when a child is thrown from a burning building.

The child may have sustained thermal injuries from the fire, penetrating injuries from shards of window glass, and blunt injuries from the sudden deceleration and impact from landing on the ground.

Penetrating injuries are less common and often the result of violence; injury patterns are directly related to the shape, force, and trajectory of the penetrating object. The anatomic structures involved determine the injury severity; considering the compact nature of the pediatric body, penetrating trauma is likely to injure a vital structure. "Blunt mechanisms of injury and children's unique physical characteristics result in multisystem injury being the rule rather than the exception. Clinicians should presume, therefore, that multiple organ systems may be injured until proven otherwise."[2(p188)] **Table 9-1** reviews common blunt mechanisms with associated traumatic injuries.

TABLE 9-1 Common Pediatric Blunt Mechanisms and Patterns of Injury	
Mechanism	**Injuries**
Pedestrian versus motor vehicle traveling at low speed	Lower extremity fractures
Pedestrian versus motor vehicle traveling at high speed	Multisystem trauma Head and neck injuries Lower extremity fractures
Motor vehicle collision, restrained occupant	Chest and abdominal injuries Lower spine fractures
Motor vehicle collision, unrestrained occupant	Multisystem trauma Head and neck injuries Scalp and facial lacerations
Seat belt injury complex associated with "seat belt sign"[14]	Abdominal wall contusion across the lap Small bowel injury Chance fracture (lumbar spine) Abdominal vasculature injuries Ureteral trauma Spleen and liver injuries
Fall from low height	Upper extremity fractures
Fall from medium height	Head and neck injuries Extremity fractures
Fall from high height	Multisystem trauma Head and neck injuries Extremity fractures
Bicycle crash, not wearing a helmet	Intracranial trauma Scalp, facial, and neck lacerations Upper extremity fractures
Bicycle crash, wearing a helmet	Upper extremity fractures
Bicycle injury involving handlebar	Intra-abdominal injuries

Data from American College of Surgeons. (2018). *Advanced trauma life support: Student course manual* (10th ed., Chapter 10); Ernst, G. (2020). Pediatric trauma. In J. E. Tintinalli, O. J. Ma, D. M. Yealy, G. D. Meckler, J. S. Stapczynski, D. M. Cline, & S. H. Thomas (Eds.), *Tintinalli's emergency medicine: A comprehensive study guide* (9th ed., pp. 789–797). McGraw Hill.

Motor Vehicle Crashes

The greatest number of trauma-related deaths in children are the result of motor vehicle crashes. Regional legislation guides and enforces the appropriate use of car seats based on the most recent safety data, but they do not guarantee that car seats will be used correctly. Ask about the type of car seat and where and how it was positioned in the car. The team can also obtain the following information when receiving a patient involved in a motor vehicle crash to better anticipate injuries based on the mechanism[2(Ch1)]:

- What was the extent of damage to the car, and was there intrusion?
- Was there a prolonged extrication?
- Were any passengers ejected?
- Was there a death of any passenger?
- Were seat belts worn, did the car have airbags, and, if so, did the airbags deploy?

Waddell's triad is a common pattern of injury sustained by children who are struck by a motor vehicle[30]:

- The triad generally involves injuries to the head, chest/abdomen, and lower extremities.
- Toddlers and preschoolers may be knocked down and dragged under the vehicle. The vehicle's front bumper may cause chest, abdomen, pelvic, or femur injuries.
- Older preschool- and school-age children may sustain femur fractures from the bumper and chest injuries from the hood.
- If the child is thrown on to the hood of the vehicle and strikes the windshield, head and facial injuries may occur.
- When the car decelerates or stops, the child slides or rolls to the street, usually striking their head on the pavement.

Falls

Falls are a frequent childhood injury mechanism requiring medical evaluation. Factors that contribute to the injuries sustained from a fall include the following[4]:

- Patient age
- Fall mechanism
- The child's body orientation at impact
- The type of impact surface

In early childhood, children are prone to falls because of their higher center of gravity, increased mobility, and limited perception of danger. It is important to relate fall injuries to a child's developmental abilities; consider whether the mechanism related in the history is consistent with what the child is physically capable of.

- Infants more commonly sustain falls from low objects, such as high-chairs, baby walkers, shopping carts, countertops, changing tables, beds, and tables.
- Toddlers and preschoolers sustain falls from low objects and falls from heights, such as windows, balconies, and stairs.
- The school-age child is often involved in a fall related to sports or recreational activities, such as tree climbing, bicycling, playground equipment, skating, and organized sporting activities.

Submersion

In the United States, drowning is second only to birth defects as the leading cause of death for children ages 1 to 4 years, and is surpassed only by motor vehicle crashes as the leading cause of unintentional traumatic death for children ages 1–14 years.[6] Children ages 1–4 most frequently drown in swimming pools, whereas two-thirds of infant drownings occur in bathtubs.[6] Note that drownings can occur in any container that holds liquid—sinks, buckets, and basins. Such drownings are attributed to the infant's inability to lift their head out of the water, lack of supervision, weak or absent swimming ability, and inadequate barriers around pools. Drownings in lakes, rivers, and oceans are more prevalent in people older than 15 years of age,[6] and are often felt to be precipitated by risk-taking behavior, which can be magnified by influences such as drugs and alcohol.

Heat, Electricity, Chemicals, and Radiation

Burns are the fifth leading cause of nonlethal injury and the 11th leading cause of death for children 1 to 9 years of age.[13] These types of injuries are sustained after exposure to heat, electricity, chemicals, or radiation. Inhalation of hot air, smoke, steam, and toxins further complicates burn trauma with airway compromise and alterations in gas exchange.

The extent of injury is influenced by the intensity and duration of the exposure. Examples of factors that alter intensity include chemical composition (dilute or concentrated), temperature of the scalding liquid or enclosed space, voltage of the electrical source, and amount of radiation. Children may lack the physical mobility or rational thought process to quickly escape a burning environment.

Thermal burns are caused by contact with a hot substance or object, steam, smoke, or flash burns. Scald burns are often more common in toddlers and preschoolers (e.g., spilling a pot of boiling water or a hot cup of coffee), whereas flame burns are more common in older children (e.g., house fire, injuries from fireworks). Burns to the hands with sharply demarcated circumferential burns to the wrists ("burn gloves"), burns to the feet with sharply demarcated circumferential burns to the ankles ("burn socks"), or burns with a pattern, such as cigarette burns or from other hot items, should raise suspicion of maltreatment.[2(Ch9)]

Initial Assessment of the Pediatric Patient with Trauma

Chapter 5, "Initial Assessment," provides a comprehensive overview of a systematic assessment process applicable to all pediatric patients. This section focuses on unique assessments and interventions for the pediatric patient with trauma. Efforts to mitigate the trauma triad of death should include keeping the patient warm and initiating resuscitation measures that address acidosis without diluting clotting mechanisms with excessive crystalloid or packed red blood cell replacement (**Figure 9-1**). Hypocalcemia is emerging as a fourth physiologic contributor to mortality in trauma.[40]

General Impression

Prehospital providers have valuable information to share about on-scene findings that can help other clinicians who are treating the patient better understand the mechanism of injury. Setting the expectation for silence and attention to the prehospital report upon patient arrival helps ensure these data are not lost. Listen to the verbal prehospital report while forming a general impression of the patient.

Alterations in the Pediatric Assessment Triangle related to trauma focus on indicators of trauma-induced inadequacies in tissue perfusion. Assess for uncontrolled external hemorrhage. While the need for massive blood transfusion is rare in pediatric patients with trauma, stopping uncontrolled external bleeding and replacing lost blood components are life-saving interventions when indicated.[15] Management of uncontrolled external hemorrhage may require direct pressure, wound packing, tourniquets, or surgical intervention. With significant blood loss, blood component replacement may be the priority intervention; a quick assessment of pulse quality and capillary refill will help the team determine the need to prioritize "C" interventions.

Alertness and Airway with Simultaneous Cervical Spine Stabilization

Maintain a high index of suspicion for cervical spine injury. Be in the patient's line of sight when assessing alertness to avoid the natural response in which the patient turns their head toward a voice. Spinal motion restriction may scare and agitate children; make nonthreatening eye contact and reassure the patient while applying manual stabilization, properly sized cervical collars, towel rolls, or other measures to limit movement of the head and neck. Place padding under the patient's shoulders and torso to maintain neutral alignment of the head if needed to accommodate a large occiput.[22,23]

Conscious children often assume a position that opens their airway and maximizes their ability to breathe. Attempt to maintain the head and neck in neutral alignment without compromising this positioning. The jaw-thrust maneuver is used in less responsive children to open and inspect the airway while stabilizing the cervical spine.

An oropharyngeal airway can be used to provide a route for air entry behind the relatively large tongue in the unresponsive child without a gag reflex. A nasopharyngeal airway can be used as long as there is no evidence of facial trauma; a basilar skull fracture provides a route of entry from the naris to the brain. Use care during insertion of either airway, as the mucous membranes lining the narrow oral and nasal passages are delicate and easily traumatized. In a patient with burns, look for singed nasal hair or eyebrows; soot around the nose or mouth; burns to the face and neck; stridor; drooling; the presence of increased secretions; a decreased or absent cough reflex; changes in voice; or a hoarse cough.

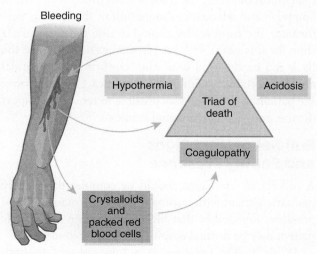

Figure 9-1 *Trauma triad of death.*

Intubation may be required to protect and maintain an open airway.

Breathing

Breath sounds can resonate throughout the child's chest, giving the false reassurance of bilateral breath sounds. Auscultate in the midaxillary area and observe for symmetric rise and fall of the chest. If breath sounds are unequal, the child may have a pneumothorax or hemothorax. One side of the chest may appear hyperinflated and not move as much as the other side in cases of a significant tension pneumothorax or hemothorax. Trauma-specific interventions may include the following:

- Prepare for and assist finger thoracostomy or chest tube insertion if a pneumothorax, tension pneumothorax, or hemothorax is present, based on findings of respiratory distress, inadequate or absent breath sounds, and/or asymmetric chest wall movement. Needle decompression is a temporizing measure for a tension pneumothorax when finger thoracostomy or chest tube insertion is not immediately available.
- Apply an appropriate vented chest seal to open wounds on the chest to prevent air entry through the wound and air trapping in the thorax with a completely occlusive dressing.
- Anticipate escharotomy of the neck or chest through circumferential burns. Burned skin can swell and lose elasticity, impairing chest wall expansion.

Circulation

Anticipate goal-directed therapy for shock (refer to Chapter 7, "The Child in Need of Stabilization"). While hypovolemia due to hemorrhage is the most likely cause, consider the possibility of neurogenic shock for patients with potential spine injuries and obstructive shock for patients with chest trauma. Use direct pressure, manual circumferential pressure around a limb, wound packing, or tourniquets to stop uncontrolled external hemorrhage. Consider sources of internal hemorrhage and anticipate the need for focused assessment with sonography for trauma (FAST) or radiographs.

Prepare for and assist with pericardiocentesis for cardiac tamponade, based on the FAST findings. Goal-directed interventions for hemorrhage control include application of a pelvic binder, administration of tranexamic acid, and preparation for interventional radiology, emergency thoracotomy, or surgery.[2(Ch10),14,21] Administer warmed intravenous crystalloids and blood products to prevent hypothermia from large amounts of room-temperature (68°F [20°C]) fluids.

Disability

Determine an age-appropriate Glasgow Coma Scale score (refer to Table 5-1 in Chapter 5, "Initial Assessment"). In an infant, bulging fontanelles are a sign of increased intracranial pressure.[36] Unequal or fixed and dilated pupils are concerning findings associated with cerebral herniation. Interventions include maintenance of cerebral perfusion by supporting the patient's airway, breathing, and circulation to avoid hypoxia and hypotension, along with administration of hypertonic saline or mannitol to decrease cerebral edema. Keep the head in neutral alignment and minimize spikes in intracranial pressure caused by vomiting, agitation, or seizures by administering ordered antiemetics, sedation, or anticonvulsants.[2(Ch10),21]

Expose

Any clothing that remains on the pediatric patient is removed for a complete assessment of all body areas for injuries. Consider the need for forensic evidence preservation. Do not cut through any defects in the clothing that might have been caused by a weapon such as a gun or knife. Warming methods may be initiated to maintain a normothermic state (e.g., increased room temperature, radiant warmer, warmed blankets, overbed warmer, fluid warming devices, or heated humidified oxygen). Remember that hypothermia is a preventable part of the trauma triad of death.

Any prehospital transport devices are removed at this time to prevent skin breakdown and promote comfort. Log rolling has been shown to cause unacceptable movement of an unstable spine and increases the risk of life-threatening hemorrhage in a patient with an unstable pelvis.[29,34] "As long as the patient's spine is protected, a detailed examination can be safely deferred until the patient is stable. Although there are often many competing clinical interests, the trauma team must ensure that a complete and adequate examination of the spine is performed. The team leader should decide the appropriate time for this exam."[2(p144)] A physical examination of the back can be deferred until after confirmation of spinal and pelvic stability with imaging studies. Carefully move the patient in the safest way possible to remove transport devices and facilitate imaging studies.

Full Set of Vital Signs and Family Presence

A full set of vital signs should be completed for every pediatric patient with trauma, including a manual blood pressure. Remember that blood pressure in a pediatric patient may be normal despite significant blood loss.

While family presence is a huge benefit to both the child and the family, balance allowing visitors unsupervised access to the patient with a healthy concern for the possibility of intentional injury. Consider the need for security, child protective services, or police involvement in cases where the assailant poses a continued threat to patient or staff safety.

Get Adjuncts and Give Comfort

Blood typing is a high priority for the injured patient; blood that has not been cross-matched can be administered emergently but is not ideal. Cardiac monitoring is useful to identify dysrhythmias or electrocardiogram changes after blunt chest trauma. When available, CO-oximetry monitoring may help identify carbon monoxide poisoning in children who were burned in an enclosed space (e.g., house fire). Pulse oximetry readings are not reliable in the presence of carbon monoxide poisoning.[13] Increased work of breathing may not be evident in patients with a spinal cord injury, as they are unable to recruit the necessary accessory muscles to increase ventilation; capnography is a useful adjunct to identify respiratory insufficiency in the absence of obvious respiratory distress. Rising end-tidal CO_2 levels indicate inadequate ventilation, which may also occur in patients with an altered mental status due to other conditions associated with trauma such as shock, head injury, or intoxication. Anticipate gastric tube insertion or vent preexisting gastric tubes to decrease gastric distention and increase diaphragmatic excursion. Do not insert nasogastric tubes in patients with any signs of facial trauma.

Traumatic injuries are frightening and painful. Assess pain using a scale appropriate for the patient's age and level of consciousness. In the unresponsive child with traumatic injuries, pain can be assumed to be present. Implement nonpharmacologic comfort measures such as distraction, family presence, padding bony prominences, repositioning, splinting, and verbal reassurance. Splint joints above and below bony deformities, and assess neurovascular status before and after splinting. Applying ice to injured areas may be appropriate for minor trauma but will contribute to hypothermia. Decrease airflow over burned areas with a sterile sheet.[13] Request an order for analgesic medication. Traumatic injury may exacerbate medications' adverse effects such as respiratory depression and hypotension, necessitating close monitoring.

History and Head-to-Toe Assessment

The prehospital report and/or description of events leading up to the injury from the patient or witnesses can help the team anticipate more subtle injuries that might be missed despite a thorough head-to-toe assessment. Which symptoms are the patient and family concerned about? Is there any past medical history that may complicate traumatic injury or otherwise impact care? Use inspection, palpation, and auscultation to identify traumatic injuries. Bruising and swelling may not be immediately apparent; it takes time to develop ecchymoses and edema as blood leaks from damaged vessels and inflammatory responses are triggered.

Do not further manipulate the pelvis if bony crepitus, pain, or instability is noted with gentle downward and medial pressure over the iliac crests. When assessing the pelvis, consider the best way to monitor urinary output. Contraindications to insertion of a urethral catheter include signs of a urethral injury such as blood at the urinary meatus and scrotal/labial/perineal swelling.[16]

Inspect Posterior Surfaces

If the patient has a suspected spinal or pelvic injury, obtain imaging studies prior to turning the patient for a full examination of the back. The log roll maneuver may cause secondary injuries including spinal cord trauma or hemorrhage.[29,34]

Additional Interventions and Diagnostics

Other trauma-specific interventions and diagnostics the nurse can anticipate based on assessment findings may include the following[14,21]:

- Antibiotics for open fractures
- Antidote therapy for toxic inhalants
- Carboxyhemoglobin and cyanide levels for patients with burns
- Calcium level
- Creatine kinase
- Do *not* remove any impaled objects.
- Escharotomies for circumferential burns to the chest or extremities associated with respiratory or neurovascular compromise
- Evaluation for child maltreatment (see Chapter 16, "The Child with a Suspicious Presentation")
- Imaging, ideally with consultation from a pediatric radiologist to minimize radiation exposure
- Preparation for radiologic or surgical intervention
- Sedation for musculoskeletal or other painful procedures
- Specialty consults
- Tetanus immunization
- Thromboelastography or thromboelastometry to evaluate the blood's ability to clot and guide blood component replacement[20]
- Transfer to regional pediatric burn and/or trauma center

Just Keep Reevaluating

Children with traumatic injuries require meticulous and frequent reassessment. Ongoing bleeding, the inflammatory response, adverse reactions to medications, or other injury sequelae can easily cause subtle or abrupt deterioration. Monitor and trend mental status, vital signs, and urinary output to assess the adequacy of resuscitation. Initial improvements may not be sustained, and additional interventions may be needed. Anticipate the need for ongoing pain management.

Tertiary Survey

Comprehensive serial reevaluations over the duration of the emergency department (ED) or hospital stay in conjunction with appropriate physical assessments and diagnostic testing will decrease the likelihood that injuries are missed.

Selected Injuries

Many trauma-specific assessments and interventions are included in the "Initial Assessment of the Pediatric Patient with Trauma" section in this chapter. Highlights of the pathophysiologic basis with additional assessment findings and interventions for selected traumatic injuries are discussed here. The Trauma Nursing Core Course provides more comprehensive information for those nurses interested in optimal care of patients with trauma.

Burns

Burns directly destroy tissue; large burns (defined as burns affecting 15% or more of the total body surface area [TBSA] in young children and 20% or more of the TBSA in older children) often trigger a systemic response.[18] Local and systemic vascular permeability increases and leads to fluid extravasation into the interstitial space, along with protein and electrolyte shifts. Airway edema and loss of intravascular volume threaten the patient's airway, breathing, and circulation. Destruction of red blood cells reduces oxygen-carrying capacity and worsens tissue perfusion. Inhalation of sooty debris, carbon monoxide, or cyanide also impairs oxygenation and ventilation.[2(Ch9),18]

Electrical burns may appear small on the surface, yet result in significant injury within the body, including long bone fractures from muscle spasm and tetany. Muscle damage from an electrical injury can trigger the release of myoglobin, resulting in myoglobinuria and kidney damage. The cardiovascular system and the nervous system are the two systems with the greatest potential to cause immediate life-threatening disruptions. Initiate cardiac monitoring to detect dysrhythmias.[1(Ch6),2(Ch2)]

Stopping the burning process through decontamination of chemicals and removal of heat-retaining items may be the first priority; continued contact with a chemical can be as damaging as contact with burning clothing. Airway edema can progress rapidly in patients with an inhalation injury; anticipate early intubation to prevent the need for a surgical airway. Closely monitor respiratory effort, chest wall expansion, and neurovascular status in patients with circumferential burns of the chest, neck, or extremities. Anticipate fluid resuscitation as intravascular volume becomes depleted with fluid shifts into the interstitial space. It is challenging to maintain adequate tissue perfusion while avoiding complications of over- and under-resuscitation in patients with burns.[1(Ch4)] Estimate total volume needs and titrate as ordered based on TBSA burned, age, weight, hemodynamics, and urine output (**Table 9-2**).

Tools used to estimate TBSA in adults have been adapted to reflect the proportion differences in children based on age. The size of the patient's palm (including the fingers) is roughly equivalent to 1% of TBSA for irregular or scattered burns. **Figure 9-2**, **Figure 9-3**, and **Figure 9-4** illustrate methods to calculate TBSA based on age and body area. When calculating the size of the burn, do not include superficial burns without blisters. The depth of the burn injury may not be completely determined in the ED. Injuries that initially appear to be partial-thickness burns may be identified as full-thickness burns days after the initial injury.[1(Ch2)]

Ensure removal of all clothing and jewelry. Cool tap water may be useful for pain control in patients with burns covering less than 5% TBSA; hypothermia is a significant risk with larger burns.[1(Ch5)] Anticipate the need for pain management with wound care. Consult with regional burn and wound care services to guide emergency care and facilitate transfer or appropriate outpatient follow-up. Burn center referral criteria are listed in **Box 9-1**.

Head Injury

Injuries to the head can threaten the airway, breathing, circulation, and disability elements, including damage to the scalp, skull, brain, vasculature, and face. Distortion of facial anatomy or damage to the cardiorespiratory center in the brain may necessitate endotracheal intubation for airway management and assisted ventilation. The scalp has a rich vascular supply that can be the source of significant hemorrhage.[33] The unfused sutures of the infant skull provide enough intracranial capacity for bleeding to cause anemia and hypotension.[2(Ch10),31]

TABLE 9-2 Fluid Resuscitation (Lactated Ringer's Solution) for Pediatric Burns

Initial Infusion Rates (Prior to TBSA Calculation)	Hourly Rate	
	Calculated Based on TBSA	**Titrate to Urine Output**
≤ 5 years of age = 125 mL/hr 6–13 years of age = 250 mL/hr ≥ 14 years of age = 500 mL/hr	Flame or scald › ≥ 14 years of age = 2 mL/kg/TBSA › < 14 years of age = 3 mL/kg/TBSA Electrical › 4 mL/kg/TBSA when possible to calculate; visible contact areas may be small and not correlate with the trajectory of electricity through the body › Add maintenance fluids with dextrose for infants and children weighing ≤ 30 kg › Consider adjusting weight if a large amount of volume has already been infused (use a recent pre-burn weight, if known)	One-half of total volume to be infused in the first 8 hours after the time of injury Remaining volume to be infused over the next 16 hours Titrate based on urine output per ideal body weight: › ≤ 30 kg: 1 mL/kg/hr › > 30 kg: 0.5 mL/kg/hr Increase hourly rate for myoglobinuria as evidenced by dark, red-tinged urine

Data from American Burn Association. (2018). Shock and fluid resuscitation. *Advanced burn life support course provider manual* (Chapter 4, pp. 31–38).

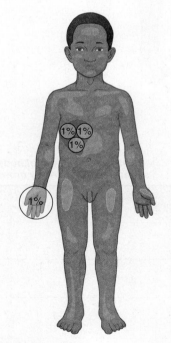

Figure 9-2 *Rule of palms.*

The brain is protected by a fibrous layer called the dura, the surrounding cerebrospinal fluid, and the skull. Traumatic brain injury is distinguished as primary or secondary. The primary injury occurs when there is direct tissue damage sustained from an impact of the brain on the skull, objects piercing the brain (e.g., depressed skull segment, bony shards, bullets), and shearing forces. For example, a coup–contrecoup injury occurs when the impact accelerates the brain enough to collide with the opposite side of the skull (**Figure 9-5**). Secondary injury results from hypoxia, cerebral edema, hemorrhage, and hypotension that compromises cerebral perfusion.[33]

After the cranial sutures fuse (i.e., closure of the fontanelles), the intracranial space is limited. Increases in volume due to cerebral edema, hemorrhage, masses, or inadequate cerebrospinal fluid drainage within this closed space will cause increased intracranial pressure. Assessment findings associated with head trauma and increasing intracranial pressure include the following[2(Ch6,Ch10),31,33]:

- Ataxia (loss of muscle control and coordination)
- Altered mental status ranging from mild confusion or sleepiness to agitation or stupor
- Amnesia, repetitive questions
- Bony crepitus or deformity
  - Note the area and avoid further palpation when bony irregularities are noted to the skull, to avoid causing further penetrating injury from depressed bony segments or shards.
- Bulging or tense fontanelle

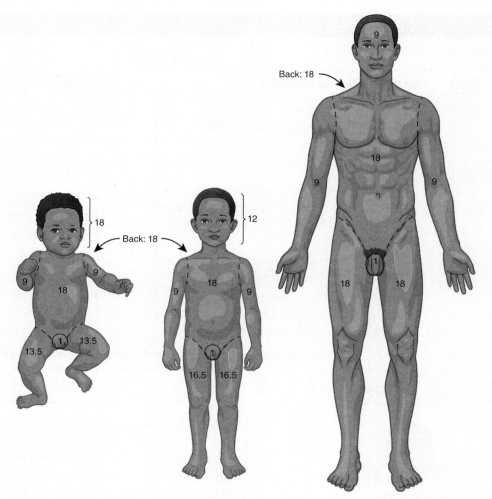

Figure 9-3 *Rule of nines.*

Region	%
Head	
Neck	
Ant. Trunk	
Post. Trunk	
Right arm	
Left arm	
Buttocks	
Genitalia	
Right leg	
Left leg	
Total burn	

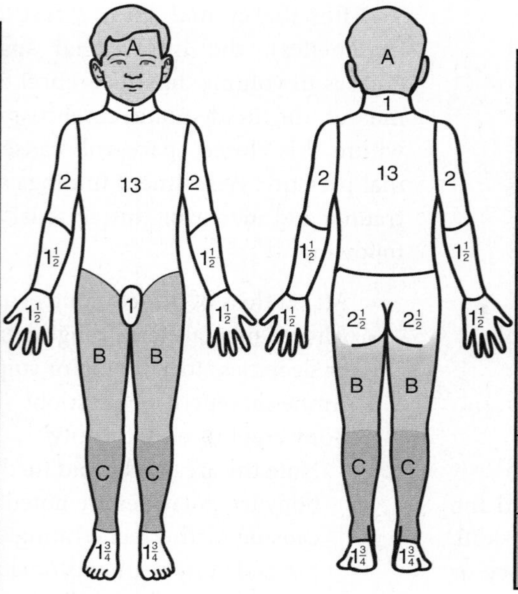

Relative percentages of body surface area affected by growth

Age (years)	A ($\frac{1}{2}$ of head)	B ($\frac{1}{2}$ of one thigh)	C ($\frac{1}{2}$ of one leg)
0	$9\frac{1}{2}$	$2\frac{3}{4}$	$2\frac{1}{2}$
1	$8\frac{1}{2}$	$3\frac{1}{4}$	$2\frac{1}{2}$
5	$6\frac{1}{2}$	4	$2\frac{3}{4}$
10	$5\frac{1}{2}$	$4\frac{1}{4}$	3
15	$4\frac{1}{2}$	$4\frac{1}{2}$	$3\frac{1}{4}$
Adult	$3\frac{1}{2}$	$4\frac{3}{4}$	3

Figure 9-4 *Lund and Browder chart.*

- Difficulty speaking or comprehending (slurred speech, expressive or receptive aphasia)
- Ecchymosis associated with basilar skull fracture
  - Battle's sign is postauricular ecchymosis (bruising behind the ears).
  - "Raccoon eyes" is an informal term used to describe periorbital ecchymosis.

BOX 9-1 Burn Center Referral Criteria

Burn center referral criteria include the following:

1. Burns of the face, hands, feet, genitalia, perineum, or major joints
2. Partial-thickness burns covering > 10% TBSA
3. Full-thickness burns
4. Electrical burns, including lightning injury
5. Chemical burns
6. Inhalation injury
7. Preexisting conditions that could complicate management, prolong recovery, or affect mortality
8. Concomitant trauma (e.g., fractures) in which the burn injury poses the greatest risk of morbidity or mortality
9. No qualified personnel or equipment for pediatric care
10. Need for social, emotional, or rehabilitative intervention

Data from American Burn Association. (2018). Initial assessment and management. *Advanced burn life support course provider manual* (Chapter 2, pp. 17–22).

- Fluid drainage from the ears or nose
  - Refer to Figure 5-3 in Chapter 5, "Initial Assessment," for the halo test, which is used to help determine whether the fluid is cerebrospinal fluid.
- Headache
- Hemiparesis
- History of loss of consciousness
- Nausea, vomiting
- Pain on palpation of the head or face
- Posturing (abnormal flexion or extension of the extremities with stimulation)
- Pupillary changes (decreased reactivity to light, unequal, or fixed and dilated)
- Redness
- Seizure activity
- Soft-tissue swelling
- Unequal grip strength or extremity movement or tone

Acutely, the priorities of care are to maintain cerebral perfusion by supporting the patient's airway, breathing, and circulation and to monitor for signs of deterioration. Hypotension will worsen cerebral perfusion. Keep the patient's head midline to facilitate venous and cerebrospinal fluid drainage. Diminish spikes in intracranial pressure caused by agitation, seizures, or vomiting by administering sedation, anticonvulsants, and sedation as ordered. Administer mannitol or hypertonic saline to shift fluid from edematous cerebral tissue into the vascular space.

Traumatic brain injury in infants and toddlers is more likely to be the result of child maltreatment. Suspicious presentations in these patients warrant further investigation.[31,33]

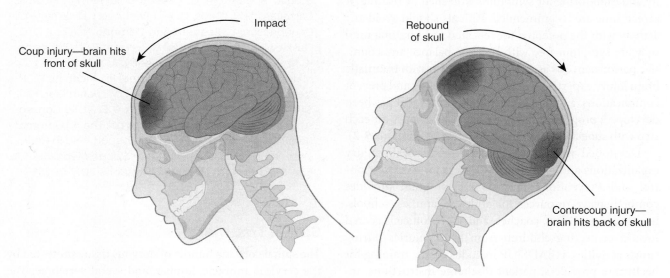

Figure 9-5 *Coup–contrecoup brain injury.*

TABLE 9-3 Symptoms of Mild Traumatic Brain Injury/Concussion			
Physical	**Thinking/Remembering**	**Social/Emotional**	**Sleep**
Bothered by light or noise	Attention or concentration problems	Anxiety or nervousness	Sleeping less than usual
Dizziness or balance problems	Feeling slowed down	Irritability or easily angered	Sleeping more than usual
Feeling tired, no energy	Foggy or groggy	Feeling more emotional	Trouble falling asleep
Headaches	Problems with short- or long-term memory	Sadness	
Nausea or vomiting	Trouble thinking clearly		
Vision problems			

Reproduced from Centers for Disease Control and Prevention. (n.d.). *Symptoms of mild TBI and concussion.* https://www.cdc.gov/traumaticbraininjury/concussion/symptoms.html

Mild Traumatic Brain Injury (Concussion)

Mild traumatic brain injury, also known as concussion, is clinically diagnosed in patients who have experienced head trauma associated with typically short-lived neurologic impairment; imaging studies, if performed, will not show any abnormalities.[25-27] Post-concussive syndrome can manifest for several days or months after the trauma. Provide anticipatory guidance to patients and caregivers (**Table 9-3**).

Second impact syndrome occurs when a child sustains a second head injury before fully recovering from the first and manifests with devastating cerebral edema.[26] There is also the concern for chronic traumatic encephalopathy that has been identified postmortem in athletes who have sustained multiple concussions.[26]

In any patient who has experienced a mild traumatic brain injury, a day or two of physical and cognitive rest with supervised resumption of noncontact aerobic activity and monitoring for symptoms worsened by reading or screen time are recommended. Patients should avoid any activity with the potential for repeated head trauma until they are symptom-free with baseline balance and cognitive performance as assessed by a clinician with traumatic brain injury expertise.[25,26] To promote healing and prevent complications, a gradual return to play protocol has been developed; progression requires at least 24 hours for each step with supervision to monitor for symptoms (**Box 9-2**).

Developed with input from traumatic brain injury organizations and experts, the Centers for Disease Control and Prevention's HEADS UP program provides comprehensive resources for athletes, families, schools, healthcare providers, coaches, and sports officials geared toward protecting children from head injuries during sports activities. HEADS UP includes online training for healthcare providers, patient discharge instructions, return to activity guidelines, and infographics (**Figure 9-6**).

BOX 9-2 Graduated Return to Play Protocol

The steps in a gradual return to play are as follows:

1. Back to regular nonathletic activities (school)
2. Light aerobic activity (walking, stationary bicycle)
3. Moderate activity (running)
4. Heavy, noncontact activity (passing drills, resistance training)
5. Full contact (normal training activities)
6. Competition

Data from Centers for Disease Control and Prevention. (n.d.). *Managing return to activities: Information for health care professionals.* https://www.cdc.gov/headsup/providers/return_to_activities.html; McCrory, P., Meeuwisse, W. H., Dvorak, J., Aubry, M., Bailes, J., Broglio, S. Cantu, R. C., Cassidy, D., Echemendia, R. J., Castellani, R. J., Davis, G. A., Ellenbogen, R., Emery, C., Engebretsen, L., Feddermann-Demont, N., Giza, C. C., Guskiewicz, K. M., Herring, S., Iverson, G. L., Johnston, K. M., Kissick, J., Kutcher, J., Leddy, J. J., Maddocks, D., Makdissi, M., Manley, G. T., McCrea, M., Meehan, W, P., Nagahiro, S., Patricios, J., Putukian, M., Schneider, K. J., Sills, A., Tator, C. H., Turner, M., & Vos, P. E. (2017). Consensus statement on concussion in sport: The 5th international conference on concussion in sport held in Berlin, October 2016. *British Journal of Sports Medicine, 51,* 838–847. https://doi.org/10.1136/bjsports-2017-097699

Spinal Trauma

The spinal cord is a bundle of nervous tissue protected by the cervical, thoracic, lumbar, and sacral vertebrae. The vertebrae are stabilized by ligaments and the surrounding

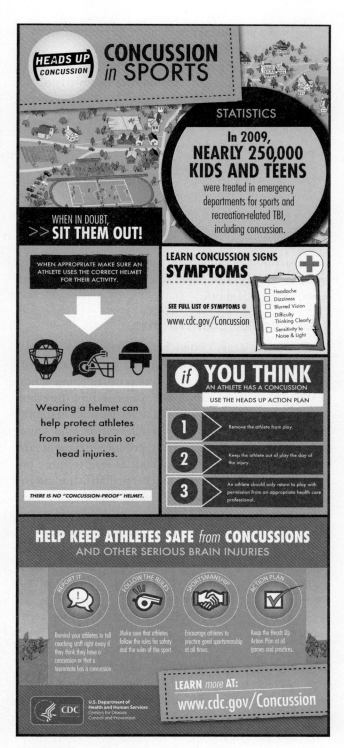

Figure 9-6 *HEADS UP infographic.*

Reproduced from Centers for Disease Control and Prevention. (n.d.). *Concussion in sports.* https://www.cdc.gov/headsup/pdfs/infographics/HU_Sports_infographic -a.pdf

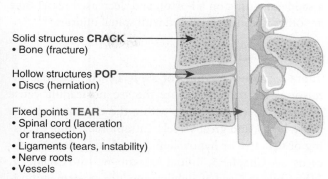

Solid structures **CRACK**
• Bone (fracture)

Hollow structures **POP**
• Discs (herniation)

Fixed points **TEAR**
• Spinal cord (laceration or transection)
• Ligaments (tears, instability)
• Nerve roots
• Vessels

Figure 9-7 *The effects of force on spinal structures.*

structures within the spine (**Figure 9-7**). Ligamentous injuries with vertebral dislocations and subluxations are more common in children younger than 8 years of age.[23]

The immediate life threat from spinal trauma is cord damage leading to loss of the ability to protect the airway or adequately ventilate. Respiratory distress will not necessarily be obvious, as the cord injury impairs muscle function needed to increase respiratory effort. An ineffective cough or increasing end-tidal carbon dioxide level may be the only signs of respiratory compromise. Neurogenic shock—a unique form of distributive shock characterized by vasodilation and bradycardia—can make circulation inadequate.

In spinal trauma, the primary cord injury (i.e., acute vertebral dislocation with spinal cord/bone impact) is exacerbated by secondary injury from hypoxia, hypotension, interruption in vascular supply to the cord, hemorrhage, edema, or additional cord trauma with movement of unstable vertebrae or penetrating objects. For this reason, it is important to prevent secondary injury with spinal motion restriction and support of airway, breathing, and circulation.[10,17,35] Take note of any spontaneous extremity movement prior to administration of paralyzing agents for intubation.

A complete spinal cord injury results in flaccid paralysis and loss of sensation below the level of the injury. An incomplete spinal cord injury presents with a wide range of sometimes subtle symptoms depending on the area of cord involved. Symptoms may be unilateral or bilateral, and may affect only the upper or lower extremities. Weakness may be appreciated only after repeated tests of strength. Assessing for loss of the ability to sense vibration and temperature, the appreciation of proprioception (is the toe up or down?), and sharp versus dull/light versus deep touch can be challenging in young children. Hyperesthesia (increased pain sensation), urinary retention, loss of bowel or bladder control, priapism, saddle paresthesias (numbness to areas that would be in contact with

musculature. The corticospinal tracts within the cord conduct motor impulses from the brain to the body; the spinothalamic tracts conduct sensory impulses from the body to the brain.[10,35] Trauma can damage multiple

a saddle if sitting on a horse), and decreased rectal tone are other findings associated with spinal injuries.[10,17,35]

Chest Trauma

Thoracic injuries account for 5% to 12% of pediatric admissions for trauma but are the second leading cause of death.[14] Vital structures within the chest include the heart, lungs, and great vessels. Intrathoracic injury causing obstructive or hypovolemic shock are primary concerns. See Chapter 5, "Initial Assessment," and Chapter 7, "The Child in Need of Stabilization," for assessment findings and interventions. Any signs of trauma to the torso are concerning for underlying organ injury even without rib crepitus or deformity; pediatric pulmonary contusions are more common than pediatric rib fractures.[2(Ch10)]

A pneumothorax is a collection of air outside the lung but within the pleural space. A hemothorax is a collection of blood within the pleural space. A pneumothorax interferes with gas exchange in the lungs and a tension pneumothorax compresses the heart and great vessels; a hemothorax interferes with gas exchange and can be a significant source of volume loss. Unequal breath sounds or asymmetric chest rise and fall are concerning for pneumothorax or hemothorax. Assessment findings can be falsely reassuring; breath sounds resonate throughout the thin pediatric chest, jugular venous distention is less prominent, and tracheal deviation might not be appreciated until very late, if at all, because of the child's more flexible trachea.[11,12,14]

Abdominal Trauma

Abdominal trauma is the third most common type of trauma in children, after the head and the extremities, and is the most common site of missed injury that results in death.[14] Commonly injured solid organs include the spleen, liver, and kidney; less commonly injured hollow injuries include the intestines (jejunum, duodenum, colon) and stomach.[14,28,32] Injury to abdominal structures can cause hemorrhage with organ lacerations or vascular disruption; bowel perforation can cause peritonitis.

The abdominal assessment of a child with an injury can be challenging because of altered mental status, distracting injuries, pain, anxiety, or lack of cooperation with the examination. Assess for the following[14,28,32]:

- Abdominal pain, tenderness, guarding, rigidity, or distention
- Respiratory distress, signs of shock
- Evisceration of abdominal organs
- Shoulder pain (Kehr's sign) due to phrenic nerve irritation caused by blood or fluid in the peritoneal cavity

- Abrasions, contusions, wounds, or ecchymosis to abdomen and/or flanks.
  - Seat belt and handlebar signs on the abdomen can indicate significant injuries to underlying structures.
- Emesis, gastric aspirate, or urine with visible or occult blood
- Dysphagia
- Rectal bleeding or blood at the urinary meatus

Families of children with blunt abdominal trauma who are discharged home are instructed to follow up with their primary care provider. Immediate care is needed for respiratory distress, worsening abdominal pain, abdominal distention, bloody/dark stools or emesis, bruising near the umbilicus or flank, jaundice, blood in the urine, fever, or signs of shock.

Musculoskeletal Trauma

Unless there is associated hemorrhage from vascular disruption, musculoskeletal injuries are not a priority during the primary survey. After life-threatening abnormalities have been addressed, consider limb-threatening conditions and perform an assessment of extremity pulses, temperature, capillary refill, motion, and sensation. Even when they do not produce neurovascular compromise, musculoskeletal injuries lead to more operative interventions than any other pediatric trauma and have the potential to result in lifelong disability if missed or mismanaged.[38]

Force applied to bony structures, muscles, tendons, and ligaments may cause fractures, sprains, strains, subluxations, and dislocations.[37,38] Fracture patterns include those shown in **Figure 9-8** and **Figure 9-9**. Pediatric bone growth and structure make torus (cortical/buckle type), greenstick, and epiphyseal–metaphyseal fractures more common in children; plastic deformation without fracture can be seen as bending or bowing of the bone.[24] A greenstick fracture can be considered analogous to a young, green tree branch that bends and splinters, but does not fully break. Epiphyseal–metaphyseal fractures (commonly referred to as Salter–Harris fractures) involve the growth plate (physis); they can be difficult to see on radiographs and impair future bone growth.[24] A slipped capital femoral epiphysis can cause pain and gait abnormalities in children with no history of trauma.[19]

Injury Prevention

Chapter 2, "Preparing for Pediatric Emergencies," describes ways to incorporate health promotion into routine ED discussions with patients and families. Regional

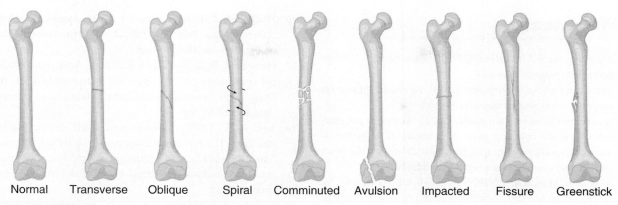

Figure 9-8 *Common types of fractures.*

Normal   Transverse   Oblique   Spiral   Comminuted   Avulsion   Impacted   Fissure   Greenstick

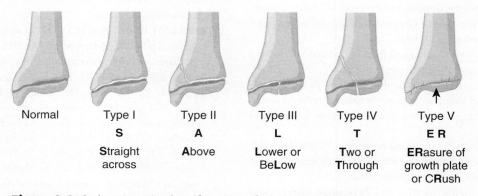

Normal   Type I   Type II   Type III   Type IV   Type V
         S   **A**   **L**   **T**   **E R**
         Straight   Above   Lower or   Two or   ERasure of
         across   BeLow   Through   growth plate
                                                    or CRush

Figure 9-9 *Salter–Harris classification of physeal fractures.*

pediatric trauma centers are resources for trauma prevention, but many initiatives can be implemented locally. Nurses who care for injured patients can be particularly impactful in these efforts.

Summary

Care of the pediatric patient with trauma requires a coordinated effort from the trauma team and the family. Collaboration by the multidisciplinary team facilitates optimal patient care and integrates the resources that are needed to care for these patients. Knowledge of normal growth and development, anatomy, mechanisms of injury, and responses to injury (physiological and psychosocial) is the foundation for providing trauma nursing care to the pediatric patient. Following a systematic approach to assessment and intervention contributes to positive patient outcomes through early identification of injuries and recognition of life-threatening conditions. Incorporating the family throughout the care process is important in meeting the psychosocial and emotional needs of the patient and the family.

References

1. American Burn Association. (2018). *Advanced burn life support course provider manual.*

2. American College of Surgeons. (2018). *Advanced trauma life support student course manual* (10th ed.).

3. American College of Surgeons. (2022). *Resources for optimal care of the injured patient: 2022 standards.* https://www.facs.org/quality-programs/trauma/quality/verification-review-and-consultation-program/standards/

4. Baalmann, M., Lu, K., Ablah, E., Lightwine, K., & Haan, J. M. (2020). Incidence and circumstances of pediatric fall-related injuries: Which fall variables matter? *American Journal of Surgery, 220*(4), 1098–1102. https://doi.org/10.1016/j.amjsurg.2020.02.030

5. Centers for Disease Control and Prevention. (n.d.). *Concussion in sports.* https://www.cdc.gov/headsup/pdfs/infographics/HU_Sports_infographic-a.pdf

6. Centers for Disease Control and Prevention. (n.d.). *Drowning facts.* https://www.cdc.gov/drowning/facts/

7. Centers for Disease Control and Prevention. (n.d.). *Managing return to activities: Information for health care professionals.* https://www.cdc.gov/headsup/providers/return_to_activities.html

8. Centers for Disease Control and Prevention. (n.d.). *Symptoms of mild TBI and concussion.* https://www.cdc.gov/traumaticbraininjury/concussion/symptoms.html

9. Centers for Disease Control and Prevention (n.d.). *Web-based Injury Statistics Query and Reporting System.* Retrieved May 12, 2022, from https://www.cdc.gov/injury/wisqars/index.html

10. Dobkin, B. H. (2022). Paraplegia and spinal cord syndromes. In J. Jankovic, J. C. Mazziotta, S. L. Pomeroy, & N. J. Newman (Eds.), *Bradley and Daroff's neurology in clinical practice* (8th ed., pp. 356–361). Elsevier.

11. Eisenberg, M. (2022). Thoracic trauma in children: Initial stabilization and evaluation. *UpToDate.* Retrieved May 15, 2022, from https://www.uptodate.com/contents/thoracic-trauma-in-children-initial-stabilization-and-evaluation

12. Eisenberg, M., & Colins, J. L. (2021). Thoracic trauma. In K. Shaw & R. Bachur (Eds.), *Fleisher & Ludwig's textbook of pediatric emergency medicine* (7th ed., pp. 1274–1289). Wolters Kluwer.

13. Ellison, A. M., & Samuels-Kalow, M. E. (2021). Burns. In K. Shaw & R. Bachur (Eds.), *Fleisher & Ludwig's textbook of pediatric emergency medicine* (7th ed., pp. 1095–1103). Wolters Kluwer.

14. Ernst, G. (2020). Pediatric trauma. In J. E. Tintinalli, O. J. Ma, D. M. Yealy, G. D. Meckler, J. S. Stapczynski, D. M. Cline, & S. H. Thomas (Eds.), *Tintinalli's emergency medicine: A comprehensive study guide* (9th ed., pp. 789–797). McGraw-Hill.

15. Evangelista, M. E., Gaffley, M., & Neff, L. P. (2020). Massive transfusion protocols for pediatric patients: Current perspectives. *Journal of Blood Medicine, 11,* 163–172. https://doi.org/10.2147/JBM.S205132

16. Haider, M. Z., & Annamaraju, P. (2021, August 22). *Bladder catheterization.* StatPearls Publishing. https://www.ncbi.nlm.nih.gov/books/NBK560748/

17. Hansebout, R. R., & Kachur, E. (2018). Acute traumatic spinal cord injury. (2018). *UpToDate.* Retrieved May 14, 2022, from https://www.uptodate.com/contents/acute-traumatic-spinal-cord-injury

18. Joffe, M. D. (2021). Moderate and severe thermal burns in children: Emergency management. *UpToDate.* Retrieved March 2, 2022, from https://www.uptodate.com/contents/moderate-and-severe-thermal-burns-in-children-emergency-management

19. Kienstra, A. J. & Macias, C. G. (2021). Evaluation and management of slipped capital femoral epiphysis (SCFE). *UpToDate.* Retrieved May 15, 2022, from https://www.uptodate.com/contents/evaluation-and-management-of-slipped-capital-femoral-epiphysis-scfe

20. Kutcher, M. E., & Cohen, M. J. (2021). Coagulopathy in trauma patients. *UpToDate.* Retrieved May 8, 2022, from https://www.uptodate.com/contents/coagulopathy-in-trauma-patients

21. Lee, L. K., & Fleisher, G. R. (2020). Trauma management: Approach to the unstable child. *UpToDate.* Retrieved May 6, 2022, from https://www.uptodate.com/contents/trauma-management-approach-to-the-unstable-child

22. Leonard, J. C. (2020). Cervical spine injury in infants and children. In J. E. Tintinalli, O. J. Ma, D. M. Yealy, G. D. Meckler, J. S. Stapczynski, D. M. Cline, & S. H. Thomas (Eds.), *Tintinalli's emergency medicine: A comprehensive study guide* (9th ed., pp. 706–709). McGraw-Hill.

23. Leonard, J. C. (2022). Evaluation and acute management of cervical spine injuries in children and adolescents. *UpToDate.* Retrieved May 14, 2022, from https://www.uptodate.com/contents/evaluation-and-acute-management-of-cervical-spine-injuries-in-children-and-adolescents

24. Mathison, D. J., & Agrawal, D. (2021). General principles of fracture management: Fracture patterns and description in children. *UpToDate.* Retrieved May 15, 2022, from https://www.uptodate.com/contents/general-principles-of-fracture-management-fracture-patterns-and-description-in-children

25. McCrory, P., Meeuwisse, W. H., Dvorak, J., Aubry, M., Bailes, J., Broglio, S., Cantu, R. C., Cassidy, D., Echemendia, R. J., Castellani, R. J., Davis, G. A., Ellenbogen, R., Emery, C., Engebretsen, L., Feddermann-Demont, N., Giza, C. C., Guskiewicz, K. M., Herring, S., Iverson, G. L., Johnston, K. M., . . . Vos, P. E. (2017). Consensus statement on concussion in sport: The 5th international conference on concussion in sport held in Berlin, October 2016. *British Journal of Sports Medicine, 51,* 838–847. https://doi.org/10.1136/bjsports-2017-097699

26. Meehan, W. P., & O'Brien, M. J. (2022). Concussion in children and adolescents: Management. *UpToDate.* Retrieved May 12, 2022, from https://www.uptodate.com/contents/concussion-in-children-and-adolescents-management

27. Misch, M. R., & Raukar, N. P. (2020). Sports medicine update: Concussion. *Emergency Medicine Clinics of North America, 38*(1), 207–222. https://doi.org/10.1016/j.emc.2019.09.010

28. Naik-Mathuria, B. (2021). Hollow viscus blunt abdominal trauma in children. *UpToDate*. Retrieved May 15, 2022, from https://www.uptodate.com/contents/hollow-viscus-blunt -abdominal-trauma-in-children

29. National Institute for Health and Care Excellence. (2017, November 13). *Fractures (complex): Assessment and management*. https://www.nice.org.uk/guidance/ng37

30. Paz, M. S., & Mendez, M. D. (2021, November 29). Waddell triad. *StatPearls*. https://www.ncbi.nlm.nih.gov/books/NBK537094/

31. Proctor, M. R. (2021). Intracranial subdural hematoma in children: Epidemiology, anatomy, and pathophysiology. *UpToDate*. Retrieved March 3, 2022, from https://www.uptodate .com/contents/intracranial-subdural-hematoma-in-children -epidemiology-anatomy-and-pathophysiology

32. Saladino, R. A., & Conti, K. (2022). Pediatric blunt abdominal trauma: Initial evaluation and stabilization. *UpToDate*. Retrieved May 15, 2022, from https://www.uptodate.com /contents/pediatric-blunt-abdominal-trauma-initial-evaluation -and-stabilization

33. Schutzman, S., & Mannix, R. (2021). Injury: Head. In K. Shaw & R. Bachur (Eds.), *Fleisher & Ludwig's textbook of pediatric emergency medicine* (7th ed., pp. 268–274). Wolters Kluwer.

34. Shodari, A. F., Almaghrabi, M. A., Basindwah, S. A., Alhazmi, B. F., & Fallatah, S. M. (2021). Techniques and tools used in trauma patients transfer: A review. *Saudi Journal of Emergency Medicine, 2*(1), 85–91. https:///doi.org/10.24911/SJEMed/72 -1598298728

35. Sjeklocha, L., & Gatz, J. D. (2021). Traumatic injuries to the spinal cord and peripheral nervous system. *Emergency Clinics of North America, 39*(1), 1–28. https://doi.org/10.1016/j .emc.2020.09.001

36. Tasker, R. C. (2022). Elevated intracranial pressure (ICP) in children: Clinical manifestations and diagnosis. *UpToDate*. Retrieved May 7, 2022, from https://www.uptodate.com /contents/elevated-intracranial-pressure-icp-in-children -clinical-manifestations-and-diagnosis

37. Walsh, C. (2020). Musculoskeletal injuries. In K. A. McQuillan & M. F. Makic (Eds.), *Trauma nursing: From resuscitation through rehabilitation* (5th ed., pp. 599–638). Elsevier.

38. Wathen, B., & Recicar, J. (2020). Trauma in the pediatric patient. In K. A. McQuillan & M. F. Makic (Eds.), *Trauma nursing: From resuscitation through rehabilitation* (5th ed., pp. 677–703). Elsevier.

39. World Health Organization. (2022, January 28). *Older children and young adolescent mortality (5 to 14 years)* [Fact sheet]. https://www.who.int/news-room/fact-sheets/detail /older-children-and-young-adolescent-mortality-(5-to -14-years)

40. Wray, J. P., Bridwell, F. E., Schauer, S. G., Schakelford, S. A., Bebarta, V. S., Wright, F. L, Bynum, J., & Long, B. (2021). The diamond of death: Hypocalcemia in trauma and resuscitation. *American Journal of Emergency Medicine, 41*, 104–109. https:// doi.org.10.1016/j.ajem.2020.12.065

References   168

The Child with a Fever

Lisa Smotrich, BSN, RN, CPEN, NPD-BC, CCRN-K

OBJECTIVES

Upon completion of this chapter, the learner will be able to:

1. Describe characteristics and selected causes of pediatric fever.
2. Discuss assessment and interventions for common pediatric febrile illnesses.
3. Apply the Pediatric Nursing Process to a febrile child.

Introduction

Fever is a normal physiologic response to certain conditions and is a physiologic expression of disease, most commonly a response to an infectious or other assault on the body. The assessment and treatment of fever have changed significantly in the past 20 years. It is now accepted that the fever itself does not require treatment; instead, the goals of intervention are to provide comfort and to identify and treat the underlying cause.[32]

Fever. which is defined as an abnormal elevation of body temperature,[32] accounts for 10% to 20% of all pediatric emergency department (ED) visits.[24] It is recognized as a sign or symptom of illness. While most fevers are caused by self-limiting viral illnesses and not inherently dangerous, this symptom itself causes anxiety in caregivers and healthcare providers alike.[8]

Normal body temperature has historically been defined as 98.6°F (37°C), but this can vary based on age, activity level, or time of day. The generally accepted normal temperature range in pediatrics is between 97.2°F (36.2°C) and 100.4°F (38°C).[13]

Anatomy and Physiology

Body temperature is regulated by the hypothalamus, which balances heat production (from metabolic activity) with heat loss (primarily from the skin and lungs). When triggered by a stressor (such as a virus, bacterium, or toxin), the hypothalamus produces prostaglandins, which increase the body's temperature "set point." The body actively generates heat by increasing the metabolic rate and muscle activity (shivering) and retains heat through vasoconstriction. The resulting increase in body temperature impairs pathogen function and improves the immune response.[32]

It is important to differentiate fever (a regulated rise in temperature controlled by the central nervous system) from hyperthermia. Hyperthermia is much more serious—even deadly. This unregulated rise in temperature is caused by external factors and cannot be controlled or compensated for by the body. Causes of hyperthermia include heat stroke (e.g., being left in a hot car), effects of some medications, and central nervous system (CNS) insults. Antipyretic medications typically used to treat fever are not effective for hyperthermia.[32]

Associated Risks of Fever

Fever is a normal physiologic response to illness that is typically not harmful in and of itself. However, children with a fever are often uncomfortable. Circulating prostaglandins may be responsible for the body aches that are often experienced during a fever. The physiologic responses that lead to increased temperature also cause an increase in metabolic rate, which leads to tachycardia, tachypnea, and increased oxygen consumption. These effects are not harmful for healthy children but could be of concern in children with complex medical issues or significant underlying illness.[32]

"Fever phobia"—the misconception that the fever itself constitutes a dangerous disease or can have life-threatening effects such as causing seizures or brain damage—is a very real phenomenon that affects caregivers as well as healthcare providers.[8] Fever phobia in caregivers results in overuse of the healthcare system and use of potentially dangerous home treatments such as incorrect or overly frequent doses of antipyretics, cold baths, or application of alcohol to the child's skin.[3] Fever phobia in healthcare providers can result in unnecessary diagnostic testing, hospitalization, and antibiotic use.[13]

It is important to reassure caregivers that in most cases fever itself does not cause adverse effects or make the illness worse, and to provide anticipatory guidance regarding appropriate care for the child with a fever. Emphasis should be placed on determining the cause of the fever and treating symptoms.[32]

Temperature Measurement

Accurate temperature measurement is crucial to identifying fever when it is present. The degree of fever may also provide a clue about the underlying etiology.[13] Controversy exists regarding the best route for temperature measurement in children. Each method has advantages and limitations that must be considered.[12,32] Other factors to consider include the reason for temperature measurement (screening versus significant illness), age, developmental level, and contraindications.[11] **Table 10-1** provides an overview of common temperature measurements.[12,32]

Focused Assessment

The approach to the pediatric patient discussed in Chapter 5, "Initial Assessment," will facilitate a thorough evaluation of the child with a fever.

History

Elicit information about the duration of fever, maximum temperature, associated signs and symptoms, and medications that have been given. General information such as recent travel, immunization status, and exposure to sick family members or other contacts can help to identify risks for specific infections and identify a need for isolation precautions. Determine whether the patient has a history of any diseases or takes any medications that put the child at increased risk for infection.[13]

Diagnostics

Diagnostic tests that are often ordered to evaluate the underlying etiology include a complete blood count (CBC), blood culture, urinalysis and urine culture, cerebrospinal fluid (CSF) studies, C-reactive protein (CRP), and chest radiograph. The patient's age, clinical condition, medical history, symptoms, and physical examination will guide which diagnostic tests should be performed.[32]

Appropriate General Interventions

Care of the febrile child is multifaceted. The goal is to identify serious conditions requiring intervention, prevent complications, and promote comfort.

Infection Control

Given that infectious agents are a common cause of fever, appropriate interventions should be put in place to prevent the spread of infection. Hand hygiene should always be performed before and after any patient contact. Other interventions to prevent the spread of infection may include the use of personal protective equipment (e.g., gloves, gowns, masks), single-patient rooms, cohorting of patients with similar symptoms, use of negative-pressure rooms or air filtration devices, and surface disinfection.[2]

Supportive Treatment

Antipyretic medications, such as acetaminophen or ibuprofen, are commonly used to treat discomfort associated with fever. It is important to obtain an accurate weight so as to dose these medications appropriately and to ensure that they are given at the appropriate intervals.[13] Given that many over-the-counter remedies contain multiple medications, it is important to counsel patients and caregivers to review the contents of all medications to avoid unintentional overdose.

Alternating acetaminophen and ibuprofen is not routinely recommended due to the risk of inaccurate dosing, increasing "fever phobia," and contributing to renal or liver injury in dehydrated children. It may be appropriate to administer the alternate antipyretic if the fever or discomfort returns before the next dose of the original

TABLE 10-1	Common Temperature Measurements	
Method	**Indications**	**Cautions**
Oral	› Appropriate for children who can follow directions and keep the thermometer under their tongue.	› Recent oral intake can cause falsely high or low readings.
Temporal artery (infrared)	› Good option for temperature screening; may not be the best option for clinical decision making.	› Accurate results rely heavily on use of good technique. › Results that do not align with other clinical findings should be rechecked using another method.
Tympanic	› Good option for temperature screening; may not be the best option for clinical decision making.	› Results that do not align with other clinical findings should be rechecked using another method.
Axillary	› Noninvasive alternative to oral temperature for children who cannot follow instructions.	› Wide variations between axillary and core/rectal temperatures are possible. For decision making or critically ill patients, the rectal route may be preferred.
Rectal	› Historically the preferred method for temperature measurement in infants and young children. › Approximates core temperature.	› Can be distressing for patients and families. › Contraindicated for patients with immune compromise. › Rectal temperature changes more slowly than true core temperature.
Other	› Caregiver report of tactile fever should be taken into consideration, especially if antipyretic medications were given before the patient's arrival at the ED. However, an appropriate quantitative method temperature measurement should be used to drive clinical decision making. › Chemical dot thermometers, "smart" devices, and other methods of temperature measurement are not recommended for use in the emergency setting.	

Data from Emergency Nurses Association. (2020). *Non-invasive temperature measurement* [Clinical practice guidelines]. https://enau.ena.org/Users/LearningActivityAssetSingleViewer.aspx?LearningActivityAssetID=TbwwtNCjqK4WlYkrLtmMkw%3d%3d; and Ward, M. A. (2020). Fever in infants and children: Pathophysiology and management. *UpToDate*. Retrieved July 29, 2021, from https://www.uptodate.com/contents/fever-in-infants-and-children-pathophysiology-and-management

antipyretic is due. Other supportive treatment includes rest and encouraging oral fluids to treat or prevent dehydration.[32]

Selected Conditions

Selected conditions covered in this section include fever in infants, immunocompromised patients, sepsis, febrile seizure, meningitis, urinary tract infection (UTI) and pyelonephritis, Kawasaki disease, and streptococcal infections.

Fever in Infants

Infants and young children are at higher risk for serious bacterial infection compared to older children.[13] Because of this heightened risk and the difficulty of accurately assessing this population, evaluation and management of infants and young children with fever are generally more aggressive than for older children.

Younger Than 3 Months

In infants younger than 3 months of age, fever is typically defined as a rectal temperature of 100.4°F (38°C) or higher.[27] For the purposes of management guidelines, this age cohort is typically divided into two groups: those who are well-appearing and those who are ill-appearing. Well-appearing infants younger than 21 days of age receive a full sepsis evaluation and are started on antibiotics; antibiotics may be discontinued if cultures are negative. Well-appearing infants 21 to 60 days of age typically do not require a lumbar puncture and may not require empiric antibiotics if other testing is reassuring.[22]

More than 10% of ill-appearing infants in this age group are found to have bacterial infections, whether or not they have a fever.[27] All ill-appearing infants younger than 3 months of age receive a full evaluation for sepsis, including blood culture, urinalysis and urine culture, CBC, CRP, and CSF evaluation.[25] Additional evaluation based on symptoms may include chest radiograph, surface cultures, electrocardiogram, echocardiogram, stool cultures, additional blood testing, and other symptom-specific diagnostic testing.

Interventions for the ill-appearing febrile infant younger than 3 months of age include supportive care and empiric antimicrobial therapy.[25] Antimicrobial therapy is started as soon as possible after cultures are obtained; do not delay starting antimicrobial therapy if the infant is too unstable to obtain CSF or other samples. Ideally, these patients will be admitted to a facility capable of providing pediatric intensive care.

Infants and Young Children 3 to 36 Months

Infants and young children 3 to 36 months of age are at lower risk for serious bacterial infection than those younger than 3 months but still require thorough assessment and evaluation. The history and/or physical examination findings will guide diagnostic testing. Children who are not immunized (or not fully immunized) and who do not have an apparent source of infection are at risk for bacteremia and are evaluated with a CBC, blood culture, urinalysis (with or without urine culture), and chest radiograph. Fully immunized children are at much lower risk for bacteremia, but UTIs are still common in this population. Bagged urine specimens may be used for urinalysis but are not appropriate for urine culture because they are often contaminated.[1]

Immunocompromised Patients

Children who are immunocompromised due to hematologic, oncologic, or autoimmune diseases are at high risk for infection. These patients can rapidly become ill and decompensate within hours.

Assessment Findings and Interventions

Chemotherapy and other cancer treatments cause neutropenia, leaving the body unable to mount a response to even a minor infection. Fever in a child undergoing cancer treatment or with a history of cancer must be considered a sign of severe infection until proven otherwise. Obtain a CBC and blood cultures (consider separate cultures from each central line lumen or port if present). Lumbar puncture or radiography is not routinely recommended unless other symptoms are present. Empiric antibiotics are ideally started within 60 minutes of the patient's arrival at the ED.[29]

Patients who receive organ transplants are treated with immunosuppressants to prevent organ rejection. Children with sickle cell disease have impaired immune function caused by damage to the spleen from sickled cells. Children post transplant or with sickle cell disease who present with fever require rapid evaluation and treatment. Evaluation includes a CBC, blood cultures, and chest radiograph (if chest pain and/or respiratory symptoms are present). Ideally, empiric antibiotics are started within 60 minutes of the patient's arrival at the ED.[29]

Sepsis

A typical infection causes a localized immune response. Sepsis occurs when the immune response to an infection escalates and begins to cause systemic effects throughout the body.[23] Symptoms can range from moderate illness to multiple organ failure and cardiovascular collapse. Early identification and rapid intervention are critical to ensuring the best possible outcome.

Assessment Findings and Interventions

Symptoms that should raise suspicion for sepsis include fever, hypothermia, tachycardia, tachypnea, weak or bounding pulses, delayed or flash capillary refill, hypotension, altered mental status, and skin abnormalities such as rash, petechiae, or purpura. Petechiae below the nipple line are more concerning because petechiae above the nipple line can occur after vomiting or coughing.[19] As sepsis progresses, signs of organ dysfunction such as hypotension, prolonged capillary refill, increased oxygen requirements, altered mental status, thrombocytopenia, increased serum creatinine, and decreased urine output develop.

Lab studies for sepsis include blood glucose, blood gas monitoring, CBC, lactate, serum electrolytes, coagulation studies, blood cultures, urinalysis, and urine culture. Additional diagnostic testing such as lumbar puncture, radiography, and additional laboratory testing may be ordered based on the patient's specific symptoms.[23]

Sepsis care bundles have been instrumental in standardizing care and improving outcomes for patients with sepsis since 2004.[9] Though these guidelines and the updates that have followed included pediatric considerations, a need was identified for a stand-alone guideline for care of pediatric sepsis. In 2020, the Surviving Sepsis Campaign and an international panel of experts published the first guidelines for management of pediatric septic shock.[33]

The goals of sepsis treatment are to reverse (or prevent) shock and restore (or maintain) tissue perfusion. Vascular access should be initiated as early as possible to facilitate fluid resuscitation and early antimicrobial therapy.[23] If hypotension or signs of decreased perfusion are present, a rapid intravenous fluid bolus of 10 to 20 mL/kg of isotonic crystalloid is administered. Additional boluses may be administered if cardiac output does not improve, up to a total of 40–60 mL/kg (as long as there are no signs of fluid overload). If fluid therapy is not effective, vasoactive medications may be required.[33] Signs of improved cardiac output and adequate tissue perfusion include strong distal pulses, capillary refill less than 2 seconds, normal mental status, urine output of at least 1 mL/kg/hr, and adequate systolic blood pressure for age.[34]

Febrile Seizure

Febrile seizures occur in 2% to 5% of children and are most common between the ages of 6 months and 5 years.[14] Most febrile seizures are benign, although they may be frightening for caregivers. Febrile seizures typically occur within the first 24 hours of an illness and are associated with the degree of fever: The higher the fever, the more likely that a febrile seizure will occur.[16] The majority of febrile seizures are classified as simple febrile seizures, characterized by loss of consciousness and generalized tonic–clonic activity that lasts less than 15 minutes (in an otherwise healthy child) and does not recur within a 24-hour period. In contrast, complex febrile seizures may be focal rather than generalized, last longer than 15 minutes, or reoccur within 24 hours.[14]

Approximately one-third of children with febrile seizures will have at least one recurrence. The younger children are when they have their first febrile seizure, the more likely they are to experience another event.[14] There is no evidence that a simple febrile seizure causes epilepsy, developmental or cognitive delay, or other neurologic concerns.[26] Antipyretic medications may reduce recurrence of febrile seizures during a current febrile event,[20] but there is no evidence that they prevent future febrile seizures.[21]

Assessment Findings and Interventions

Care of the child with a febrile seizure focuses on maintaining airway patency and breathing effectiveness, identifying the source of fever, and supporting caregivers. The most common assessment findings are a child who is postictal, lethargic, irritable, or confused after resolution of the seizure. A history of the event should be obtained from the parent or caregiver, including a description of the seizure, length of the seizure, history of current febrile illness, patient or family history of febrile seizures, exposure to illness, and immunization status. Most children who experience a simple febrile seizure do not require extensive diagnostic testing. Urinalysis, lumbar puncture, electroencephalogram, and imaging are not indicated unless the history or physical assessment raises concerns for serious illness.[6]

If the patient is well-appearing and has returned to baseline after a simple febrile seizure, the child may be discharged home.[14] Discharge teaching should include the following items:

- Reassurance for caregivers that, in many cases, febrile seizures do not recur
- Reassurance for caregivers that seizures do not cause neurologic damage
- Instructions on how to take the child's temperature and how to respond to a fever
- Dosing and administration of appropriate antipyretic medication
- When to call the doctor or seek emergency care

Meningitis

Meningitis is an inflammation of the meninges that may be caused by bacteria, viruses, or fungi. Its presentation and prognosis will vary based on the patient's age, the causative organism, and the severity of illness. Viral meningitis is typically less severe than bacterial meningitis and has become less common as *Haemophilus influenzae* type B immunization rates have increased. Bacterial meningitis tends to produce more severe symptoms and has the potential to cause long-term neurologic sequelae.[15]

Assessment Findings and Interventions

One challenge in identifying meningitis is the wide range of symptoms and presentations. Fever is common and may be the only symptom in the first 24 hours of illness, particularly in neonates and young infants.[10] Other symptoms vary by the age of the child.

Neonates and young infants may present with the following symptoms[17]:

- Fever or hypothermia
- Poor feeding, lethargy, and listlessness
- Irritability, shrill cry, difficult to console
- Bulging or tense fontanelle
- Irregular breathing patterns or apnea

Older infants and children may present with the following symptoms[17]:

- Fever (usually present, although critically ill children may present with hypothermia)
- Headache

- Nausea and vomiting
- Nuchal rigidity
- Photophobia

Children of any age may present with the following symptoms[17]:

- Petechiae and purpura (nonblanching)
- Signs of disseminated intravascular coagulation
- Pallor, weak central pulse, decreased capillary refill
- Seizures or coma

Diagnostic testing should include blood cultures, CBC, lactate, and metabolic panel. Performing a lumbar puncture is important to identify the causative organism; however, if signs of increased intracranial pressure are present, a head computed tomography (CT) scan should be performed prior to the lumbar puncture. Antibiotic administration is a priority, and should not be delayed while waiting for the head CT. If signs of decreased perfusion are present, administer fluid boluses and vasopressors as indicated. Children with cardiovascular or neurologic compromise should be admitted to a pediatric intensive care unit for ongoing care and monitoring.[17]

Urinary Tract Infection and Pyelonephritis

UTIs are a common cause of fevers in the pediatric population. If not diagnosed and treated promptly, a UTI can progress to the kidneys (pyelonephritis) and can cause permanent renal damage.

Assessment Findings and Interventions

In young children, a fever may be the only apparent symptom of a UTI. Other nonspecific symptoms may include irritability, vomiting, and foul-smelling urine. Incontinence in a toilet-trained child warrants evaluation for UTI. Older children may complain of symptoms such as painful urination, urgency, frequency, or pain in the abdomen or flanks.[13] Rates of UTIs are higher in females older than 1 year of age (in children younger than 1 year, the incidence is the same for boys and girls), in uncircumcised males, and in children with a history of a prior UTI.[31]

Diagnosis of UTI requires laboratory confirmation of bacteria in the urine. The most appropriate method for sample collection will depend on the patient's age, developmental level, and clinical condition. Suprapubic bladder aspiration performed by a trained clinician provides an excellent sample with minimal risk of contamination, but this method is painful and invasive. Urinary catheterization will provide a sterile sample with less discomfort. Clean catch urine specimens are typically acceptable for children who are old enough to follow the instructions for sample collection.

Most children with a UTI will be discharged home on antibiotics with instructions to follow up with a primary care provider. Infants younger than 2 months of age and ill-appearing children may require hospital admission. Children with recurrent UTIs may require outpatient follow-up evaluation to determine the cause.[13]

Kawasaki Disease

Kawasaki disease (KD) is an acute febrile illness that can occur in children of any age but is most common in children younger than 5 years. It is the most common cause of acquired heart disease in children.[18] The underlying etiology of KD remains unknown despite decades of study. Patients with this disease develop vasculitis (particularly of medium-sized arteries) and inflammation of multiple organs and other tissues. The coronary arteries are particularly susceptible to damage from KD vasculitis, and between 15% and 20% of children who do not receive treatment will go on to develop coronary artery aneurysms, which can contribute to development of arrhythmias, myocardial infarction, heart failure, and death.[4] Early recognition and treatment of KD is critical to avoid or minimize long-term sequelae.

Assessment Findings and Interventions

The hallmark symptom of KD is a fever, usually greater than 102.2°F (39°C). Diagnosis of "classic" KD requires the presence of fever that lasts for at least 5 days and at least four of the following symptoms[18]:

- Bilateral conjunctivitis without drainage
- Erythema of the lips, oral, and/or pharyngeal mucosa, or "strawberry tongue" (**Figure 10-1**)
- Erythema and/or edema of the hands and/or feet (during the acute phase) or peeling of the skin around the fingernails and toenails (after the acute phase)
- Erythematous maculopapular rash (**Figure 10-2**), most commonly on the torso and groin
- Cervical lymphadenopathy (> 1.5 cm)

If fewer than four of these symptoms are present, further evaluation via echocardiogram and laboratory studies may lead to a diagnosis of "incomplete" KD. Findings that support a diagnosis of incomplete KD are outlined in **Table 10-2**.[18] Nonspecific assessment findings may include cough, diarrhea, vomiting, arthralgia, and irritability. Incomplete KD is most common in infants younger than 6 months of age.[4]

Treatment of KD is aimed at decreasing inflammation and preventing cardiovascular complications.

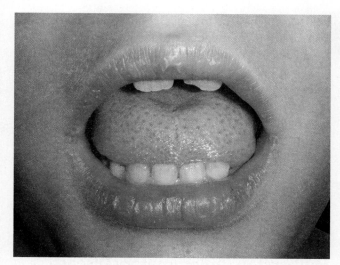

Figure 10-1 *Strawberry tongue from Kawasaki disease.*
© ISM/ISM/Medical Images.

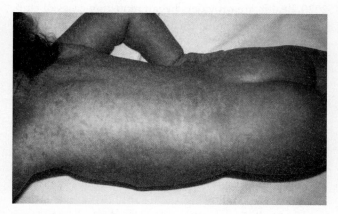

Figure 10-2 *Erythematous maculopapular rash.*
© Biophoto Associates/Science Source.

TABLE 10-2	Evaluation of Incomplete Kawasaki Disease
Type of Test	**Findings**
Laboratory studies	C-reactive protein (CRP) ≥ 3.0 mg/dL **and/or** erythrocyte sedimentation rate ≥ 40 mm/hr **And** three or more of the following: › Anemia › Platelet count ≥ 450,000 after day 7 of fever › Albumin < 3.0 g/dL › Elevated alanine aminotransferase (ALT) › White blood cell (WBC) count ≥ 15,000/mm³ › Urine ≥ 10 WBC/hpf
Echocardiogram	› Increased diameter of left anterior descending or right coronary artery (for age) › Presence of coronary artery aneurysm › Decreased left ventricular function › Mitral regurgitation › Pericardial effusion

Data from McCrindle, B. W., Rowley, A. H., Newburger, J. W., Burns, J. C., Bolger, A. F., Gewitz, M., Baker, A. L., Jackson, M. A., Takahashi, M., Shah, P. B., Kobayashi, T., Wu, M. H., Saji, T. T., & Pahl, S. E. (2017). Diagnosis, treatment, and long-term management of Kawasaki Disease: A scientific statement for health professionals from the American Heart Association. *Circulation, 135*(17), e927–e999. https://doi.org/10.1161/CIR.0000000000000484

Intravenous immunoglobulin (IVIG) has been shown to decrease the incidence of coronary artery abnormalities when administered within 10 days of the onset of illness. High-dose aspirin is administered until at least 48 to 72 hours after fever has resolved, followed by low-dose aspirin for several weeks. Corticosteroids may be given to patients who do not respond to IVIG treatment. Alternative treatments such as infliximab (a monoclonal antibody), cyclosporine, and anakinra are also being studied. Follow-up evaluation is required for several weeks after the initial treatment to monitor the patient's cardiovascular status.[18]

Streptococcal Infections

Streptococci are a group of gram-positive bacteria that cause of a variety of infections in both children and adults. The strains most commonly seen in children are Group A (*Streptococcus pyogenes*) and Group B (*Streptococcus agalactiae*). Vertical transmission of Group B strep is a major cause of sepsis and meningitis in neonates.[30]

Prevention measures include routine screening of pregnant women and treatment with prophylactic antibiotics prior to delivery. Group A streptococci (GAS) can cause several types of infections, including pharyngitis (strep throat), scarlet fever, toxic shock syndrome, and skin infections. Untreated GAS infection can lead to development of acute rheumatic fever.[5]

Pharyngitis

As many as 40% of pharyngitis cases in children are caused by GAS. Pharyngitis is spread through direct contact with oral and nasal secretions, and occurs most commonly among children ages 5 to 15, particularly during the first few years of elementary school.[5] Symptoms include sore throat, difficulty swallowing, fever,

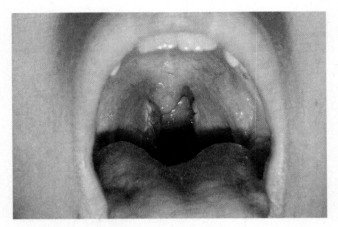

Figure 10-3 *Enlarged tonsils with exudate.*
© Scott Camazine/Medical Images.

and malaise. Physical exam findings include redness of the oropharynx, enlarged tonsils with exudate (**Figure 10-3**), and enlarged submandibular lymph nodes. Rapid antigen testing can accurately identify many cases of GAS pharyngitis, but negative rapid antigen tests should be followed up with more sensitive throat culture testing. Antibiotic treatment is not recommended until a positive result is confirmed.[30]

Scarlet Fever

Scarlet fever is most common in children between 2 and 8 years of age. The initial presentation of scarlet fever is similar to GAS pharyngitis but is followed 1 to 2 days later by a rash that begins on the trunk and spreads to the limbs. Initially the rash is made up of small, blanchable red macules; as it spreads, it changes to a papular rash that is classically described as feeling like sandpaper. Other symptoms may include fever, flushed cheeks, and a "strawberry tongue" appearance similar to that associated with KD. The rash typically resolves in about a week and is often followed by peeling skin that starts on the palms and soles and lasts for several weeks. Scarlet fever is treated with antibiotics.[5]

Acute Rheumatic Fever

Acute rheumatic fever (ARF) is a systemic inflammatory response that can occur approximately 2 weeks after an acute GAS infection that is not effectively treated. Pharyngitis and scarlet fever are the most common infections preceding development of ARF, with two-thirds of patients reporting a history of recent pharyngitis.[5] ARF is most common in areas with crowded living conditions and low access to healthcare; the highest prevalence is in South Asia and central sub-Saharan Africa.[30]

Symptoms of ARF include fever, joint pain, carditis, subcutaneous nodules, involuntary body movements (chorea), and a pink blanching rash on the trunk and

limbs. Cardiac effects include electrocardiogram changes, heart murmur, and damage to the heart valves.[30] Treatment consists of long-term antibiotics to treat the underlying GAS infection and several weeks of nonsteroidal anti-inflammatory drugs or aspirin for management of inflammation. Steroids may be required in severe cases. Most symptoms resolve with treatment, but cardiac damage may lead to long-term health effects such as congestive heart failure or chronic rheumatic heart disease.[5]

Emerging Trends

The emerging trend discussed in this section is multisystem inflammatory disease in children (MIS-C).

Multisystem Inflammatory Disease in Children

During the first peak of the SARS-CoV-2 pandemic in 2020, healthcare providers began reporting cases of children with severe inflammatory illnesses that presented similarly to KD. This condition was dubbed multisystem inflammatory syndrome in children, or MIS-C.[7] The Centers for Disease Control and Prevention (CDC) diagnostic criteria for MIS-C are as follows[28]:

- Age younger than 21 years
- Fever lasting 24 hours or longer
- Laboratory evidence of inflammation (e.g., erythrocyte sedimentation rate, CRP, D-dimer)
- Symptoms involving two or more organ systems, such as the following:
  - Cardiovascular (e.g., shock, arrhythmia, abnormal echocardiogram)
  - Respiratory (e.g., pneumonia, acute respiratory distress syndrome, pulmonary embolism)
  - Renal (e.g., acute kidney injury, renal failure)
  - Neurologic (e.g., seizure, stroke)
  - Hematologic (e.g., coagulopathy)
  - Gastrointestinal (e.g., vomiting, diarrhea, abdominal pain)
  - Dermatologic (e.g., rash, mucositis)
- Severe illness requiring hospitalization
- Recent or current SARS-CoV-2 infection or exposure (may or may not be confirmed with lab testing)
- No other plausible diagnoses

Clinical management of MIS-C is evolving as we learn more about the condition. Patients should be placed on continuous cardiorespiratory monitoring. Vital signs and lab test results are also monitored closely. Treatment with IVIG is recommended for all patients who meet the MIS-C diagnostic criteria. Steroids may be indicated for patients who require care in the pediatric intensive care unit or who do not respond to IVIG. Anticoagulation therapy may be considered for patients who are at risk for thrombus formation. Epinephrine or norepinephrine infusions are used to manage refractory shock caused by vasodilation, while milrinone, dopamine, and dobutamine may be used to support cardiac function. Extracorporeal membrane oxygenation (ECMO) may be used for critically ill patients who are not responding to other treatments. At this time, overall mortality is low (1% to 2%), with higher mortality rates noted among children with comorbidities. Some case studies report prolonged symptoms, but hospital readmission rates are low. Ongoing surveillance and research are needed to better understand the long-term outcomes of MIS-C and guide treatment protocols.[28]

Summary

Fever is a common symptom in children and is usually a normal physiologic process to fight infection. Although frequently benign, it can be indicative of serious illness, especially in neonates, in children with chronic illnesses, and in children with a history of very high fever or fever that has lasted more than 5 days. Discharge education includes temperature measurement, appropriate use of antipyretics, importance of proper hydration, dispelling of common myths, and knowing when to contact the primary care provider or return to the ED.

References

1. Allen, C. H. (2020). Fever without a source in children 3 to 36 months of age: Evaluation and management. *UpToDate*. Retrieved October 2, 2021, from https://www.uptodate.com/contents/fever-without-a-source-in-children-3-to-36-months-of-age-evaluation-and-management

2. Almeida, S.-L. (2020). Communicable diseases and organisms in the health care setting. In V. Sweet & A. Foley (Eds.), *Sheehy's emergency nursing* (7th ed., pp. 183–192). Elsevier.

3. Arias, D., Chen, T. F., & Moles, R. J. (2019). Educational interventions on fever management in children: A scoping review. *Nursing Open, 6*(3), 713–721. https://doi.org/10.1002/nop2.294

4. Becker, T. M., & Hazen, M. (2021). Rheumatologic emergencies. In K. Shaw & R. Bachur (Eds.), *Fleisher & Ludwig's textbook of pediatric emergency medicine* (8th ed., pp. 991–1028). Wolters Kluwer.

5. Bryant, A. E., & Stevens, D. L. (2020). *Streptococcus pyogenes*. In J. E. Bennett, R. Dolin, & M. J. Blaser (Eds.), *Mandell, Douglas, and Bennett's principles and practice of infectious diseases* (9th ed., pp. 2446–2461). Elsevier.

6. Carapetian, S., Hageman, J., Lyons, E., Leonard, D., Janies, K., Kelley, K., & Fuchs, S. (2015). Emergency department evaluation and management of children with simple febrile seizures. *Clinical Pediatrics, 54*(10), 992–998. https://doi.org/10.1177/0009922815570623

7. Centers for Disease Control and Prevention. (2020, May 14). *Multisystem inflammatory syndrome in children (MIS-C) associated with coronavirus disease 2019 (COVID-19)*. https://emergency.cdc.gov/han/2020/han00432.asp

8. Clericetti, C. M., Milani, G. P., Bianchetti, M. G., Simonetti, G. D., Fossali, E. F., Balestra, A. M., Bozzini, M., Agostoni, C., & Lava, S. A. G. (2019). Systematic review finds that fever phobia is a worldwide issue among caregivers and healthcare providers. *Acta Paediatrica, 108*(8), 1393–1397. https://doi.org/10.1111/apa.14739

9. Dellinger, R. P., Carlet, J. M., Masur, H., Gerlach, H., Calandra, T., Cohen, J., Gea-Banacloche, J., Keh, D., Marshall, J. C., Parker, M. M., Ramsay, G., Zimmerman, J. L., Vincent, J. L., Levy, M. M., & Surviving Sepsis Campaign Management Guidelines Committee. (2004). Surviving Sepsis Campaign guidelines for management of severe sepsis and septic shock. *Critical Care Medicine, 32*(6), 858–873. https://pubmed-ncbi-nlm-nih-gov.proxy1.library.jhu.edu/15090974/

10. Edwards, B. L., & Dorfman, D. (2020). High-risk pediatric emergencies. *Emergency Medicine Clinics of North America, 38*(2), 383–400. https://www.clinicalkey.com/nursing/#!/content/journal/1-s2.0-S0733862720300043

11. Emergency Nurses Association. (2018). *Pediatric fever* [Topic brief]. https://enau.ena.org/Users/LearningActivityAssetSingleViewer.aspx?LearningActivityAssetID=LgNJrMgTXT1H%2bmoRSFxUmg%3d%3d

12. Emergency Nurses Association. (2020). *Non-invasive temperature measurement* [Clinical practice guideline]. https://enau.ena.org/Users/LearningActivityAssetSingleViewer.aspx?LearningActivityAssetID=TbwwtNCjqK4WIYkrLtmMkw%3d%3d

13. Florin, T. A., Cohn, K. A., & Alpern, E. R. (2021). Fever. In K. Shaw & R. Bachur (Eds.), *Fleisher & Ludwig's textbook of pediatric emergency medicine* (8th ed., pp. 194–205). Wolters Kluwer.

14. Kimia, A. A., & Chiang, V. W. (2021). Seizures. In K. Shaw & R. Bachur (Eds.), *Fleisher & Ludwig's textbook of pediatric emergency medicine* (8th ed., pp. 491–499). Wolters Kluwer.

15. Ledford, L. (2020). Neurologic emergencies. In V. Sweet & A. Foley (Eds.), *Sheehy's emergency nursing* (7th ed., pp. 249–259). Elsevier.

16. Leung, A. K., Hon, K. L., & Leung, T. N. (2018). Febrile seizures: An overview. *Drugs in Context, 7*, Article 212536. https://doi.org/10.7573/dic.212536

17. Logee, K. (2020). Pediatric emergencies. In V. Sweet & A. Foley (Eds.), *Sheehy's emergency nursing* (7th ed., pp. 556–575). Elsevier.

18. McCrindle, B. W., Rowley, A. H., Newburger, J. W., Burns, J. C., Bolger, A. F., Gewitz, M., Baker, A. L., Jackson, M. A., Takahashi, M., Shah, P. B., Kobayashi, T., Wu, M. H., Saji, T. T., & Pahl, S. E. (2017). Diagnosis, treatment, and long-term management of Kawasaki disease: A scientific statement for

health professionals from the American Heart Association. *Circulation, 135*(17), e927–e999. https://doi.org/10.1161/CIR .0000000000000484

19. McGrath, A., & Barrett, M. J. (2021, September 13). Petechiae. *StatPearls.* https://www.ncbi.nlm.nih.gov/books/NBK482331/

20. Murata, S., Okasora, K., Tanabe, T., Ogino, M., Yamazaki, S., Oba, C., Syabana, K., Nomura, S., Shirasu, A., Inoue, K., Kashiwagi, M., & Tamai, H. (2018). Acetaminophen and febrile seizure recurrences during the same fever episode. *Pediatrics, 142*(5), Article e20181009. https://doi.org/10.1542 /peds.2018-1009

21. Offringa, M., Newton, R., Nevitt, S. J., & Vraka, K. (2021). Prophylactic drug management for febrile seizures in children. *Cochrane Database of Systematic Reviews, 6*(6), Article CD003031. https://doi.org/10.1002/14651858.cd003031.pub4

22. Pantell, R. H., Roberts, K. B., Adams, W. G., Dreyer, B. P., Kuppermann, N., O'Leary, S. T., Okechukwu, K., Woods, C. R., Jr., & Subcommittee on Febrile Infants. (2021). Evaluation and management of well-appearing febrile infants 8 to 60 days old. *Pediatrics, 148*(2), Article e2021052228. https:// pediatrics.aappublications.org/content/148/2/e2021052228

23. Pomerantz, W. J., & Weiss, S. L. (2020). Systematic inflammatory response syndrome (SIRS) and sepsis in children: Definitions, epidemiology, clinical manifestations, and diagnosis. *UpToDate.* Retrieved October 13, 2021, from https://www .uptodate.com/contents/systemic-inflammatory-response -syndrome-sirs-and-sepsis-in-children-definitions-epidemiology -clinical-manifestations-and-diagnosis

24. Rose, E. (2021). Pediatric fever. *Emergency Medicine Clinics of North America, 39*(3), 627–639. https://doi.org/10.1016/j .emc.2021.04.011

25. Scarfone, R. J., & Cho, C. S. (2021). Approach to the ill-appearing infant (younger than 90 days of age). *UpToDate.* Retrieved October 2, 2021, from https://www.uptodate.com /contents/approach-to-the-ill-appearing-infant-younger-than -90-days-of-age

26. Smith, D. K., Sadler, K. P., & Benedum, M. (2019). Febrile seizures: Risks, evaluation, and prognosis. *American Family Physician, 99*(7), 445–450. https://www.aafp.org/afp/2019/0401 /p445.html

27. Smitherman, H. F., & Macias, C. G. (2021). Febrile infant (younger than 90 days of age): Management. *UpToDate.* Retrieved October 2, 2021, from https://www.uptodate .com/contents/febrile-infant-younger-than-90-days-of-age -management

28. Son, M. B. F., & Friedman, K. (2021). COVID-19: Multisystem inflammatory syndrome in children (MIS-C) management and outcome. *UpToDate.* Retrieved December 21, 2021, from https://www.uptodate.com/contents/covid-19-multisystem -inflammatory-syndrome-in-children-mis-c-management -and-outcome

29. Stephanos, K., & Dubbs, S. B. (2021). Pediatric hematologic and oncologic emergencies. *Emergency Medicine Clinics of North America, 39*(3), 555–571. https://doi.org/10.1016/j .emc.2021.04.007

30. Stevens, D. L. (2020). Nonpneumococcal streptococcal infections and rheumatic fever. In L. Goldman, A. I. Schafer, & R. L. Cecil (Eds.), *Goldman-Cecil medicine* (26th ed., 1871–1878). Elsevier.

31. Tullus, K., & Shaikh, P. N. (2020). Urinary tract infections in children. *Lancet, 395*(10237), 1659–1668. https://doi .org/10.1016/s0140-6736(20)30676-0

32. Ward, M. A. (2020). Fever in infants and children: Pathophysiology and management. *UpToDate.* Retrieved July 29, 2021, from https://www.uptodate.com/contents/fever-in-infants -and-children-pathophysiology-and-management

33. Weiss, S. L., Peters, M. J., Alhazzani, W., Agus, M., Flori, H. R., Inwald, D. P., Nadel, S., Schlapbach, L. J., Tasker, R. C., Argent, A. C., Brierley, J., Carcillo, J., Carrol, E. D., Carroll, C. L., Cheifetz, I. M., Choong, K., Cies, J. J., Cruz, A. T., De Luca, D., Deep, A., … Tissieres, P. (2020). Executive summary: Surviving Sepsis Campaign international guidelines for the management of septic shock and sepsis-associated organ dysfunction in children. *Pediatric Critical Care Medicine, 21*(2), 186–195. https://www .sccm.org/SurvivingSepsisCampaign/Guidelines/Pediatric-Patients

34. Weiss, S. L., & Pomerantz, W. J. (2020). Septic shock in children: Rapid recognition and initial resuscitation (first hour). *UpToDate.* Retrieved October 13, 2021, from https://www .uptodate.com/contents/septic-shock-in-children-rapid -recognition-and-initial-resuscitation-first-hour

The Child with Vomiting

Margaret M. Dymond, BSN, RN, ENC(C), DCS, FAEN

OBJECTIVES

Upon completion of this chapter, the learner will be able to:

1. Describe characteristics and selected causes of pediatric vomiting.
2. Apply the Pediatric Nursing Process to a child experiencing a gastrointestinal (GI) emergency.
3. Describe GI and non-GI causes of vomiting.
4. Discuss selected medical and surgical conditions related to vomiting.

Introduction

Vomiting is a common concern for caregivers who are seeking emergency care for their child. The clinical presentation may range from a self-limiting, benign course of illness to a life-threatening condition, and from mild dehydration to shock. Vomiting can occur as a single symptom or in combination with other symptoms and can represent a multitude of clinical disorders, from gastrointestinal (GI) conditions to various non-GI causes. See Chapter 12, "The Child with Abdominal Pain," for conditions that may cause vomiting but are more commonly associated with abdominal pain.

Pathophysiology and Pediatric Considerations

This section begins with the general pathophysiology of vomiting and then turns to application of the Pediatric Nursing Process to a child with vomiting.

Pathophysiology of Vomiting

The process of vomiting and stimulation of the emetic reflex (i.e., ejection of the stomach contents through the mouth) is the result of activation of four main pathways: mechanical, bloodborne toxins, motion, and emotional response. More than one pathway can be stimulated at the same time (**Table 11-1**).[14] Understanding the mechanisms that potentiate vomiting can assist with determining the cause and the most appropriate interventions to alleviate it.[44]

Assessment Related to Vomiting in a Pediatric Patient

The initial assessment using the Pediatric Nursing Process determines the child's need for immediate stabilization. A thorough history and physical assessment will provide information needed to develop a plan of care. This section highlights abnormalities and precautions for the vomiting child.

TABLE 11-1	Pathophysiology Pathways of Vomiting		
Pathway	**Pathophysiology**	**Example**	**Treatment**
Mechanical	Stimulation of intestinal mechanoreceptors Stimulation of chemoreceptors	Child eats too much Appendicitis Foreign body Pyloric stenosis Malrotation with or without volvulus Intussusception Toxin ingestion	Ondansetron Ginger Metoclopramide
Bloodborne	Stimulation of the chemoreceptor trigger zone in the brainstem	Chemotherapy agents Alcohol Opioids Pregnancy	Ondansetron Dexamethasone
Motion	Body motion stimulates the vestibular response and triggers the emetic reflex	Motion sickness Cyclic vomiting syndrome Abdominal migraine	Dimenhydrinate
Emotional	Response to strong emotions	Fear and anxiety Strong smells/tastes Eating disorder	Cognitive behavioral therapy

Data from Di Lorenzo, C. (2021). Approach to the infant or child with nausea and vomiting. *UpToDate*. Retrieved July 4, 2021, from https://www.uptodate.com/contents/approach-to-the-infant-or-child-with-nausea-and-vomiting; and Shields, M. T., & Lightdale, J. R. (2018). Vomiting in children. *Pediatrics in Review, 39*(7), 342–358. https://doi.org/10.1542/pir.2017-0053

Primary Survey

The primary survey assesses and intervenes for any life-threatening conditions.

Alertness and Airway

Alertness and airway considerations include the following:

- Altered mental status may lead to inability to maintain the airway and predispose the patient to aspiration due to vomiting.
- The pediatric airway is more cephalad and anterior than in adults, which increases the child's risk for aspiration following vomiting.
- Suctioning can stimulate the gag reflex, potentially causing vomiting and bradycardia.
- The size of a child's head is disproportionately larger than the rest of the body. Placing a child in the supine position without a towel roll or support under the shoulders may occlude or partially occlude the airway, leading to increased risk of choking and aspiration with vomiting.

Breathing and Ventilation

Breathing considerations include the following:

- Tachypnea may indicate a compensatory response to hypovolemic shock and acidosis.
- Bradypnea may indicate loss of the gag reflex, increased risk of aspiration, and impending respiratory arrest.
- Faster respiratory rates increase insensible fluid losses through the respiratory tract, increasing volume loss and worsening dehydration.
- Respiratory distress may be present if aspiration has occurred from vomiting.
- Respiratory distress may indicate a respiratory infection as a cause of vomiting.
- Assisted ventilation increases the risk of gastric distention, regurgitation, and aspiration.
- Insertion of a nasogastric or orogastric tube or venting of a preexisting feeding tube, particularly after assisted ventilation and/or endotracheal intubation, decompresses the stomach to reduce vomiting and aspiration risk.
- Coughing may induce post-tussive vomiting.

Circulation

Circulation considerations include the following:

- Their greater relative body surface area predisposes children to increased insensible fluid loss through the skin, adding to dehydration and volume losses from vomiting.
- Children's greater water to body mass ratio increases their risk for dehydration.
- Younger children cannot concentrate urine efficiently, which increases volume loss through voiding.
- Tachycardia is an early indicator of volume loss and an early sign of shock. Bradycardia is a late and ominous finding in shock.
- Delayed capillary refill and weak peripheral pulses are indicators of compensation for hypovolemia.
- Hypotension is associated with significant volume loss and decompensated or irreversible shock.

Disability

Disability considerations include the following:

- Altered mental status may indicate altered cerebral perfusion from hypovolemic shock.
- Altered mental status and pupil changes may indicate increased intracranial pressure.
- Infants and younger children have lower glycogen stores, which can exacerbate hypoglycemia in the setting of increased metabolic demand and decreased oral intake.
- Assess the patient's blood glucose level with any change in mental status.

Exposure and Environmental Control

Exposure and environment considerations include the following:

- Fever may indicate an infectious cause of vomiting.
- Fever may lead to a greater insensible fluid loss, exacerbating volume loss from vomiting and diarrhea.
- Rash may indicate an infectious or allergic cause of vomiting.

Full Set of Vital Signs and Family Presence

A full set of vital signs is one way to evaluate the child's clinical response and stability after primary survey interventions. Caregivers can provide comfort and support. They are also necessary to help the clinician obtain a complete history in the secondary survey.

Get Adjuncts and Give Comfort

Adjuncts to the primary survey include the following:

- Laboratory analysis to identify contributing or resulting abnormalities, including electrolyte abnormalities, organ function and perfusion, hydration status, infection severity/source, toxicology, and pregnancy
- Monitoring of cardiac rhythm and trending of vital signs to identify improvement or decompensation
- Nasogastric or orogastric tube insertion for gastric decompression
- Oxygenation and ventilatory monitoring including oximetry, capnography, and co-oximetry (as available) with interventions as indicated
- Pain assessment and management

Secondary Survey

The secondary survey uses a thorough history and physical assessment to identify all abnormalities and determine the need for further diagnostics.

History

The history may need to involve the caregivers and may help with determining etiology.

- Sources include the child's self-report, caregivers, medical records, bystanders, prehospital providers, and any referring facility.
- The history may help determine whether the vomiting is acute, chronic, or cyclic, assisting with establishing its cause. **Box 11-1** describes common patterns of vomiting[14,44] and **Table 11-2** outlines a SAMPLE history that includes vomiting-specific questions.[14,34]

BOX 11-1 Patterns of Vomiting

Patterns of vomiting can be described as follows[14,44]:

- **Acute onset:** Presents within 24–28 hours
- **Chronic pattern:** Vomiting, usually intermittent, for more than 1 week
- **Episodic vomiting:** Cycles of vomiting, often severe, followed by asymptomatic periods

Data from Di Lorenzo, C. (2021). Approach to the infant or child with nausea and vomiting. *UpToDate.* Retrieved July 4, 2021, from https://www.uptodate.com/contents/approach-to-the-infant-or-child-with-nausea-and-vomiting; and Shields, M. T., & Lightdale, J. R. (2018). Vomiting in children. *Pediatrics in Review, 39*(7), 342–358. https://doi.org/10.1542/pir.2017-0053

TABLE 11-2	SAMPLE History for a Patient with Vomiting
SAMPLE History	**Vomiting-Specific Questions**
Signs and symptoms	› When did the vomiting begin?
	› How many episodes of vomiting have occurred—over hours, days, weeks?
	› Are there any factors that trigger or relieve the vomiting?
	› Does the vomiting awaken the child from sleep?
	› Is there a pattern of vomiting at certain times of the day?
	› What color is the vomitus?
	› Is the vomiting forceful or effortless?
	› Are there any other associated symptoms? Pain, fever?
	› Presence of diarrhea? Number, color, consistency of stools?
Allergies	› Exposure to foods causing the vomiting—food intolerance, allergy, anaphylaxis
Medications	› Medication history
	› Are there any new medications or changes to medication doses/routes/ frequency?
	› Consider all medications, including prescription, nonprescription, herbs, supplements, traditional remedies
	› Ingestions (alcohol, drugs, toxins)
Past medical history	› Past illnesses, surgeries, health conditions
Past surgical history	› Immunization status (recent immunizations or under-immunized)
Past immunizations	
Last meal/oral intake	› Refusal to eat or drink, refusal to breastfeed
Last urine output	› Is the patient drinking any fluids and, if so, what type of fluid?
Last bowel movement	• Free water: may lead to hyponatremia
Last menstrual period	• Formula preparation: under-dilution may lead to hypernatremia, over-dilution may lead to hyponatremia (parent mistakenly thinks less fluid will decrease vomiting while maintaining nutrition or more fluid will increase hydration)
	› Estimated urinary output and number of diarrhea stools
	› Color and odor of urine
	› Consistency, color, and odor of stools
	› Estimated number of diaper changes
	› Sexual health history—pregnancy-capable patient?
Events	› Any contacts with similar symptoms?
	› Does the child attend daycare or preschool?
	› Recent travel history
	› Any history of trauma or head injury
	› "What do we need to know about your child?"
	› What are the caregiver's concerns?

Data from Di Lorenzo, C. (2021). Approach to the infant or child with nausea and vomiting. *UpToDate*. Retrieved July 4, 2021, from https://www.uptodate.com/contents/approach-to-the-infant-or-child-with-nausea-and-vomiting; and Mier, M., Nelson, A., & Finkel, L. (2020). Vomiting children: It's not always gastroenteritis. *Pediatric Annals, 49*(5), e233–e241. https://doi.org/10.3928/19382359-20200416-01

Developmental Dehydration Risks

Infants, toddlers, and children with certain disabilities cannot communicate their hydration needs or access fluids freely.

Head-to-Toe

Table 11-3 identifies abnormal findings of importance in the head-to-toe assessment of a child with vomiting.

General Diagnostics

Children may require few, if any, diagnostic studies following a general physical assessment and history if their clinical status is stable. Based on the assessment findings and history, some children may require further laboratory and imaging tests depending on the clinical evaluation of the pediatric patient and suspected cause of the vomiting.

General diagnostics for vomiting include the following[14,32]:

- Labs
  - Amylase, lipase, liver and renal function

TABLE 11-3	Head-to-Toe Assessment: Focused Findings Related to Vomiting	
Assessment	**Focus**	**Potential Relevance**
Head and neck	Evidence of trauma Fontanelle Pupils Neck	Vomiting due to elevated intracranial pressure (ICP) Sunken fontanelle: dehydration Bulging fontanelle: elevated ICP, meningitis Unequal pupils: elevated ICP Pinpoint pupils: opiate, sedative, or toxin exposure Dilated pupils: stimulant or toxin exposure Nuchal rigidity: meningeal irritation
Respiratory exam	Rate/pattern Lung sounds	Rapid breathing: compensation for hypovolemic shock and acidosis Crackles, rales, rhonchi: aspiration, pneumonia Wheeze: allergic reaction
Cardiovascular	Central/peripheral pulses: rate, presence, quality Skin: color, temperature, moisture	Weak, cool, diaphoretic: hypovolemic shock
Abdominal exam	Rigid, distended abdomen, masses, protrusions, visible bowel loops Pain, tenderness, guarding Bowel sounds: absent, faint, or high-pitched	Bowel obstruction Pyloric stenosis (olive-shaped mass) Signs of peritonitis/sepsis
Flanks	Pain, tenderness	Renal colic, pyelonephritis
Perineum	Excoriation, bruising, bleeding, discharge	Irritation of perineum from urine/stool, infection, sexually transmitted infection, signs of child maltreatment
Extremities	Quality of pulses, capillary refill, temperature	Hypovolemia, shock
Posterior surfaces	Evidence of injury, wound, or rash	Trauma, infection, or sepsis

- Blood cultures, lactate, and procalcitonin if sepsis is suspected
- C-reactive protein to identify an acute inflammatory process
- Electrolytes and anion gap
- Pregnancy testing as appropriate for age and history
- Type and screen for suspected GI bleeding or anemia
- Urinalysis for presence of infection, specific gravity for degree of dehydration
- Urine culture if urinary tract infection suspected
- Stool cultures
- Imaging studies (while minimizing unnecessary radiation exposure)
  - Chest and/or abdominal radiographs
  - Ultrasound
  - Computed tomography
  - Magnetic resonance imaging
  - Endoscopy

Dehydration Assessment and Management

Signs and symptoms of hypovolemia (dehydration) include the following[47]:

- Altered mental status: irritability, inconsolability, confusion, lethargy
- Presence of thirst
- Absence of tears
- Poor skin turgor
- Delayed capillary refill
- Dry mucous membranes
- Increasing respiratory and heart rates
- Hypotension
- Low urinary output

Determining the degree of dehydration is challenging, as some tools use weight loss as a marker of severity of dehydration. In many cases, the child's weight is not known prior to the onset of illness. A clinical evaluation may offer a practical approach to assessing for the presence of mild, moderate, or severe dehydration in addition to estimating weight loss to determine the degree of dehydration. Typically, weight loss of less than 3–5% of total body weight is considered mild dehydration, 6–9% weight loss is considered moderate dehydration, and 10% or greater weight loss is considered severe dehydration. In severe cases, untreated dehydration may cause electrolyte imbalances, hypovolemic shock, and cardiorespiratory failure.[15,43]

The Clinical Dehydration Scale is a popular tool that involves assessing four parameters for degree of dehydration. It is practical to apply in the clinical setting and has been validated in children 1–36 months of age (**Table 11-4**).[19,20,25] A limitation of the Clinical Dehydration Scale is that it relies on the clinician's subjective assessment.[15,41]

Interventions

Treating dehydration involves a combination of rehydration protocols, replacement of ongoing fluid losses, antiemetic therapy, and continuing feeding or normal diet as tolerated when feasible. The goal is to replace fluid volume deficits in the least invasive manner possible based on the child's clinical status. The approach to

CLINICAL PEARL

Clinical Signs Helpful in Assessing for Dehydration Resulting in Greater than 5% Loss of Body Weight

· Prolonged capillary refill
· Abnormal skin turgor
· Abnormal respiratory pattern
· Cool extremities
· Weak pulse
· Lack of tears

Data from Santillanes, G., & Rose, E. (2018). Evaluation and management of dehydration in children. *Emergency Medicine Clinics of North America, 36*, 259–273. https://doi.org/10.1016/j.emc.2017.12.004

TABLE 11-4	Clinical Dehydration Scale for Children Ages 1–36 Months		
Characteristic	**0**	**1**	**2**
General appearance	Normal	Thirsty, restless, or lethargic, but irritable when touched	Drowsy, limp, cold, or sweaty, possibly comatose
Eyes	Normal	Slightly sunken	Deeply sunken
Mucous membranes	Moist	Sticky	Dry
Tears	Present	Decreased	Absent

Score of 0, no dehydration, < 3%; score of 1–4, mild dehydration, < 6%; score of 5–8, moderate to severe dehydration, > 6%.

Data from Freedman, S. B., Vandermeer, B., Milne, A., & Hartling, L. (2015). Diagnosing clinically significant dehydration in children with acute gastroenteritis using noninvasive methods: A meta-analysis. *Journal of Pediatrics, 166*(4), 908–916.e6. https://doi.org/10.1016/j.jpeds.2014.12.029; Friedman, J. N., Goldman, R. D., Srivastava, R., & Parkin, P. C. (2004). Development of a clinical dehydration scale for use in children between 1 and 36 months of age. *Journal of Pediatrics, 145*(2), 201–207. https://doi.org/10.1016/j.jpeds.2004.05.035; and Henicksen, M. A., Zaremba, J., Wey, A. R., Gaillard, P. R., & Kharbanda, A. B. (2018). The use of a triage-based protocol for oral rehydration in a pediatric emergency department. *Pediatric Emergency Care, 34*(4), 227–232. https://doi.org/10.1097/pec.0000000000001070

TABLE 11-5	Comparison of Oral Fluids			
Solution	**Carbohydrate (g/L)**	**Sodium (mmol/L)**	**Potassium (mmol/L)**	**Osmolality (mmol/L)**
Pedialyte	25	45	20	250
Enfalyte	30	50	25	200
Sports drink	45	20	3	330
Coca-Cola Classic	112	2	0	750
Apple juice, full strength	120	3	32	730

Modified from Santillanes, G., & Rose, E. (2018). Evaluation and management of dehydration in children. *Emergency Medicine Clinics of North America, 36*, 259–273. https://doi.org/10.1016/j.emc.2017.12.004

patient management is determined following the clinical assessment and determining the degree of dehydration. Fluid replacement therapy may include one or more of the following[43,48]:

- Oral methods, including drinking, syringe feeding, spoon feeding, or administration via gastric tube
- Subcutaneous fluid administration
- Intravenous fluid administration

Oral Rehydration Therapy

For mild to moderate dehydration, oral rehydration therapy (ORT) with an electrolyte solution is preferred. Plain water alone is inappropriate for ORT and may lead to hyponatremia and hypoglycemia. Solutions low in carbohydrate and higher in sodium are most effectively absorbed. Drinks high in osmolality often increase diarrhea, so avoid giving patients full-strength juice or soft drinks.[18] **Table 11-5** compares the osmolality, carbohydrate, and electrolyte composition of commercial oral rehydration solutions with those of other fluids that are commonly used but not recommended for dehydration.[40]

ORT can be delivered by mouth or gastric tube. The recommended amount of oral electrolyte solution is 50–100 mL/kg over 2–4 hours. Small amounts of fluids (around 5–10 mL) are administered every 5 minutes, with the amounts being increased as tolerated. Administration can be facilitated via spoon, oral syringe, or medication dropper if the child will not or cannot drink. Frozen electrolyte solutions are commercially available and may be well tolerated in young children. Administration via gastric tube is useful for infants in respiratory distress who might not otherwise feed.[43]

If vomiting and/or diarrhea persists, an additional replenishment ORT should be considered—2 mL/kg for each vomiting episode and 10 mL/kg for each diarrhea stool. Infants may continue to nurse and most children can eat solids, if tolerated. Oral fluids and foods high in simple sugars should be avoided, as their ingestion may increase diarrhea. ORT may take 2–4 hours and likely requires less time for staff to administer than subcutaneous or intravenous fluid infusions. Parents and caregivers can participate in the ORT administration and be taught to administer the fluids orally. ORT is not appropriate for patients with an altered mental status, paralytic ileus, or severe dehydration and shock.[18]

ORT with an Antiemetic

While not routinely recommended, some children may benefit from administration of an antiemetic prior to starting ORT or after failed ORT. Ondansetron has been shown to be effective in reducing or stopping vomiting episodes by reducing the stimulation of the mechanoreceptors and halting the emetic reflex from the stomach. ORT can proceed about 10–15 minutes post medication administration. Ondansetron is not contraindicated but is used with caution in children and patients with diarrhea.[12,43]

Other types of antiemetics are associated with unacceptable adverse reactions in children and are not recommended. These antiemetics cause drowsiness and sedation and interfere with ORT. Extrapyramidal symptoms such as dystonia and dyskinesia are associated with promethazine and metoclopramide. Promethazine is contraindicated in children younger than 2 years of age because it can cause fatal respiratory depression.[44]

Subcutaneous Fluid Therapy

Subcutaneous fluid therapy may be an option if ORT is not tolerated or is contraindicated in children who are unable to have oral fluids or have difficult venous access. This method of rehydration is not recommended for severely dehydrated children. Its advantages include less pain, no limb immobility required, and low incidence of infection. Its disadvantages include a longer administration time, delayed fluid overload, and tissue inflammation.[42] To promote fluid absorption, a recombinant human hyaluronidase may be instilled into the patient's subcutaneous tissue.[23,43]

Intravenous Fluid Therapy

Intravenous crystalloid solutions are administered based on the patient's weight and clinical condition. Consideration of the patient's degree of dehydration and cardiorespiratory status is needed to guide rehydration. There is no consensus on the exact rate of delivery. Severely dehydrated children with signs of shock are treated with 20 mL/kg of fluid over 5–10 minutes. Reevaluate the patient's status after administration. If the child is still exhibiting signs of shock but has no signs of volume overload, the bolus may be repeated two more times within the first hour. Moderately dehydrated children may need only 10 mL/kg over 30–60 minutes. Depending on the patient's response and ability to tolerate oral fluids, maintenance fluids that take into consideration any electrolyte imbalances and glucose needs may be administered orally or intravenously.[1,14,28,43,48,50]

CLINICAL PEARL

Monitoring During Rehydration

Electrolyte imbalances, hypoglycemia, and fluid volume overload may occur during rehydration. Monitor patients for the following signs and symptoms[16,45]:

- Abdominal distention
- Altered mental status
- Bulging fontanelle
- Confusion
- Crackles, rales, or diminished breath sounds
- Edema
- Electrocardiogram morphology and rhythm changes
- Headache
- Heart murmur or gallop
- Hepatomegaly
- Increased intracranial pressure
- Irritability/fussiness
- Lethargy
- Muscle cramps
- Respiratory distress
- Tachypnea

Selected Conditions

The plan of care will depend on the suspected cause of the vomiting.

Vomiting Without Diarrhea: Non-GI Conditions

Presentation of a patient with vomiting in the emergency department can occur from a non-GI cause. Such a clinical presentation can be associated with a wide range of disorders, requiring a thorough clinical examination and history to determine the most appropriate interventions. The vomiting may be due to an acute, chronic, or cyclic cause.[34] **Table 11-6** lists non-GI causes of vomiting by body system.[27,34]

Gastroenteritis: Vomiting with or Without Diarrhea

Acute gastroenteritis is defined as an infection in the GI tract caused by a viral, bacterial, or parasitic pathogen. Bacterial and parasitic infections may cause longer, more

TABLE 11-6 Non-GI Causes of Vomiting		
System	**Condition**	**Other Signs**
Head and neck	Pharyngitis/sore throat	Sore throat, assess for dehydration
	Foreign body	Choking, gagging, drooling
		Speech difficulty
		Change in voice
Neurologic	Head injury	Headache, altered mental status, pupillary changes
	Central nervous system infections	Fever, altered mental status, pupils
	Mass-occupying lesions (tumors)	Headache
	Headache	Change in behavior, loss of consciousness, pupillary changes
Respiratory	Respiratory infections	Post-tussive vomiting, alterations in breath sounds, rhinorrhea, fever
Renal	Renal colic	Flank/abdominal pain, hematuria
	Urinary tract infection	Fever, abdominal/flank pain, dysuria, urinary urgency, urinary frequency
Gynecologic	Pregnancy	Hyperemesis
Endocrine	Diabetic ketoacidosis	Polyuria, polydipsia, altered mental state
	Adrenal insufficiency	Weight loss
		Hypotension
Metabolic	Inborn errors of metabolism	Failure to thrive
Toxic ingestion	Alcohols	Observe for altered mental status
	Accidental/intentional	Signs and symptoms of toxidromes
	Drugs of abuse	Observe for altered mental status
	Cannabis	Hyperemesis
Psychogenic	Eating disorders	Unexplained weight loss
	Anxiety, stress	Refusal or inability to eat
	Factitious disorder (formerly known as Munchausen syndrome/Munchausen by proxy)	Blood in vomit or stool
		History of enteral or parenteral nutrition
Infection	Sepsis	Fever, diarrhea, altered mental status, pain, altered vital signs, signs of shock

Data from Hornor, G. (2021). Medical child abuse: Essentials for pediatric health care providers. *Journal of Pediatric Health Care, 35*(6), 644-650. https://doi.org/10.1016/j.pedhc.2021.01.006; and Mier, M., Nelson, A., & Finkel, L. (2020). Vomiting children: It's not always gastroenteritis. *Pediatric Annals, 49*(5), e233–e241. https://doi.org/10.3928/19382359-20200416-01

severe symptoms and are treated with medications based on stool culture results.[14] A vaccine is available to prevent gastroenteritis caused by rotavirus. Common viruses causing acute gastroenteritis in rotavirus-immunized children living in the United States include adenovirus, arbovirus, and sapovirus. Norovirus is highly contagious and causes gastroenteritis in all age groups.[2,39]

Acute viral gastroenteritis occurs predominately in the fall and winter, but some viral strains are seen year-round. Symptoms in general have an acute onset and resolve within 1 to 10 days depending on the type of viral infection.[39] These symptoms may include a combination of vomiting, diarrhea, abdominal cramping or pain, and fever that may lead to dehydration. The pediatric patient has a greater risk for volume loss due to vomiting and diarrhea as well as insensible fluid loss through the skin and respiratory tract.

Food Reactions

Adverse pediatric reactions to food range from mild GI discomfort to anaphylaxis. Various reaction descriptions and definitions include allergy, immunoglobulin E (IgE)-mediated, non-IgE-mediated, intolerance, non-allergic, nonimmunologic, and sensitivity. It is not always possible to determine the precise etiology of an adverse food reaction in the emergency department. The recognition of life-threatening presentations and anticipation of life-saving interventions associated with adverse food reactions and reinforcement of the need for follow-up is more important than an exact diagnosis. Be attentive for signs of airway obstruction, anaphylactic shock, hypoglycemia, and hypovolemic shock. Referrals to an allergist, gastroenterologist, and/or epinephrine auto-injector instructions may be warranted.[8]

The prevalence of IgE-mediated pediatric food reactions with the potential to cause anaphylaxis is approximately 8%.[40,46] Regional variations exist in causative agents (e.g., sesame in Israel and seafood in China), but milk, egg, peanuts, and tree nuts are common culprits.[35,46] GI symptoms such as nausea, vomiting, cramping, and diarrhea are frequently associated with food allergies.[7,46]

Food-Induced Anaphylaxis

The GI signs of food-induced anaphylaxis are more common and pronounced than the typical signs of anaphylaxis. Nausea, vomiting, diarrhea, and abdominal cramping with hypotension may be the only indications of anaphylaxis.[11] Skin symptoms may have resolved or may not manifest in as many as 10% of anaphylactic presentations.[11] Other signs of anaphylaxis include the following[46]:

- Anxiety/panic
- Cough

- Difficulty swallowing
- Drooling
- Edema
- Flushing
- Hives
- Hypotension
- Increased work of breathing
- Itching
- Rhinorrhea
- Swelling to the face (eyes, mouth, ears, tongue)
- Tachycardia
- Tachypnea
- Voice changes
- Wheezing

Other signs of pediatric anaphylaxis or symptom descriptions from children may include the following[17]:

- Putting their hands in their mouths
- Pulling or scratching at their tongues
- Slurring their words
- Voice changes (e.g., becomes hoarse or squeaky)
- "This food is too spicy."
- "My tongue [or mouth] is hot [or burning, tingling, itching]."
- "It [my tongue] feels like there is hair on it."
- "My tongue feels full [or heavy or funny]."
- "There's something stuck in my throat."
- "It feels like a bump is on the back of my tongue [throat]."
- "My lips feel tight."
- "It feels like there are bugs in there." (to describe itchy ears)
- "My eyes are burning [or itchy]."
- "My skin feels itchy."
- "My stomach [or tummy] hurts."
- "My chest is tight."
- "Something is wrong" or "Something bad is happening."

RED FLAG

Consider anaphylaxis early when children present with vomiting, abdominal cramping, diarrhea, and hypotension.

The priority intervention is administration of intramuscular epinephrine. Airway management including intubation, inhaled albuterol, and intravenous fluids may be required. Adjunctive treatments include antihistamines and steroids but are *not* life-saving interventions.[1(Pa10),10]

Other food reactions do not carry a risk of anaphylaxis but can cause vomiting, diarrhea, blood-streaked stools, abdominal pain, and malabsorption.[7,8,13] These reactions can lead to hypovolemic shock, failure to thrive, and hypoglycemia. Their pathophysiology varies, but includes enzyme deficiency (such as a deficiency of the lactase needed to break down lactose in dairy) or immune (but not IgE-mediated) responses to specific proteins (such as gluten in celiac disease).[24,26] Food protein-induced enterocolitis syndrome (FPIES) is another example of a non-IgE-mediated response commonly associated with milk, soy, rice, oat, egg, and fish that may present with profuse vomiting and dehydration.[13,36]

Some food reactions may resolve over time; others will require lifelong food avoidance. Food avoidance has both social and psychological ramifications.[37] Preparing patients and their families to respond to anaphylactic symptoms is important, but close follow-up with allergists and/or gastroenterologists is also necessary to determine the best way to evaluate the reaction, ensure adequate nutrition, and prevent unnecessary food avoidance.[29]

Surgical Abdomen

Potentially surgical conditions that may present with vomiting are covered in this section. Discuss allowing any oral intake with the physician or advanced practice provider. It is usually best not to offer any food or fluids to patients with vomiting until a medical evaluation has been completed, so as to prevent anesthesia-related aspiration if emergent surgical intervention is required.

Appendicitis

Appendicitis is the most common abdominal surgical emergency in childhood. This condition is more frequently seen in the second decade of life, and its incidence peaks between the ages of 9 and 12.[5,32] While rare in this population, appendicitis is more dangerous in infants. A much higher perforation rate (70–85%) is seen in infants than in children 5–12 years of age (7% perforation rate).[3] Vague presentations and delays in seeking care may lead to a perforated appendix, septic shock, and death.[5,32]

Assessment Findings

Fever, vomiting, abdominal pain, anorexia, irritability, grunting respirations, and difficulty ambulating are common findings with appendicitis. Pediatric abdominal pain may be difficult to pinpoint, often starts in the periumbilical area, and does not always migrate to the right lower quadrant.[5] **Table 11-7** describes findings related to

presentation of appendicitis per age group. Adolescents tend to present with the classic signs and symptoms as seen in adult appendicitis.[3,5]

Interventions

The physical exam, history, and laboratory results are used in combination with clinical decision-making tools such as the Pediatric Appendicitis Score (**Table 11-8**) to evaluate the likelihood of appendicitis.[4,22] Ultrasound has emerged as the preferred imaging study to minimize radiation exposure and simultaneously evaluate for the presence of potential gynecologic etiologies; ensuring pain management prior to this procedure is vital.[5,32]

Surgical management or a nonoperative approach may be an option depending on the patient's clinical status, early versus late appendicitis, actual or likely perforation, and patient/family preference. Appendectomy offers a curative approach, and surgical exploration can also determine whether other conditions are present but not seen on imaging. Nonoperative management is an option for low-risk patients with no signs of perforation and for patients who have comorbidities that increase the risks associated with a surgical intervention. A nonsurgical approach, when appropriate, involves treating the patient with intravenous antibiotics and clinical observation as an inpatient until the clinical condition stabilizes, the child is pain free, and the white blood cell count has normalized.[6,21,32]

Pyloric Stenosis

The pyloric sphincter is a muscular ring that controls passage of stomach contents into the duodenum. Hypertrophy of this smooth muscle (**Figure 11-1**) causes inadequate stomach emptying after feeding. Symptoms of pyloric stenosis typically present between 2 to 5 weeks of age and are rare after 3 months of age.[32,38] The classic presentation is an infant who is persistently hungry despite forceful, nonbilious vomiting after feeding. Varying degrees of dehydration, weight loss, and electrolyte abnormalities may be noted depending on symptom duration and stenosis severity. The upper abdominal examination may reveal a palpable olive-shaped mass and visible peristaltic waves. Diagnosis is usually confirmed by ultrasound but may require endoscopy. Surgical intervention is highly effective, with a low rate of complications.[14,32,38]

Intussusception

Intussusception develops as the bowel telescopes into itself (**Figure 11-2**), leading to intestinal edema, bowel

TABLE 11-7   Appendicitis Signs and Symptoms by Age Group

Age Group	Signs and Symptoms	Other Conditions and Considerations
Neonates	› Abdominal distention › Bilious emesis › Vomiting › Decreased oral intake › Abdominal tenderness › Sepsis › Temperature instability › Lethargy, irritability › Abdominal wall cellulitis › Respiratory distress › Abdominal mass › Blood in stools	Bowel obstruction Inguinal hernia Malrotation, volvulus Necrotizing enterocolitis

Children < 5 years	› Abdominal pain
	› Fever
	› Vomiting
	› Food avoidance
	› Abdominal exam
	  · Rebound tenderness
	  · Guarding
	  · Generalized tenderness
	  · Point tenderness
	  · Distention
	› Diarrhea
		Intussusception
		Gastroenteritis
		Hemolytic uremic syndrome
		Streptococcal pharyngitis
		Pneumonia
		Urinary tract infection

Children 5–12 years	› Anorexia › Vomiting › Fever › Diarrhea › Nausea › Right lower quadrant abdominal pain › Difficulty walking › Pain with coughing or hopping	Bowel obstruction Diabetic ketoacidosis Gastroenteritis
Children 13 years or older	› Fever › Anorexia › Periumbilical pain with migration to right lower quadrant › Nausea and vomiting	Ectopic pregnancy Ovarian torsion Pelvic inflammatory disease Testicular torsion

Data from Bence, C. M., & Densmore, J. C. (2020). Neonatal and infant appendicitis. *Clinics in Perinatology, 47*(1), 183–196. https://doi.org/10.1016/j.clp.2019.10.004; and Brandt, M. L., & Lopez, M. E. (2021). Acute appendicitis: Clinical manifestations and diagnosis. *UpToDate*. Retrieved March 3, 2022, from https://www.uptodate.com/contents/acute-appendicitis-in-children-clinical-manifestations-and-diagnosis

TABLE 11-8 Pediatric Appendicitis Score	
Symptoms	**Score**
Anorexia	1
Vomiting	1
Migration of pain	1
Fever: temperature > 38°C (100.5°F)	1
Pain with coughing, percussion or hopping	2
Right lower quadrant tenderness	2
White blood cell count > 10,000 cells/mL	1
Absolute neutrophil count > 7500 cells/mL	1
Total	

Scores can be interpreted as follows:

PAS ≤ 2 to 3 = low likelihood, associated with a 0–2% frequency of appendicitis

PAS 3 to 6 = inconclusive, associated with an 8–48% frequency of appendicitis

PAS ≥ 7 = high likelihood, associated with a 78–96% frequency of appendicitis

Data from Brandt, M. L., & Lopez, M. E. (2021). Acute appendicitis: Clinical manifestations and diagnosis. *UpToDate*. Retrieved March 3, 2022, from https://www.uptodate.com/contents /acute-appendicitis-in-children-clinical-manifestations-and -diagnosis; and Goldman, R. D., Carter, S., Stephens, D., Antoon, R., Mounstephen, W., & Langer, J. C. (2008). Prospective validation of the pediatric appendicitis score. *Journal of Pediatrics, 153*(2), 278–282. https://doi.org/10.1016/j.jpeds.2008.01.033

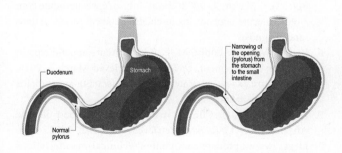

Figure 11-1 *Pyloric stenosis.*
© Designua/Shutterstock.

obstruction, and ischemia. Bowel necrosis, perforation, and peritonitis may occur if the condition goes undetected. The most commonly affected patients are younger than 1 year of age, with an average age of 6–36 months.[32,49]

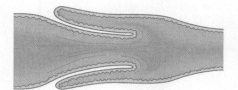

Figure 11-2 *Intussusception.*

Most cases of intussusception are without a confirmed etiology, but viral illnesses or mechanical obstructions (such as Meckel diverticulum and polyps) may be present prior to the onset of symptoms.[9,33,49] Henoch-Schönlein purpura, celiac disease, Crohn's disease, and cystic fibrosis have also been associated with an increased incidence of intussusception.[26,30,31,49]

Assessment Findings

Assessment findings may include the following[30, 44,49]:

- Crampy, intermittent, severe abdominal pain. Nonverbal children may become irritable and draw up their legs toward the abdomen. Inconsolable episodes may be followed by normal activity as the bowel self-reduces.
- Occult blood in stool.
- Vomiting initially nonbilious but then becomes bilious as the obstruction progresses.
- Lethargy.
- Fever may be present but also indicates a concurrent infection.
- Sausage-shaped abdominal mass on palpation.
- Although rare, currant jelly-like stools (blood mixed with mucus) may be present and indicate bowel ischemia.

Interventions

Ultrasound is highly effective in identifying intussusception and other potential etiologies while minimizing radiation exposure. Abdominal radiographs are used to evaluate for perforation. If perforation is present, operative intervention is required. Otherwise, nonoperative reduction options include hydrostatic (saline, contrast) or air enema with fluoroscopy or ultrasound guidance.[32,49]

Malrotation and Volvulus

Malrotation with volvulus (**Figure 11-3**) is a pediatric surgical emergency. Most cases present within the first year of life, but as many as one-fourth of cases involve patients older than 5 years of age.[4] Malrotation is a fetal growth anomaly in which an abnormal fixation of

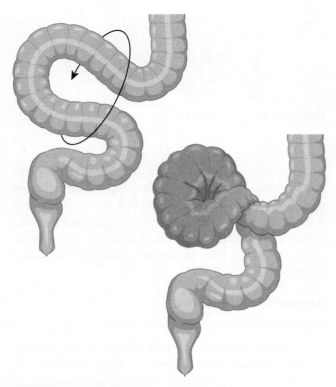

Figure 11-3 *Malrotation with volvulus.*

the intestine to the mesentery predisposes patients to the development of volvulus (twisting of the intestine). Bowel ischemia occurs as the mesenteric blood supply is compromised.[14]

Assessment Findings

Assessment findings may include the following[4,32]:

- Bilious vomiting
- Hypovolemic or septic shock
- Abdominal distention and pain
- Peritonitis
- Occult or frank blood in stool
- Nonbilious vomiting
- Feeding problems with intermittent bilious vomiting
- Failure to thrive with feeding intolerance

Interventions

Immediate resuscitation and surgical intervention are required for unstable patients. Ultrasound, abdominal radiographs, and endoscopy may be anticipated for stable patients.[51] Gastric tube insertion facilitates GI decompression and potentially aids diagnosis when abnormal tube placement is noted on imaging studies.[4,32]

Summary

Vomiting can be a sign of a multitude of clinical conditions stemming from both GI and non-GI causes. Patient age, a thorough history, and a physical exam will aid in identifying abnormal assessment findings and planning effective interventions. The child's clinical condition, general appearance, and vital signs determine the appropriate approach. Necessary interventions range from basic handwashing and anticipatory guidance education to resuscitation measures. Recognition of red flags during the assessment is vital to early identification and management of life-threatening conditions. Delayed recognition often results in poor patient outcomes. Early recognition and intervention promote optimal pediatric patient care and outcomes.

References

1. American Heart Association. (2020). *Pediatric advanced life support provider course manual.*
2. Bányai, K., Estes, M. K., Martella, V., & Parashar, U. D. (2018). Viral gastroenteritis. *Lancet, 392*(10142), 175–186. https://doi.org/10.1016/s0140-6736(18)31128-0
3. Bence, C. M., & Densmore, J. C. (2020). Neonatal and infant appendicitis. *Clinics in Perinatology, 47*(1), 183–196. https://doi.org/10.1016/j.clp.2019.10.004
4. Brandt, M. L. (2021). Intestinal malrotation in children. *UpToDate.* Retrieved March 5, 2022, from https://www.uptodate.com/contents/intestinal-malrotation-in-children
5. Brandt, M. L., & Lopez, M. E. (2021). Acute appendicitis in children: Clinical manifestations and diagnosis. *UpToDate.* Retrieved March 3, 2022, from https://www.uptodate.com/contents/acute-appendicitis-in-children-clinical-manifestations-and-diagnosis
6. Brandt, M. L., & Lopez, M. E. (2021). Acute appendicitis in children: Management. *UpToDate.* Retrieved March 5, 2022, from https://www.uptodate.com/contents/acute-appendicitis-in-children-management
7. Burks, W. (2021). Clinical manifestations of food allergy: An overview. *UpToDate.* Retrieved March 2, 2022, from https://www.uptodate.com/contents/clinical-manifestations-of-food-allergy-an-overview
8. Burks, W. (2021). History and physical examination in the patient with possible food allergy. *UpToDate.* Retrieved March 1, 2022, from https://www.uptodate.com/contents/history-and-physical-examination-in-the-patient-with-possible-food-allergy
9. Burnett, E., Parashar, U. D., & Tate, J. E. (2020). Associations of intussusception with adenovirus, rotavirus, and other pathogens: A review of the literature. *Pediatric Infectious Diseases Journal, 39*(12), 1127–1130. https://doi.org/10.1097/inf.0000000000002860

10. Campbell, R. L. (2021). Anaphylaxis: Emergency treatment. *UpToDate*. Retrieved February 22, 2022, from https://www.uptodate.com/contents/anaphylaxis-emergency-treatment

11. Campbell, R. L., & Kelso, J. M. (2020). Anaphylaxis: Acute diagnosis. *UpToDate*. Retrieved March 4, 2022, from https://www.uptodate.com/contents/anaphylaxis-acute-diagnosis

12. Carter, B., & Seupaul, R. A. (2021). Update: Antiemetics for vomiting associated with acute gastroenteritis in children. *Annals of Emergency Medicine, 60*(3), 5–6. https://doi.org/10.1016/j.annemergmed.2012.01.031

13. Connors, L., O'Keefe, A., Rosenfield, L, & Kim, H. (2018). Non-IGE-mediated food hypersensitivity. *Allergy, Asthma, and Clinical Immunology, 14*(suppl 2). Article 56. https://doi.org/10.1186/s13223-018-0285-2

14. Di Lorenzo, C. (2021). Approach to the infant or child with nausea and vomiting. *UpToDate*. Retrieved July 4, 2021, from https://www.uptodate.com/contents/approach-to-the-infant-or-child-with-nausea-and-vomiting

15. Falszewska, A., Dziechciarz, P., & Szajewska, H. (2017). Diagnostic accuracy of clinical dehydration scales in children. *European Journal of Pediatrics, 176*(8), 1021–1026. https://doi.org/10.1007/s00431-017-2942-8

16. Feld, L. G., Neuspiel, D. R., Foster, B. A., Leu, M. G., Garber, M. D., Austin, K., Basu, R. K., Conway, E. E., Fehr, J. J., Hawkins, C., Kaplan, R. L., Rowe, E. V., Waseem, M., & Moritz, M. L. (2018). Clinical practice guideline: Maintenance intravenous fluids in children. *Pediatrics, 142*(6), Article e20183083. https://doi.org/10.1542/peds.2018-3083

17. Food Allergy Research and Education. (2022). *How a child might describe a reaction*. https://www.foodallergy.org/resources/how-child-might-describe-reaction

18. Freedman, S. (2022). Oral rehydration therapy. *UpToDate*. Retrieved February 27, 2022, from https://www.uptodate.com/contents/oral-rehydration-therapy

19. Freedman, S. B., Vandermeer, B., Milne, A., & Hartling, L. (2015). Diagnosing clinically significant dehydration in children with acute gastroenteritis using noninvasive methods: A meta-analysis. *Journal of Pediatrics, 166*(4), 908–916.e6. https://doi.org/10.1016/j.jpeds.2014.12.029

20. Friedman, J. N., Goldman, R. D., Srivastava, R., & Parkin, P. C. (2004). Development of a clinical dehydration scale for use in children between 1 and 36 months of age. *Journal of Pediatrics, 145*(2), 201–207. https://doi.org/10.1016/j.jpeds.2004.05.035

21. Georgiou, R., Eaton, S., Stanton, M. P., Pierro, A., & Hall, N. J. (2017). Efficacy and safety of non-operative treatment for acute appendicitis: A meta-analysis. *Pediatrics, 139*(3), Article e20163003. https://doi.org/10.1542/peds.2016-3003

22. Goldman, R. D., Carter, S., Stephens, D., Antoon, R., Mounstephen, W., & Langer, J. C. (2008). Prospective validation of the pediatric appendicitis score. *Journal of Pediatrics, 153*(2), 278–282. https://doi.org/10.1016/j.jpeds.2008.01.033

23. Gorski, L. A., Hadway, L., Hagle, M. E., Broadhurst, D., Clare, S., Kleidon, T., Meyer, B. M., Nickel, B., Rowley, S., Sharpe, E., & Alexander, M. (2021). Infusion therapy standards of practice, 8th edition. *Journal of Infusion Nursing, 44*(1s), S1–S224. https://doi.org/10.1097/NAN.0000000000000396

24. Hammer, H. F., & Högenauer, C. (2022). Lactose intolerance and malabsorption: Clinical manifestations, diagnosis, and management. *UpToDate*. Retrieved March 3, 2022, from https://www.uptodate.com/contents/lactose-intolerance-and-malabsorption-clinical-manifestations-diagnosis-and-management

25. Henicksen, M. A, Zaremba, J., Wey, A. R., Gaillard, P. R., & Kharbanda, A. B. (2018). The use of a triage-based protocol for oral rehydration in a pediatric emergency department. *Pediatric Emergency Care, 34*(4), 227–232. https://doi.org/10.1097/pec.0000000000001070

26. Hill, I. D. (2021). Epidemiology, pathogenesis, and clinical manifestations of celiac disease in children. *UpToDate*. Retrieved March 3, 2022, from https://www.uptodate.com/contents/epidemiology-pathogenesis-and-clinical-manifestations-of-celiac-disease-in-children

27. Hornor, G. (2021). Medical child abuse: Essentials for pediatric health care providers. *Journal of Pediatric Health Care, 35*(6), 644–650. https://doi.org/10.1016/j.pedhc.2021.01.006

28. Iro, M. A., Sell, T., Brown, N., & Maitland, K. (2018). Rapid intravenous rehydration of children with acute gastroenteritis and dehydration: A systematic review and meta-analysis. *BMC Pediatrics, 18*(1), Article 44. https://doi.org/10.1186/s12887-018-1006-1

29. Krajewski, G. S., & Krajewski, T. (2022). Evaluation and management of food allergies in the emergency department. *Emergency Medicine Clinics of North America, 40*(1), 57–67. https://doi.org/10.1016/j.emc.2021.08.009

30. Levinson, H., Rimon, A., Scolnik, D., Amarilyio, G., & Glatstein, M. (2019). Fever as a presenting symptom in children evaluated for ileocolic intussusception: The experience of a large tertiary care pediatric hospital. *Pediatric Emergency Care, 35*(2), 121–124. https://doi.org/10.1097/pec.0000000000001391

31. Lin, X. K., Xia, Q. Z., Huang, X. Z., Han, Y. J., He, G. R., & Zheng, N. (2017). Clinical characteristics of intussusception secondary to pathologic lead points in children: A single-center experience with 65 cases. *Pediatric Surgery International, 33*(7), 793–797. https://doi.org/10.1007/s00383-017-4101-8

32. Lipsett, S. C, & Bachur, R. G. (2021). Abdominal emergencies. In K. Shaw & R. Bachur (Eds.), *Fleisher & Ludwig's textbook of pediatric emergency medicine* (7th ed., pp. 1290–1312). Wolters Kluwer.

33. Lu, H. L., Ding, Y., Goyal, H., & Xu, H. G. (2019). Association between rotavirus vaccination and risk of intussusception among neonates and infants: A systematic review and meta-analysis. *JAMA Network Open, 2*(10), Article e1912458. https://doi.org/10.1001/jamanetworkopen.2019.12458

34. Mier, M., Nelson, A., & Finkel, L. (2020). Vomiting children: It's not always gastroenteritis. *Pediatric Annals, 49*(5), e233–e241. https://doi.org/10.3928/19382359-20200416-01

35. Motosue, M. S., Bellolio, M. F., Van Houten, H. K., Shah, N. D., & Campbell, R. L. (2018). National trends in emergency department visits and hospitalizations for food-induced anaphylaxis in US children. *Pediatric Allergy Immunology, 29*(5), 538–544. https://doi.org/10.1111/pai.12908

36. Nowak-Wegrzyn, A. (2021). Food protein-induced entero-colitis syndrome (FPIES). *UpToDate.* Retrieved March 15, 2022, from https://www.uptodate.com/contents/food-protein -induced-enterocolitis-syndrome-fpies

37. Nowak-Wegrzyn, A., Hass, S. L., Donelson, S. M., Robison, D., Cameron, A., Etschmaier, M., Duhig, A., & McCann, W. A. (2021). The Peanut Allergy Burden Study: Impact on the qual-ity of life of patients and caregivers. *World Allergy Organiza-tion Journal, 14*(2), Article 100512. https://doi.org/10.1016/j .waojou.2021.100512

38. Olivé, A. P., & Endom, E. E. (2020). Infantile hypertrophic pyloric stenosis. *UpToDate.* Retrieved March 15, 2022, from https://www.uptodate.com/contents/infantile-hypertrophic -pyloric-stenosis

39. O'Ryan, M. G. (2021). Acute viral gastroenteritis in children in resource-rich countries: Clinical features and diagno-sis. *UpToDate.* Retrieved March 15, 2022, from https://www .uptodate.com/contents/acute-viral-gastroenteritis-in-children -in-resource-rich-countries-clinical-features-and-diagnosis

40. Österlund, J., Winberg, A., & West, C. E. (2019). A 10-year review found increasing incidence trends of emergency egg allergy reactions and food-induced anaphylaxis in children. *Acta Paediatrica, 108*(2), 314–320. https://doi.org/10.1111 /apa.14464

41. Pringle, K., Shah, S. P., Umulisa, I., Munyaneza, R. M., Dushimiyimana, J. M., Stegman, K., Musavuli, J., Ngabitsinze, P., Stulac, S., & Levine, A. C. (2011). Comparing the accuracy of three popular clinical dehydration scales in children with diar-rhea. *International Journal of Emergency Medicine, 4*, Article 58. https://doi.org/10.1186/1865-1380-4-58

42. Saganski, G. F., & De Souza Freire, M. H. (2019). Safety and ef-fectiveness of hypodermoclysis compared to intravenous fluid infusion for rehydrating children with mild to moderate dehy-dration: A systematic review protocol. *JBI Database of System-atic Reviews and Implementation Reports, 17*(7), 1270–1276. https://doi.org/10.11124/jbisrir-2017-003696

43. Santillanes, G., & Rose, E. (2018). Evaluation and manage-ment of dehydration in children. *Emergency Medicine Clin-ics of North America, 36*, 259–273. https://doi.org/10.1016/j .emc.2017.12.004

44. Shields, M. T., & Lightdale, J. R. (2018). Vomiting in children. *Pediatrics in Review, 39*(7), 342–358. https://doi.org/10.1542 /pir.2017-0053

45. Shrimanker, I., & Bhattarai, S. (2021, July 26). *Electrolytes.* StatPearls Publishing. https://pubmed.ncbi.nlm.nih.gov/3108 2167/

46. Sicherer, S. H. (2022). Food-induced anaphylaxis. *UpToDate.* Retrieved March 1, 2022, from https://www.uptodate.com /contents/food-induced-anaphylaxis

47. Somers, M. J. (2020). Clinical assessment and diagnosis of hypovolemia (dehydration) in children. *UpToDate.* Re-trieved February 27, 2022, from https://www.uptodate.com /contents/clinical-assessment-and-diagnosis-of-hypovolemia -dehydration-in-children

48. Somers, M. J. (2020). Treatment of hypovolemia (dehy-dration) in children. *UpToDate.* Retrieved February 27, 2022, from https://www.uptodate.com/contents/treatment-of -hypovolemia-dehydration-in-children

49. Vo, N., & Sato, T. T. (2020). Intussusception in children, *UpToDate,* Retrieved June 8, 2021, from https://www.uptodate .com/contents/intussusception-in-children?search= intussusception%20in%20children&source=search_result& selectedTitle=1~120&usage_type=default&display_rank=1

50. Waltzman, M. (2020). Initial management of shock in chil-dren. *UpToDate.* Retrieved February 28, 2022, from https:// www.uptodate.com/contents/initial-management-of -shock-in-children

51. Wong, K., Van Tassel, D., Lee, J., Buchmann, R., Riemann, M., Egan, C., & Youssfi, M. (2020). Making the diagnosis of mid-gut volvulus: Limited abdominal ultrasound has changed our clinical practice. *Journal of Pediatric Surgery, 55*(12), 2614–2617. https://doi.org/10.1016/j.jpedsurg.2020.04.012

CHAPTER
12

The Child with Abdominal Pain

Margaret M. Dymond, BSN, RN, ENC(C), DCS, FAEN

OBJECTIVES

Upon completion of this chapter, the learner will be able to:

1. Describe a focused assessment and history for a child presenting with abdominal pain.
2. Apply the Pediatric Nursing Process to a child experiencing a gastrointestinal or genitourinary emergency.
3. Describe selected gastrointestinal and genitourinary emergencies and interventions.

Introduction

Abdominal pain accounts for approximately 5–10% of all emergency department visits annually in the pediatric population and is a frequent complaint in school-aged children.[42] In many instances, the cause of abdominal pain is benign and self-limiting, requiring few, if any, interventions. However, evaluation should include assessing for any potential presence of a life-threatening condition that requires urgent or emergent interventions. **Appendix 12-1** lists common causes of abdominal pain in children.

Abdominal pain may be associated with the gastrointestinal (GI), genitourinary (GU), or another body system. Causes of abdominal pain can be linked to a change in eating habits, medical illness, trauma, travel, medications, or exacerbation of a chronic ongoing disease process (e.g., vaso-occlusive crisis in sickle cell disease).

General Assessment

Use the Pediatric Nursing Process to prioritize initial assessments and interventions. The history and head-to-toe examination in the secondary survey are often key to developing a plan of care for the child experiencing abdominal pain.

History

For young or nonverbal children, history may be available only from the caregivers. Children older than age 5 can usually provide information regarding their symptoms. In nonverbal children, caregivers may observe and report behavioral changes and other symptoms that appear different from the child's baseline behavior. The description of pain, location of pain, and other history can help the clinician determine the potential cause of abdominal pain and clinical urgency (**Table 12-1**).[32]

TABLE 12-1   Characteristics of Abdominal Pain

Characteristics	Condition
Periumbilical, migrating to right lower quadrant	Appendicitis
Peritoneal signs: abdominal rigidity, guarding	Peritonitis, intra-abdominal source of sepsis
Acute onset, severe, unilateral lower quadrant	Ovarian torsion, ovarian cyst, ectopic pregnancy
Intermittent, colicky, knees to chest	Intussusception
Diffuse, vague	Gastroenteritis, hepatitis, diabetic ketoacidosis
Right upper quadrant pain	Cholecystitis
Left upper quadrant pain	Mononucleosis, splenic sequestration
Epigastric	Gastritis, peptic ulcer disease
Steady periumbilical/subxiphoid, radiates to back	Pancreatitis
Flank pain radiating to lower abdomen or groin	Renal colic
Intermittent, often left-sided	Constipation

Data from Neuman, M. (2021). Emergency evaluation of the child with acute abdominal pain. *UpToDate*. Retrieved August 13, 2021, from https://www.uptodate.com/contents/emergency-evaluation-of-the-child-with-acute-abdominal-pain

The history for a child with abdominal pain may include the following information:

- **S**igns and symptoms
  - When did the pain start? Does the pain radiate to another region of the body?
  - Description of the pain: Is it constant or intermittent? Is it sharp or dull? Where does it hurt most?
  - Any associated signs and symptoms: fever, vomiting, nausea, diarrhea, last bowel movement, urinary tract symptoms, GI bleeding?
  - What, if anything, makes the pain better or worse?
- **A**llergies
  - Medications and foods, food intolerances
- **M**edications
  - Current medications, including any recent changes
  - Birth control
- **P**ast medical history
  - Medical and surgical conditions
  - Immunizations
  - Sexual health history, including safer sexual health practices for older children
- **L**ast oral intake, last output, and last menstrual period
  - Last meal, child's recent food and fluid intake
  - Last bowel movement, last void
  - Menstrual history and last normal menstrual period

- **E**vents leading up to the illness
  - What was the child doing at onset of pain?
  - Any changes to the child's routines?

Clinical Assessment

In the Pediatric Nursing Process, the primary survey is meant to identify and address immediately life-threatening conditions. Performing a thorough head-to-toe assessment, augmented by the patient history, may reveal other significant findings[42]:

- Assess appearance and hydration status.
- Assess for abnormal vital signs and presence of hypovolemic or septic shock.
  - Presence of a fever
  - Tachypnea—pneumonia, diabetic ketoacidosis, compensation for altered tissue perfusion
  - Tachycardia—pain, compensation for altered tissue perfusion
  - Hypotension—hypovolemia
  - Altered mental status—poor perfusion, ingestions, hypoglycemia
  - Exposure—presence of rash, signs of trauma
- A full system assessment is needed to evaluate for causes of abdominal pain.
  - A sore throat with abdominal pain may be noted with mononucleosis.

Confidentiality, Sexual Health, Gender Identity, and Pediatric Abdominal Pain

Before you ask any questions, share any facility- or legislative-specific privacy practices so the patient knows what can and cannot be kept confidential.

Conducting a sexual health history in a standardized, matter-of-fact, normalizing manner increases the likelihood of obtaining complete information. Ask specific questions, because some sexual acts that place the patient at risk for infection are not perceived as "having sex."

With lower abdominal pain, asking about the patient's gender is a priority. Lower abdominal complaints can be life-threatening (ectopic pregnancy) or fertility-threatening (ovarian or testicular torsion). Asking inappropriate questions about genitalia or surgical status is a form of harassment. However, in some cases it is directly relevant to patient care.

These questions may help the clinician obtain an accurate medical and sexual health history:

- "We ask all patients some sensitive questions that are important to your health. Some patients your age are sexually active. Have you started having sex?"
  - "What kind of sexual contact have you had? Some examples are penis in or on the vagina; penis in or on the anus; mouth on penis, vagina, or anus; and finger in the vagina or anus."
  - "Have you done anything to prevent pregnancy or sexually transmitted infections?"
  - "Who are your sexual partners?"
- "Because you are having abdominal pain, I will need to ask some questions related to your sexual history and any transition-related procedures or therapies. There are potentially serious causes of your pain that we would miss if we did not ask. Have you started any medical or surgical interventions as part of your gender affirmation process?"

- Upper abdominal pain is relatively common in pediatric pneumonia.
- Assess the abdomen:
  - Inspect
    - Assess for abdominal distention, masses, rash, bruising, and signs of trauma.
  - Auscultate
    - Assess bowel sound quality—normal, high-pitched (obstruction), absence (peritonitis, shock).
  - Palpate
    - Palpate the least painful area(s) first.
    - Note the location of maximum tenderness, masses, guarding, or firmness.
    - Gently palpate to identify the liver and spleen, assessing for enlargement, masses, or tenderness.
  - Genitourinary exam
    - Assess for bleeding, discharge, genital lesions, presence of foreign objects, genital trauma, and pain.
    - A rectal exam and testing for fecal occult blood may be required.
    - A pelvic exam may be required.

General Interventions and Diagnostics

The child's age, clinical examination, and history can assist with planning care and interventions, as certain conditions are more prevalent in particular age groups (see Appendix 12-1). General interventions based on the child's clinical status include assessing hydration status and need for intravenous fluid therapy, managing shock, blood component therapy, antibiotic therapy if sepsis is a concern, and symptom management. Diagnostic evaluation may assist in determining medical versus surgical causes of abdominal pain. Consider the risk associated with radiation exposure during imaging versus the benefit in children experiencing abdominal pain.[20]

Selected Conditions

Selected conditions covered in this section include constipation, foreign body ingestion, incarcerated hernia, GI bleeding, and GU issues.

Constipation

Constipation in children is largely attributed to a functional or benign problem but can be associated with certain pathologies such as Hirschsprung disease. Constipation is one of the most common causes of abdominal pain in children.[58] It is especially common around the time of toilet training and starting school. Infants may experience constipation when solid foods are introduced. Causes of constipation can be multifactorial. Chronic constipation may lead to loss of anal sensation and awareness of the urge to defecate.[27]

Assessment Findings and Interventions

In general, assess the number of bowel movements per week; presence of hard, difficult-to-pass stools; presence of anal bleeding; loss of appetite; presence of abdominal distention and pain; presence of fecal incontinence; and any recent changes to diet or fluid intake. The Rome criteria (**Box 12-1**)[21,27,39] can be used to determine whether constipation is present but only after medical causes have been ruled out (**Box 12-2**).[44]

BOX 12-1 Rome Criteria Constipation and No Pathologic Cause

Presence of two or more of the following criteria in a month:

- Two or fewer bowel movements in a week
- History of hard, painful bowel movements
- History of retentive posturing or excessive volitional stool retention
- History of large-caliber stools that can block the toilet
- Presence of a large fecal mass in the rectum
- One or more episodes of fecal incontinence in a week

Infants and toddlers:

- Two or fewer bowel movements in a week
- History of hard or painful bowel movements
- History of excessive stool retention
- History of large-caliber stools in toilet-trained children
- History of large-diameter stools that can obstruct the toilet
- Presence of a fecal mass in the rectum
- One or greater episodes of fecal incontinence per week

Data from Hyams, J. S., Di Lorenzo, C., Saps, M., Shulman, R. J., Staiano, A., & van Tilburg, M. (2016). Childhood functional gastrointestinal disorders: Child/adolescent. *Gastroenterology, 150*(6), 1456–1468.E2. https://doi.org/10.1053/j.gastro.2016.02.015; Leung, A. K. C., & Hon, K. L. (2021). Paediatrics: How to manage functional constipation. *Drugs in Context, 10*, Article 2020-11-2. https://doi.org/10.7573/dic.2020-11-2; and Robin, S. G., Keller, C., Zwiener, R., Hyman, P. E., Nurko, S., Saps, M., Di Lorenzo, C., Shulman, R. J., Hyams, J. S., Palsson, O., & van Tilburg, M. A. (2018). Prevalence of pediatric functional gastrointestinal disorders utilizing the Rome IV criteria. *Journal of Pediatrics, 195*, 134–139. https://doi.org/10.1016/j.jpeds.2017.12.012

BOX 12-2 Organic Causes of Constipation

Although functional constipation is far more common, pathologic etiologies are responsible for less than 5% of cases of pediatric constipation. These etiologies include the following:

- Anorectal anomalies (imperforate anus, anal fissures)
- Cow's-milk intolerance
- Cystic fibrosis
- Hirschsprung disease
- Meconium ileus in neonate
- Medications: opiates, iron supplementation
- Metabolic and endocrine disorders (hypothyroidism)
- Muscular dystrophy
- Myopathies
- Spinal cord injury

Data from Sood, M. R. (2021). Constipation in infants and children: Evaluation. *UpToDate.* Retrieved August 8, 2021, from https://www.uptodate.com/contents/constipation-in-infants-and-children-evaluation

---

Factors and behaviors to consider asking the child or caregiver about when constipation is suspected include the following[45]:

- Presence of screaming before defecation, anticipating pain when passing stools
- Withholding behaviors—crying, sweating, stiffening of legs, rocking back and forth, crossing ankles, squatting, or hiding in a corner during defecation
- Irregular bowel habits—environmental influences such as privacy and sanitary conditions may lead to stool holding
- Toilet phobia—introducing toilet training too early, causing stress and anxiety in the child
- Switching from breast milk to cow's milk
- Prolonged period of using pureed food after infancy
- Excessive intake of refined-sugar foods
- High-protein and high-fat foods
- Low dietary fiber intake
- Decreased fluid intake
- Decreased physical activity
- Eating disorders
- Stress and anxiety

Diagnostic interventions may be ordered based on findings in the history and physical examination[44]:

- Electrolytes, thyroid function testing, serology for celiac disease

- Urinalysis and culture—fecal impaction may impair bladder emptying, predisposing the child to a urinary tract infection
- Radiography
  - Abdominal radiographs to determine fecal load in the bowel
  - Barium enema if Hirschsprung disease is suspected

Dietary modifications, medications to treat constipation, procedures such as enemas and manual disimpaction, or a combination of these interventions may be required to treat constipation, with the goal of treatment being achievement of normal stool patterns and soft, easy-to-pass stools. Surgical interventions may be required in extreme cases. Selected treatments for constipation to be considered include the following[27,46,47]:

- Dietary modifications—provide parents with guidance on dietary changes to treat constipation:
  - Prune, apple, or pear juices that contain sorbitol.
  - Foods that are high fiber purees—cereal containing barley or multigrain cereal.
  - Optimize fiber intake and ensure adequate fluid intake.
  - Fiber supplements can be considered and are safe for older children.
- Laxatives
  - Can be used if dietary measures are unsuccessful at achieving daily stools. Oral medications may take a few days to work. A combination of dietary modifications, oral, and rectal treatments may be needed.
  - Oral laxatives
    - Lactulose can be added to infant formula.
    - Polyethylene glycol 3350.
    - Mineral oil is not recommended in infancy or for children with a neurologic impairment or gastroesophageal reflux due to the risk of pneumonitis if aspirated.
  - Rectal treatments are more invasive and can cause more abdominal and anal discomfort.
    - Enemas may be required in older children. Examples include mineral oil, sodium phosphate, or saline enemas.
    - Sodium phosphate enemas are contraindicated in children younger than 2 years due to the potential for hyperphosphatemia, hypocalcemia, and bowel perforation.[27,46]
    - Glycerin suppositories are safe for infants but may cause anal irritation.
- Behavioral modification
  - Regular routines like sitting on the toilet at regular intervals
  - Rewarding and praising the child for defecation

- Other interventions
  - Rectal stimulation with a lubricated rectal thermometer may be considered, but parental teaching is required to ensure no anal or bowel trauma.
  - Disimpaction may be required. In severe cases, sedation may be required for comfort and pain management.

Foreign Body Ingestion

Foreign body (FB) ingestions are more prevalent in children between 6 months and 3 years of age and are usually a one-time occurrence. Repeated episodes are seen in children who have developmental delays or behavioral health issues.[14] Coins are the most frequent FB ingestion.[15] Other items commonly ingested include button batteries, small toy parts, jewelry, screws, pins, marbles, food bolus, and laundry detergent packets.[3,15,36] Body packing or stuffing for illicit drug smuggling sometimes involves children and adolescents and becomes a high-risk situation should the packets rupture.[53]

Many foreign ingestions may not cause symptoms and likely will pass through the GI tract over time. Special risks include the following:

- Sharp objects increase the risk of GI perforation.
- Food impaction may be seen in children with esophageal disease. Swallowing can be reported as painful.
- Ingested superabsorbent polymers will expand in size due to the water content in the stomach and bowel and can lead to bowel obstruction.[31,56]
- Batteries and magnets.
- Long objects such as forks and spoons can cause GI obstruction.
- Objects containing lead, such as fishing weights, can lead to acute lead poisoning.
- Retention of a FB in the esophagus is possible due to congenital defects present in the esophagus and the smaller diameter of the esophagus in children.
- Body packing or stuffing of drugs with potential rupture of the packets can cause acute drug toxicity.[53]

Assessment Findings and Interventions

Children may present to the emergency department because the ingestion was witnessed but may not be having symptoms. Signs and symptoms of a FB ingestion may include the following[24]:

- Abdominal pain—may indicate perforation and sepsis, bowel obstruction
- Airway—choking, cough, dysphagia, drooling indicating airway obstruction

CLINICAL PEARL

Superabsorbent Polymers

Toys with superabsorbent polymers are products that, when exposed to water, increase in size. When ingested, they can absorb the water content of the GI tract and grow to 10 times their original size. If ingested, they can result in bowel obstruction and possible perforation, leading to sepsis.

Superabsorbent polymers are found in many types of toys and products:

· Expandable water bath toys
· Balls
· Diapers and disposable hygiene products
· Beads used in decorative flower arrangements that resemble candy and are enticing to small children
· Craft products such as clay

Data from Zamora, I. J., Vu, L. T., Larimer, E. L., & Olutoye, O. O. (2012). Water-absorbing balls: A "growing" problem. *Pediatrics*, *130*(4), e1011–e1014. https://doi.org/10.1542/peds.2011-3685

- Respiratory symptoms—wheezing and/or stridor if the foreign body was aspirated
- In older children, a sensation that the object is stuck in the neck or chest
- Chest pain
- Subcutaneous emphysema—may be palpated if the esophagus was perforated
- Vomiting
- Refusal to eat

Interventions for FB ingestion may include the following[14]:

- Nothing by mouth unless cleared by the physician or advanced practice provider
- Chest and abdominal radiographs to determine the location of the FB[16]
- Abdominal ultrasonography to determine the location of the FB or to determine other causes of abdominal pain
- Computed tomography (CT) or magnetic resonance imaging (MRI) of the abdomen if the patient is symptomatic
- Consultation with a pediatric GI specialist or surgeon for FB removal—via endoscopy or surgery
- High-risk considerations:
  - Airway compromise

- Inability to swallow secretions
- Long, sharp objects
- Superabsorbent polymers
- Magnets or batteries
- Presence of peritonitis

A period of observation may be considered if the child is asymptomatic, the situation is not high risk, and there is no evidence of bowel obstruction or airway compromise. Discharge teaching includes teaching caregivers to observe whether the foreign object is passed in the stool, to ensure safety in the home, and to watch for any change in the child's clinical condition.[14]

Button Batteries and Magnets

Button battery ingestions have the potential to cause serious sequelae leading to death. Injuries due to ingestion include esophageal burns, perforation, fistula development, and major bleeding from the erosion of the chemical leak from the source through the blood vessels in the esophagus resulting in rupture. Button batteries may also be inserted in other body orifices, such as the ear and nose.[41]

The frequency of these ingestions has increased due to the more common use of button batteries in household, personal use, and recreational products (e.g., toys, watches, flashlights, hearing aids, remotely operated household devices). The button batteries are small enough to resemble a pill and can be accidentally ingested. The age group in which these ingestions occur is primarily younger than 6 years of age.[41]

The damage to mucosal tissue and injury from a button battery ingestion occurs from the following mechanisms[41]:

- Electrical discharge from the battery
- Leaking battery fluids, causing ulceration and necrosis of tissue
- Tissue erosion into other tissue or blood vessels, resulting in fistula formation
- Absorption of the solution containing metals, leading to lead or mercury poisoning

Magnets are also a component of many household appliances and toys and are more dangerous if multiple magnets have been ingested. Magnets—especially high-powered magnets—can cause pressure necrosis and fistula formation between magnets in adjacent loops of bowel, which may result in bowel obstruction, perforation, and peritonitis. Even a single high-powered magnet ingestion can be harmful if it attaches to external metals such as body jewelry, zippers, buttons, or belt buckles.[14]

Important Considerations for the SAMPLE History

Important points to cover in the SAMPLE history for battery and magnet ingestion include the following:

- Time of ingestion.
- Number of batteries or magnets ingested.
- New or older batteries—new batteries may have a higher electrical discharge.
- Packaging, if available, may provide information on the battery type. Each letter or number is significant for identifying the actual product composition.
- Presence of other symptoms:
  - Airway considerations—drooling, dysphagia, black flecks in the saliva
  - Respiratory symptoms—cough, wheeze, choking, gagging
  - Signs of shock if bleeding occurs
  - Fever
  - Chest or abdominal pain
  - Vomiting and/or hematemesis
  - Blood in stools
  - Pain, discharge, or bleeding from the nose or ears

Approach to Management: Button Battery

The approach to management of ingestion of button batteries is as follows[26,41]:

- Provide first aid.
  - The poison control center may recommend that the patient consume 5–10 mL of honey at home, followed by repeated doses in the emergency department every 10 minutes for up to six doses if the patient is asymptomatic. The honey neutralizes the chemical exposure at the site if impaction in the esophagus is a risk, leading to less esophageal tissue trauma and burns. Follow local protocols.
  - NPO except honey if appropriate.
  - NPO if symptomatic; do not give honey.
  - In the emergency department, a dose of oral sucralfate may be given.
- Stabilize the child if they present with shock. Intravenous access and resuscitation may be required.
- For stable patients (asymptomatic) after first aid measures, localization of the battery is the priority.
  - Perform chest and abdominal radiographs to determine the location of the button battery (**Figure 12-1**).
- Consult with a pediatric ear/nose/throat surgeon if the airway is involved and/or a pediatric gastroenterologist.

- Consult with a pediatric cardiothoracic surgeon if hematemesis is present. See **Box 12-3** for possible complications post-button battery ingestion.[41]
  - Insertion of an esophageal balloon device may be considered to temporalize the esophageal bleeding.

CLINICAL PEARL

National Battery Ingestion Hotline (United States)

The National Capital Poison Center maintains a call center and web page specifically for battery ingestions or insertions.

- Call **800-498-8666** for guidance if a child (or anyone) swallows a battery.
- Access the web page at https://www.poison.org/battery.

- Children with esophageal burns are hospitalized.
- Discharge home may be indicated post endoscopy if there is no indication of esophageal damage.
- Discharge home may be indicated if the patient has no symptoms or the button battery has passed through the stomach. Parents need to observe for passage of the battery in stool and to return to the emergency department if the child experiences signs of peritonitis, fever, and/or abdominal pain.
- Parent teaching regarding safety practices in the home is appropriate to prevent future exposures.
- Observe for complications from button battery ingestion (Box 12-3).

Approach to Management: Magnets

Determine the strength (if possible), number, location, and size of ingested magnets. If the magnet is still in the esophagus or stomach, endoscopy is used to facilitate its removal. Magnets that are past the stomach may be evaluated with serial radiographs and physical examinations. Radiographs will not usually show bowel compression. If the magnet is not moving down the GI tract or the patient becomes symptomatic, removal via surgery or lower GI endoscopy may be required.[14]

Incarcerated Hernia

A hernia occurs when an organ or fatty tissue protrudes through a weak spot in the cavity that normally contains it. Often hernias manifest as intestinal protrusion in the

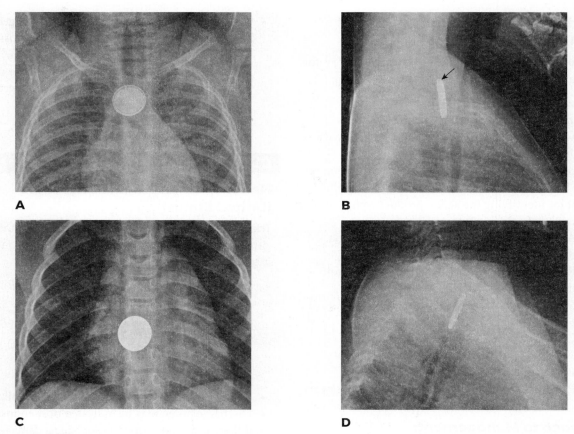

Figure 12-1 *Anteroposterior (AP) and lateral chest x-rays of a button battery (A, B) and a coin (C, D). **A.** AP x-ray demonstrating the "halo" sign of a radiolucent ring inside the outer edge of the battery. **B.** Lateral x-ray demonstrating the "step-off" sign (indicated by arrow). **C.** AP x-ray demonstrating a coin with no "halo" sign. **D.** Lateral x-ray demonstrating the smooth edges around the coin with no "step-off" sign.*

Reproduced from Hamour, A. F., Ostrow, O., James, A. L., & Wolter, N. E. (2021). Practical tips for paediatricians: Esophageal button battery impaction in children. *Paediatrics & Child Health, 27*(2), 72–74. https://doi.org/10.1093/pch/pxab078

BOX 12-3 Possible Complications of Button Battery Ingestion

- Tracheoesophageal fistula
- Vocal cord paralysis
- Aortic arch perforation
- Esophageal perforation
- Esophageal stenosis
- Mediastinitis
- Spondylodiscitis
- Aspiration pneumonia
- Gastric hemorrhage and perforation
- Intestinal perforation

Reproduced from Sinclair, K., & Hill, I. D. (2021). Button and cylindrical battery ingestion: Clinical features, diagnosis, and initial management. *UpToDate.* Retrieved August 8, 2021, from https://www.uptodate.com /contents/button-and-cylindrical-battery-ingestion -clinical-features-diagnosis-and-initial-management

---

inguinal (groin) or umbilical area. Hernias are a common pediatric surgical condition, which present more frequently in infants younger than 1 year.[2] The main concern is an incarcerated hernia, defined as entrapment of the peritoneal contents that cannot be reduced back into the abdomen; this condition may lead to strangulation and/or compromise of the vascular supply of the bowel, and subsequently to bowel ischemia and necrosis.[1,34,37,54]

Assessment Findings and Interventions

Males tend to have a higher incidence of hernia, but females have a higher incidence of incarceration. The incarceration may also involve the ovary.[37,54] Signs and symptoms of an incarcerated hernia include the following[37,54]:

- Abrupt bulging mass that may be more prevalent when the child cries, coughs, or strains
- Tender mass on palpation, signs of inflammation over the mass

- Bowel sounds auscultated in the mass if the bowel has not strangulated
- Decreased appetite
- Irritability
- Inconsolability (likely with strangulated/incarcerated hernias)
- Abdominal distention if obstruction is present
- Bloody stools—indicate bowel ischemia
- Bilious emesis—indicates obstruction

The clinical examination and history will determine the interventions required. If the hernia has self-reduced, a period of observation may be required before discharge from the emergency department. The diagnosis is often made clinically, but ultrasound may show other pathology and reveal whether reproductive organs are involved. Children with no mass or a reducible mass are referred for surgical follow-up. Bedside manual reduction may require procedural sedation. Consultation with a pediatric surgeon may be required if bedside reduction is not possible.[37,54]

Gastrointestinal Bleeding

Upper and lower GI bleeding in children can indicate a benign condition or a life-threatening hemorrhage. Occasionally the presence of GI bleeding can be misinterpreted as stemming from a GI source when the source is actually not GI—for example, the child swallowed blood from an epistaxis and then vomits the blood.[51] Some GI bleeding conditions are more prevalent in certain age groups (**Table 12-2**).[35,51] Abnormal vital signs, presence of tachycardia and/or hypotension, and delayed capillary refill are indicators of significant bleeding.

Assessment and interventions will be based on the clinical evaluation and assessment and the information obtained in the SAMPLE history. Examine the abdomen for distention, rigidity, guarding, and pain. Presence of fever may indicate an infectious cause of the bleeding. Any history of jaundice and easy bruising may indicate a hepatic cause of the bleeding. Review the child's recent medications. Take note of any substance or medication use that may cause GI bleeding, including nonsteroidal anti-inflammatory drugs, corticosteroids, tetracyclines, aspirin, alcohol, tobacco, and caffeinated beverages.[51]

While not a definitive sign, the color of the emesis and stool can help indicate the source of the bleeding. Hematemesis (blood in the vomitus) that is bright red indicates new or brisk bleeding from the esophagus or stomach. Coffee-ground emesis indicates slower bleeding. Upper GI bleeding or lower GI bleeding from

TABLE 12-2	Gastrointestinal Bleeding by Typical Age Group
Cause of Bleeding	**Age Group**
Swallowed maternal blood	Neonates, nursing infants
Necrotizing enterocolitis	Neonates
Hemophilia/coagulopathy	Neonates, infants, toddlers
Intussusception	Infants, toddlers
Meckel's diverticulum	All age groups
Bowel obstruction	All age groups
Hemolytic uremic syndrome	Preschoolers, school-age children, adolescents
Henoch-Schönlein purpura	Preschoolers, school-age children, adolescents
Inflammatory bowel disease	School-age children, adolescents
Foreign body	Preschoolers, school-age children, adolescents
Caustic ingestion	Preschoolers, school-age children, adolescents
Esophagitis	All age groups
Infectious colitis	All age groups

Data from Patel, N., & Kay, M. (2021). Lower gastrointestinal bleeding in children: Causes and diagnostic approach. *UpToDate*. Retrieved August 10, 2021, from https://www.uptodate.com/contents/lower-gastrointestinal-bleeding-in-children-causes-and-diagnostic-approach; and Villa, X. (2022). Approach to upper gastrointestinal bleeding in children. *UpToDate*. Retrieved April 15, 2022, from https://www.uptodate.com/contents/approach-to-upper-gastrointestinal-bleeding-in-children

the small intestine may produce melena (sticky, dark red or black stools). Hematochezia (fresh, bright red blood in the stool) is typically associated with lower GI bleeding.[51]

General Interventions

General interventions include the following, as indicated by the patient's condition[35,51]:

- Stabilization of the child's clinical condition, including administration of intravenous fluids and blood products

- Testing of vomitus and/or stool for blood
  - Some medications and food can cause the vomit and/or stool to appear bloody.
- Lab work
  - Complete blood count, blood typing, coagulation studies
  - Inflammatory markers
  - Electrolytes, amylase, lipase
  - Renal and liver function tests
  - Stool samples—for presence of an infectious cause or inflammatory bowel disease
- Imaging—abdominal radiography, ultrasonography, CT scan of the abdomen, MRI
- Insertion of a gastric tube to confirm and monitor bleeding
- Oral or intravenous medications—pediatric data are often limited; treatment may be based on adult studies.
  - Proton pump inhibitor (e.g., pantoprazole, omeprazole) or histamine receptor antagonist (e.g., famotidine) to reduce gastric acid production
  - Octreotide to reduce portal blood flow and variceal pressure
- Consultation with a pediatric GI specialist or surgeon
- Upper and lower endoscopy to identify the bleeding source and facilitate therapeutic interventions such as banding, clips, or cautery
- Surgical repair or resection

Meckel's Diverticulum

Meckel's diverticulum is a congenital outpouching of the intestine near the area where the small and large intestines join (**Figure 12-2**). It is more commonly seen in males. The diverticulum may have gastric ectopic tissue that secretes acid, causing ulceration of the mucosa, which then leads to bleeding. This defect may be present in children with other GI tract malformations. The malformation may be asymptomatic and found incidentally during a surgical procedure or on an imaging test.[17,23]

Meckel's diverticulum can cause mild to severe GI bleeding, bowel obstruction, perforation, and intussusception. Bleeding can be mild to severe or intermittent. Other signs and symptoms include the following[17,23]:

- Painless GI bleeding
  - Stools are dark red or maroon in color.
- Abdominal pain
- Vomiting
- Fever

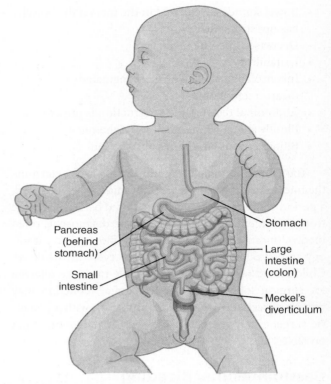

Figure 12-2 *Meckel's diverticulum.*

- Shock from severe bleeding or peritonitis after perforation
- Anemia

Inflammatory Bowel Disease

Crohn's disease (CD) and ulcerative colitis (UC) are the major types of inflammatory bowel disease (IBD). CD can involve any part of the GI tract from the oral cavity to the anus, and affects all layers of the bowel. Healthy intestine is interspersed with inflamed areas. UC is limited to the innermost layer of the colon, but the entire colon is involved.[33]

The peak incidence of IBD occurs in individuals between 15 and 30 years of age. IBD occurs rarely in school-age children, though there are some reports of such disease in infants.[19] The rate of this disease is rising worldwide, even in countries where the prevalence was previously low. Canada has the highest incidence of IBD worldwide.[10] There is theoretical speculation that the increased incidence is due to urbanization, modernization, Western diets, and genetics that interfere with the gut microbiome that maintains bowel health throughout life.[10,25]

GI symptoms prompting an emergency department visit may lead to a new diagnosis of IBD. Patients with known IBD may present with a symptom flare-up.

General GI symptoms for IBD include bloody diarrhea or frequent loose stools, abdominal pain, the sensation of needing to pass stool despite an empty bowel (tenesmus), and perianal disease (fistula, skin tags, or fissures).[19] Non-GI symptoms may include fever, fatigue, rash, eye inflammation, growth failure, and anemia.[19]

In addition to the general interventions listed previously, interventions for IBD include the following[6,7,19,57]:

- Pain and antiemetic medications
- Anti-inflammatory/immunosuppressant therapy
  - Aminosalicylates (sulfasalazine, mesalamine)
  - Corticosteroids
  - Thiopurines (mercaptopurine, azathioprine)
  - Tumor necrosis factor (TNF) blockers (infliximab, adalimumab)
- Antibiotics for abscess or infection
- Enteral nutrition
- Surgical resection (CD) or colectomy (UC)

Genitourinary Conditions

GU conditions include ovarian torsion, ectopic pregnancy, testicular torsion, priapism, and sexually transmitted infections (STIs). **Box 12-4** identifies other conditions associated with pelvic pain in females, along with general interventions for them. Chapter 10, "The Child with a Fever," offers more information on urinary tract infections and pyelonephritis.

Ovarian Torsion

Ovarian torsion occurs in females of all pediatric age groups. In this condition, the ovary rotates on itself, obstructing venous, arterial, and lymphatic flow. The ovary becomes engorged and edematous, causing pain.[42] Ovarian torsion is more common in adolescent females and is often associated with a history of ovarian cysts. Neonates and infants may present with vague nonspecific findings that require a high index of suspicion and imaging to detect the ovarian pathology.[28] There is some evidence that ovarian torsion may be associated with inguinal hernias.[30] Prompt recognition is key to prevent necrosis of the ovary and maintain ovarian viability.

Assessment Findings and Interventions

Symptoms can be nonspecific and include fever, nausea, vomiting, and dysuria. The pain is often described as developing acutely, with intermittent colicky-type pain in the right lower quadrant often mimicking the pain associated with appendicitis. Pain may radiate to the back, flank, or groin and mimic symptoms of renal colic and pyelonephritis.[38] The patient with ovarian torsion will

BOX 12-4 Pelvic Pain in Adolescent Females

Other conditions associated with pelvic pain in females include the following:

- Appendicitis
- Dysmenorrhea
- Endometriosis
- Foreign body
- Kidney stone
- Ovarian cyst
- Pelvic inflammatory disease
- Pregnancy-related issues
- Sexual abuse/assault
- Tubo-ovarian abscess
- Urinary tract infection

General interventions for female pelvic pain include the following:

- Cervical cultures, STI testing
- Complete blood count, inflammatory markers
- Gynecology consult
- Pelvic exam
- Pregnancy test
- Ultrasound
- Urinalysis

Data from Bhavsar, A. K., Gelner, E. J., & Shorma, T. (2016). Common questions about the evaluation of acute pelvic pain. *American Family Physician, 93*(1), 41–48A. https://www.aafp.org/afp/2016/0101/p41.html; and Brown, K., & Lee, J. A. (2022). Evaluation of acute pelvic pain in the adolescent female. *UpToDate.* Retrieved April 15, 2022, from https://www.uptodate.com/contents/evaluation-of-acute-pelvic-pain-in-the-adolescent-female

require pain management and a referral to a gynecologic specialist, along with preparation for laparoscopic repair or oophorectomy.[28]

Ectopic Pregnancy

Ectopic pregnancy occurs when a pregnancy becomes implanted outside the uterine cavity. The majority of ectopic pregnancies are found in the fallopian tube. This condition can lead to tubal rupture. Ruptured ectopic pregnancy results in life-threatening pelvic bleeding and accounts for 4% of the overall mortality of pregnancy.[22] There is a higher rate of ectopic pregnancy in females who smoke.[18] Ectopic pregnancy can also affect the overall health of the ovary and future fertility.

> ### RED FLAG
>
> Unilateral lower abdominal pain is considered an emergency from the age of menarche, which varies widely but is trending younger.[29,55] Patients as young as 8 years of age are at risk for life-threatening hemorrhage from a ruptured fallopian tube until a negative pregnancy test has been confirmed.

Assessment Findings and Interventions

Patients usually experience pelvic pain and vaginal bleeding 6–8 weeks after their last menstrual period. The pregnancy may or may not be known to the patient. Other symptoms of pregnancy may be present, including nausea, vomiting, and breast tenderness. Vaginal bleeding ranges from minor spotting to brisk vaginal bleeding. Pelvic pain can be diffuse or localized, and may be described as mild to severe. Referred pain felt in the shoulder (Kehr sign) may be present if rupture occurs and the intraperitoneal bleeding reaches the diaphragm. If blood pools posteriorly in the abdominal cavity, the patient may complain of the urge to defecate.[48]

The appropriate interventions depend on the patient's clinical stability. Hemodynamically unstable patients will require resuscitation and operative care. For hemodynamically stable patients, interventions can include the following[18,48–50]:

- Blood typing with administration of Rho(D) immune globulin if the patient is Rh negative
- Nonoperative management with methotrexate
  - Considered in patients at low risk for imminent rupture
    - Hemodynamically stable
    - Low quantitative human chorionic gonadotropin (hCG) levels
    - No fetal cardiac activity on ultrasound
    - Low-volume tubal mass
    - Patient able to comply with post-treatment follow-up
  - Baseline renal and liver function tests are required
  - Patient instruction to return to the emergency department should symptoms of rupture occur
- Surgical consultation for operative management
- Provision of information and support for pregnancy loss as applicable

Testicular Torsion

Testicular torsion is an ischemic event; it entails twisting of the spermatic cord that blocks blood supply to

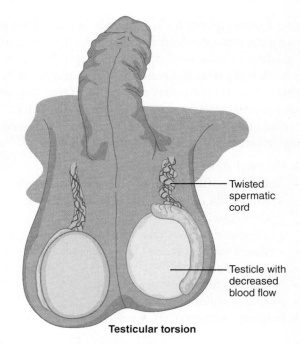

Figure 12-3 *Testicular torsion.*

the testes (**Figure 12-3**). The highest incidence of this condition is usually noted at two life points: during the neonatal period and during puberty.[8] Without prompt identification and intervention, the testicle may be lost.

Assessment Findings and Interventions

The classic finding with testicular torsion is acute onset of severe testicular or scrotal pain. Some patients will complain of inguinal or lower abdominal pain, which may awaken them at night. A small number of patients may report previous episodes of testicular pain.[42] The pain can be intermittent if the testis twists/untwists. In these cases, the testis might be horizontal or unusually mobile with a bulky spermatic cord. Most patients will experience nausea and vomiting. Other assessment findings include the following[4,8]:

- Swollen, red scrotum
- Tender, swollen, hard testis
- Elevated or horizontal-lying testis
- Cremasteric reflex absent—the testicle does not retract upward when the inner thigh is stroked

Use of a clinical scoring system (**Table 12-3**) can assist with validating the presence of testicular torsion.[4]

Interventions for scrotal pain include the following[8]:

- Urinalysis
- Evaluation for STIs, cultures
- Intravenous maintenance fluids

TABLE 12-3 Clinical Scoring System for Testicular Torsion

Symptom	Points
Nausea and vomiting	1 point
Testicular swelling	2 points
Hard testis on palpation	2 points
High-riding testis	1 point
Absent cremasteric reflex	1 point

A score of 5 or greater indicates a likelihood of testicular torsion. A score less than 2 excludes testicular torsion.

Data from Barbosa, J. A., Tiseo, B. C., Barayan, G. A., Rosman, B. M., Torricelli, F. C., Passerotti, C. C., Srougi, M., Retik, A. B., & Nguyen, H. T. (2013). Development and initial validation of a scoring system to diagnose testicular torsion in children. *Journal of Urology, 189*(5), 1859–1864. https://doi.org/10.1016/j.juro.2012.10.056

- Symptom management for pain and nausea/vomiting
- Ultrasound to assess testicular blood flow and/or identify changes consistent with torsion

An immediate urology consultation and surgery is required for confirmed testicular torsion. Fewer than 61% of torsed testicles will be viable after 12 hours of torsion. After 24 hours, testicular viability is less than 24%. When immediate operative management is not available, manual detorsion with procedural sedation may be attempted.[8]

Priapism

Priapism is defined as a persistent and painful penile erection not associated with sexual stimulation. Sustained engorgement of the clitoris is also possible. Priapism can occur in any age group and be either ischemic or non-ischemic. Priapism is primarily seen in children with sickle cell disease, which usually causes ischemic priapism. Other causes include spinal cord injury, penile trauma, cancer, hematologic conditions, prescription medications (anticoagulants, antipsychotics, trazodone), and recreational substance use.[12,40]

Assessment Findings and Interventions

The following assessment findings are associated with priapism[12,40]:

- Painful sustained rigid erection
- Prior history of priapism
- History of penile trauma
- History of sickle cell disease
- Urinary retention

Rapid interventions are needed to prevent future erectile dysfunction and may include the following measures[12,40]:

- Assessment for and treatment of dehydration and infection
- Pain management
- Blood work to evaluate for hematologic disease
- Toxicology screen
- Penile blood gases
    - Ischemic priapism is associated with dark to black blood that is hypoxic, hypercarbic, and acidotic.
    - Non-ischemic priapism is associated with red blood and normal blood gas results.
- Ultrasound
    - Evaluate blood flow to differentiate between ischemic and non-ischemic priapism.
    - Identify structural abnormalities.
- Injection of phenylephrine into the penis to reduce arterial flow
    - Monitor for hypertension and dysrhythmias.
- Needle aspiration of blood with or without sodium chloride irrigation
- Surgical referral if medical management is not effective
- Discharge teaching
    - Prophylactic medical management for patients with sickle cell disease
    - When to seek medical attention
    - Need for urology follow-up

Sexually Transmitted Infections

STIs may occur in all age groups, but predominately appear in the adolescent years. In the neonate, an STI may be passed in utero to the fetus or during a vaginal delivery if the mother has an STI. The infection may occur during consensual sexual activity, but sexual abuse, assault, and trafficking are always concerns in the pediatric population. In the United States, 50% of STIs occur in adolescents (15–24 years) and about 25% of sexually active adolescent females have had an STI.[13] Complications from an STI in females include pelvic inflammatory disease, which could result in septic shock and scar tissue formation in the fallopian tubes, predisposing the patient to an ectopic pregnancy, chronic pelvic pain, and infertility. Complications of a chlamydial infection in pregnancy can lead to premature rupture of the membranes, preterm delivery, and low-birth-weight newborns.[11]

Confidentiality and consent for treatment of STIs in pediatric patients may be challenging, as parents may have access to their child's health records. Healthcare professionals may be mandated to contact parents, depending on local practices and laws. Laws regarding reportable STIs and age of consent for sex vary. Treatment can be complicated by delays in seeking care, self-treatment with homemade therapies, coinfection with more than one STI, or infection with an STI that is highly resistant to first-line medication treatment.[13] **Appendix 12-2** identifies common STIs, their signs and symptoms, and the recommended treatments.

Assessment Findings and Interventions

Assessment for STI will include taking a history and a clinical examination, including examining the genitalia and rectum and a pelvic exam for females. The assessment should include the following components:

- Pain; discharge from the perineal area, vagina, penis, or anus; other body lesions
- Perineal, genital, rectal, and pelvic exam:
  - Presence of discharge, foul odors, (use of) foreign bodies
  - Presence of lesions: type, discharge
- Urinary tract symptoms: dysuria, pyuria, hematuria, frequency, fever
- Fever; abdominal, inguinal, or pelvic pain
- Menstrual history and last normal menstrual period
- History of physical and dating violence
- Sexual health history (**Box 12-5**)[52]

BOX 12-5 The "Ps" of a Sexual Health History for STI

The Ps of a sexual health history for any type of STI include the following:

- Partners—type of sex, gender(s) of partners
- Practices—type of sexual contact (vaginal, rectal, oral)
- Protection from STIs—use of condoms external and internal, tested for STI and human immunodeficiency virus (HIV)
- Past history of STIs—history of STI, type and treatment, partner testing, intravenous drug injection, sexual health concern
- Pregnancy intention—use of contraception, birth control practices

Data from Workowski, K. A., Bachmann, L. H., Chan, P. A., Johnston, C. M., Muzny, C. A., Park, I., Reno, H., Zenilman, J. M., & Bolan, G. A. (2021). Sexually transmitted infections treatment guidelines, 2021. *Morbidity and Mortality Weekly Report: Recommendations and Reports*, 70(4), 1–187. https://doi.org/10.15585/mmwr.rr7004a1

- Head-to-toe exam
  - Head and neck: oral lesions, cervical lymph node swelling
  - Dermatologic exam
  - Systems assessment for other signs of trauma—wounds, lacerations, injuries

Interventions may include the following[11,13,52]:

- Specimen collection for suspected STI
- Serological testing—syphilis
- Lumbar puncture—evaluation for neurosyphilis
- Counseling
- Treatment
  - For suspected or actual STI management
  - Post-exposure prophylaxis for HIV
- Contact tracing and treatment of sex partners
- Follow-up testing may be required
- Considerations for primary prevention:
  - Human papillomavirus (HPV) vaccine, hepatitis A and B vaccines, cervical screening for HPV
  - Pre-exposure prophylaxis for HIV
  - Cervical screening for cancer
  - Safer sex practices
- Intimate partner violence screening
- Reporting to child protective services

Summary

Abdominal pain in children is a frequently encountered concern. Children can present with a non-acute concern or a potentially life-threatening condition. Some clinical conditions are more prevalent in younger age groups, which assists with developing a plan of care and determining the appropriate interventions. Many children will be discharged home, and some will require pediatric specialty care.

References

1. Abdulhai, S. A., Glenn, I. C., & Ponsky, T. A. (2017). Incarcerated pediatric hernias. *Surgery Clinics of North America, 97*(1), 129–145. https://doi.org/10.1016/j.suc.2016.08.010

2. Aboagye, J., Goldstein, S. D., Salazar, J. H., Papandria, D., Okoye, M. T., Al-Omar, K., Stewart, D., Lukish, J., & Abdullah, F. (2014). Age at presentation of common pediatric surgical conditions: Reexamining dogma. *Journal of Pediatric Surgery, 49*(6), 995–999. https://doi.org/10.1016/j.jpedsurg.2014.01.039

3. American Association of Poison Control Centers. (2018, January 22). *High alert: Intentional exposures among teens to single-load laundry packets continue to rise* [Press release]. https://piper.filecamp.com/uniq/c97oWbhLAMICZTi9.pdf

4. Barbosa, J. A., Tiseo, B. C., Barayan, G. A., Rosman, B. M., Torricelli, F. C., Passerotti, C. C., Srougi, M., Retik, A. B., & Nguyen, H. T. (2013). Development and initial validation of a scoring system to diagnose testicular torsion in children. *Journal of Urology, 189*(5), 1859–1864. https://doi.org/10.1016/j.juro.2012.10.056

5. Bhavsar, A. K., Gelner, E. J., & Shorma, T. (2016). Common questions about the evaluation of acute pelvic pain. *American Family Physician, 93*(1), 41–48. https://www.aafp.org/afp/2016/0101/p41.html

6. Bousvaros, A., Setty, M., & Kaplan, J. L. (2021). Management of severe or refractory ulcerative colitis in children and adolescents. *UpToDate*. Retrieved April 15, 2022, from https://www.uptodate.com/contents/management-of-severe-or-refractory-ulcerative-colitis-in-children-and-adolescents

7. Bousvaros, A., Setty, M., & Kaplan, J. L. (2022). Management of mild to moderate ulcerative colitis in children and adolescents. *UpToDate*. Retrieved April 15, 2022, from https://www.uptodate.com/contents/management-of-mild-to-moderate-ulcerative-colitis-in-children-and-adolescents

8. Brenner, J. S., & Ojo, A. (2022). Causes of scrotal pain in children and adolescents. *UpToDate*. Retrieved April 17, 2022, from https://www.uptodate.com/contents/causes-of-scrotal-pain-in-children-and-adolescents

9. Brown, K., & Lee, J. A. (2022). Evaluation of acute pelvic pain in the adolescent female. *UpToDate*. Retrieved April 15, 2022, from https://www.uptodate.com/contents/evaluation-of-acute-pelvic-pain-in-the-adolescent-female

10. Carroll, M. W., Kuenzig, M. E., Mack, D. R., Otley, A. R., Griffiths, A. M., Kaplan, G. G., Bernstein, C. N., Bitton, A., Murthy, S. K., Nguyen, G. C., Lee, K., Cooke-Lauder, J., & Benchimol, E. I. (2019). The impact of inflammatory bowel disease in Canada 2018: Children and adolescents with IBD. *Journal of the Canadian Association of Gastroenterology, 2*(suppl 1), S49–S67. https://doi.org/10.1093/jcag/gwy056

11. Centers for Disease Control and Prevention. (n.d.). *STDs during pregnancy: CDC fact sheet (detailed)*. https://www.cdc.gov/std/pregnancy/stdfact-pregnancy-detailed.htm#

12. Deveci, S. (2022). Priapism. *UpToDate*. Retrieved April 17, 2022, from https://www.uptodate.com/contents/priapism

13. Fortenberry, J. D. (2021). Sexually transmitted infections: Issues specific to adolescents. *UpToDate*. Retrieved April 17, 2022, from https://www.uptodate.com/contents/sexually-transmitted-infections-issues-specific-to-adolescents

14. Gilger, M. A., & Jain, A. K. (2022). Foreign bodies of the esophagus and gastrointestinal tract in children. *UpToDate*. Retrieved April 13, 2022, from https://www.uptodate.com/contents/foreign-bodies-of-the-esophagus-and-gastrointestinal-tract-in-children

15. Gurevich, Y., Sahn, D., & Weinstein, T. (2018). Foreign body ingestion in pediatric patients. *Current Opinion in Pediatrics, 30*(5), 677–682. https://doi.org/10.1097/mop.0000000000000670

16. Hamour, A., Ostrow, O., James, A., & Wolter, N. (2021). Practical tips for paediatricians: Esophageal button battery impaction in children, *Paediatrics & Child Health*, Article pxab078. https://doi.org/10.1093/pch/pxab078

17. Hansen, C. C, & Søriede, K. (2018). Systemic review of epidemiology, presentation, and management of Meckel's diverticulum in the 21st century. *Medicine, 97*(35), Article e12154. https://doi.org/10.1097/md.0000000000012154

18. Hendriks, E., Rosenburg, R., & Prine, L. (2020). Ectopic pregnancy: Diagnosis and management. *American Family Physician, 101*(10), 599–606. https://www.aafp.org/afp/2020/0515/p599.html

19. Higuchi, L. M., & Bousvaros, A. (2022). Clinical presentation and diagnosis of inflammatory bowel disease in children. *UpToDate*. Retrieved April 15, 2022, from https://www.uptodate.com/contents/clinical-presentation-and-diagnosis-of-inflammatory-bowel-disease-in-children

20. Hijaz, N. M., & Friesen, C. A. (2017). Managing acute abdominal pain in pediatric patients: Current perspectives. *Pediatric Health, Medicine and Therapeutics, 8*, 83–91. https://doi.org/10.2147/phmt.s120156

21. Hyams, J. S., Di Lorenzo, C., Saps, M., Shulman, R. J., Staiano, A., & Tilburg, M. (2016). Childhood functional gastrointestinal Disorders: Child/adolescent. *Gastroenterology, 150*(6), 1456–1468. https://doi.org/10.1053/j.gastro.2016.02.015

22. Islam, A., Farwad, A., Shah, A. A., Jadoon, H., Sarwar, I., & Abbasi, A. N. (2017). Analysis of two years cases of ectopic pregnancy. *Journal of Ayub Medical College, Abbottabad, 29*(1), 65–67. https://jamc.ayubmed.edu.pk/jamc/index.php/jamc/article/view/473/868

23. Javid, P. J., & Pauli, E. M. (2022). Meckel's diverticulum. *UpToDate*. Retrieved April 15, 2022, from https://www.uptodate.com/contents/meckels-diverticulum

24. Khorana, J., Tantivit, Y., Phiuphong, C., Pattapong, S., & Siripan, S. (2019). Foreign body ingestion in pediatrics: Distribution, management and complications. *Medicina, 55*(10), Article 686. https://doi.org/10.3390%2Fmedicina55100686

25. Laharie, D., Debeugny, S., Peeters, M., Van Gossum, A., Gower-Rousseau, C., Bélaïche, J., Fiasse, R., Dupas, J. L., Lerebours, E., Piotte, S., Cortot, A., Vermeire, S., Grandbastien, B., & Colombel, J. F. (2001). Inflammatory bowel disease in spouses and their offspring. *Gastroenterology, 120*(4), 816–819. https://doi.org/10.1053/gast.2001.22574

26. Lerner, D. G., Brumbaugh, D., Lightdale, J. R., Jatana, K. R., Jacobs, I. N., & Mamula, P. (2020). Mitigating risks of swallowed button batteries: New strategies before and after removal. *Journal of Pediatric Gastroenterology and Nutrition, 70*(5), 542–546. https://doi.org/10.1097/mpg.0000000000002649

27. Leung, A. K. C., & Hon, K. L. (2021). Paediatrics: How to manage functional constipation. *Drugs in Context, 10*, Article 2020-11-2. https://doi.org/10.7573/dic.2020-11-2

28. Li, D., Zhang, J., Kiryu, S., Zhang, X., & Wang, F. (2021). Clinical and CT features of ovarian torsion in infants, children, and adolescents. *International Journal of Gynecology and Obstetrics, 156*(3), 444–449. https://doi.org/10.1002/ijgo.13657

29. Martinez, G. M. (2020). Trends and patterns in menarche in the United States: 1995 through 2013–2017. *National Health Statistics Reports, 146*. https://www.cdc.gov/nchs/data/nhsr/nhsr146-508.pdf

30. Merriman, T. E., & Auldist, A. W. (2000). Ovarian torsion in inguinal hernias. *Pediatric Surgery International, 16*(5–6), 383–385. https://doi.org/10.1007/s003830000428

31. Missouri Poison Center. (2018, April 9). *Super-absorbent polymers (SAP) ingestion.* https://missouripoisoncenter.org/super-absorbent-polymers/

32. Neuman, M. I. (2021). Emergency evaluation of the child with acute abdominal pain. *UpToDate.* Retrieved August 11, 2021, from https://www.uptodate.com/contents/emergency-evaluation-of-the-child-with-acute-abdominal-pain

33. North American Society for Pediatric Gastroenterology, Hepatology, and Nutrition, Colitis Foundation of America, Bousvaros, A., Antonioli, D. A., Colletti, R. B., Dubinsky, M. C., Glickman, J. N., Gold, B. D., Griffiths, A. M., Jevon, G. P., Higuchi, L. M., Hyams, J. S., Kirschner, B. S., Kugathasan, S., Baldassano, R. N., & Russo, P. A. (2007). Differentiating ulcerative colitis from Crohn disease in children and young adults: Report of a working group of the North American Society for Pediatric Gastroenterology, Hepatology, and Nutrition and the Crohn's and Colitis Foundation of America. *Journal of Pediatric Gastroenterology and Nutrition, 44*(5), 653–674. https://doi.org/10.1097/MPG.0b013e31805563f3

34. Palazzi, D. L., & Brandt, M. L. (2021). Care of the umbilicus and management of umbilical disorders. *UpToDate.* Retrieved April 14, 2022, from https://www.uptodate.com/contents/care-of-the-umbilicus-and-management-of-umbilical-disorders#H17

35. Patel, N., & Kay, M. (2021). Lower gastrointestinal bleeding in children: Causes and diagnostic approach. *UpToDate.* Retrieved August 10, 2021, from https://www.uptodate.com/contents/lower-gastrointestinal-bleeding-in-children-causes-and-diagnostic-approach

36. Orsagh-Yentis, D., McAdams, R. J., Roberts, K. J., & McKenzie, L. B. (2019). Foreign-body ingestions of young children treated in US emergency departments: 1995–2015. *Pediatrics, 143*(5), Article e20181988. https://doi.org/10.1542/peds.2018-1988

37. Ramsook, C. (2022). Inguinal hernia in children. *UpToDate.* Retrieved April 13, 2022, from https://www.uptodate.com/contents/inguinal-hernia-in-children

38. Robertson, J., Long, B., & Koyfman, A. (2017). Myths in the evaluation and management of ovarian torsion. *Journal of Emergency Medicine, 52*(4), 449–456. https://doi.org/10.1016/j.jemermed.2016.11.012

39. Robin, S. G., Keller, C., Zwiener, R., Hyman, P. E., Nurko, S., Saps, M., Di Lorenzo, C., Shulman, R. J., Hyams, J. S., Palsson, O., & van Tilburg, M. A. L. (2018). Prevalence of pediatric functional gastrointestinal disorders utilizing the Rome IV criteria. *Journal of Pediatrics, 195*, 134–139. https://doi.org/10.1016/j.jpeds.2017.12.012

40. Silberman, M., Stormont, G., & Hu, E. W. (2021). *Priapism.* StatPearls Publishing. https://www.ncbi.nlm.nih.gov/books/NBK459178/

41. Sinclair, K., & Hill, I. D. (2021). Button and cylindrical battery ingestion: Clinical features, diagnosis, and initial management. *UpToDate.* Retrieved August 8, 2021, from https://www.uptodate.com/contents/button-and-cylindrical-battery-ingestion-clinical-features-diagnosis-and-initial-management

42. Smith, J., & Fox, S. M. (2016). Pediatric abdominal pain: An emergency medicine perspective. *Emergency Medicine Clinics of North America, 34*, 341–361. https://doi.org/10.1016/j.emc.2015.12.010

43. Sood, M. R. (2021). Chronic functional constipation and fecal incontinence in infants, children, and adolescents: Treatment. *UpToDate.* Retrieved December 8, 2021, from https://www.uptodate.com/contents/chronic-functional-constipation-and-fecal-incontinence-in-infants-children-and-adolescents-treatment

44. Sood, M. R. (2021). Constipation in infants and children: Evaluation. *UpToDate.* Retrieved August 8, 2021, from https://www.uptodate.com/contents/constipation-in-infants-and-children-evaluation

45. Sood, M. R. (2021). Functional constipation in infants, children, and adolescents: Clinical features and diagnosis. *UpToDate.* Retrieved December 8, 2021, from https://www.uptodate.com/contents/functional-constipation-in-infants-children-and-adolescents-clinical-features-and-diagnosis

46. Sood, M. R. (2021). Recent-onset constipation in infants and children. *UpToDate.* Retrieved December 7, 2021, from https://www.uptodate.com/contents/recent-onset-constipation-in-infants-and-children

47. Southwell, B. R. (2020). Treatment of childhood constipation: A synthesis of systematic reviews and meta-analyses. *Expert Review of Gastroenterology & Hepatology, 14*(3), 163–174. https://doi.org/10.1080/17474124.2020.1733974

48. Tulandi, T. (2022). Ectopic pregnancy: Choosing a treatment. *UpToDate.* Retrieved April 15, 2022, from https://www.uptodate.com/contents/ectopic-pregnancy-choosing-a-treatment

49. Tulandi, T. (2022). Ectopic pregnancy: Clinical manifestations and diagnosis. *UpToDate.* Retrieved April 15, 2022, from https://www.uptodate.com/contents/ectopic-pregnancy-clinical-manifestations-and-diagnosis

50. Tulandi, T. (2022). Ectopic pregnancy: Methotrexate therapy. *UpToDate.* Retrieved April 15, 2022, from https://www.uptodate.com/contents/ectopic-pregnancy-methotrexate-therapy

51. Villa, X. (2022). Approach to upper gastrointestinal bleeding in children. *UpToDate.* Retrieved April 15, 2022, from https://www.uptodate.com/contents/approach-to-upper-gastrointestinal-bleeding-in-children

52. Workowski, K. A., Bachmann, L. H., Chan, P. A., Johnston, C. M., Muzny, C. A., Park, I., Reno, H., Zenilman, J. M., & Bolan, G. A. (2021). Sexually transmitted infections treatment guidelines, 2021. *Morbidity and Mortality Weekly Report: Recommendations and Reports, 70*(4), 1–187. https://doi.org/10.15585/mmwr.rr7004a1

53. Yasuda, J. L., & Manfredi, M. A. (2021). Caustic ingestion and foreign bodies. In R. Wyllie, J. S. Hyams, & M. Kay (Eds.), *Pediatric gastrointestinal and liver disease* (6th ed., pp. 179–192). Elsevier. https://doi.org/10.1016/B978-0-323-67293-1.00018-9

54. Yeap, E., Nataraja, R., & Pacilli, M. (2020). Inguinal hernias in children. *Australian Journal of General Practice, 49*(1–2), 38–43. https://doi.org/10.31128/AJGP-08-19-5037

55. Yu, E. J., Choe, S., Yun, J., & Son, M. (2020). Association of early menarche with adolescent health in the setting of rapidly

decreasing age at menarche. *Journal of Pediatric and Adolescent Gynecology, 33*(3), 264–270. https://doi.org/10.1016/j.jpag.2019.12.006

56. Zamora, I. J., Vu, L. T., Larimer, E. L., & Olutoye, O. O. (2012). Water-absorbing balls: A "growing" problem. *Pediatrics, 130*(4), e1011–e1014. https://doi.org/10.1542/peds.2011-3685

57. Zitomersky, N., & Bousvaros, A. (2021). Overview of the management of Crohn disease in children and adolescents. *UpToDate*. Retrieved April 14, 2022, from https://www.uptodate.com/contents/overview-of-the-management-of-crohn-disease-in-children-and-adolescents

58. Zurynski, Y., Churruca, K., Arnolda, G., Dalton, S., Ting, H. P., Hibbert, P. D., Molloy, C., Wiles, L. K., de Wet, C., & Braithwaite, J. (2020). Quality of care for acute abdominal pain in children. *BMJ Quality & Safety, 29*(6), 509–516. https://doi.org/10.1136/bmjqs-2019-010088

Appendix 12-1

Common Causes of Abdominal Pain in Children by Age

Neonate	1 month–2 years	2–5 years	Older Than 5 years
Adhesions	Adhesions	Adhesions	Adhesions
NEC	Foreign body ingestion	Appendicitis	Appendicitis
Volvulus	HUS	Foreign body ingestion	DKA
Colic	Hirschsprung disease	HUS	HUS
Dietary protein allergy	Incarcerated hernia	Intussusception	Myocarditis
Testicular torsion	Intussusception	Primary bacterial peritonitis	Perforated ulcer
	Abdominal trauma	Trauma	Trauma
	Inflammatory bowel disease	Gastroenteritis	Constipation
	Meckel's diverticulum	Constipation	Gastroenteritis
	Sickle cell vaso-occlusive crisis	HSP	Cholecystitis
	UTI	Inflammatory bowel disease	HSP
	Gastroenteritis	Meckel's diverticulum	Inflammatory bowel
	Dietary protein allergy	UTI	Meckel's diverticulum
		Ovarian torsion	Ovarian torsion
		Sickle cell vaso-occlusive crisis	Testicular torsion
			Sickle cell vaso-occlusive crisis
			UTI

Data from Neuman, M. I. (2021). Emergency evaluation of the child with acute abdominal pain. *UpToDate*. Retrieved August 11, 2021, from https://www.uptodate.com/contents/emergency-evaluation-of-the-child-with-acute-abdominal-pain

Abbreviations: NEC, necrotizing enterocolitis; HUS, hemolytic uremic syndrome; UTI, urinary tract infection; HSP, Henoch-Schönlein purpura; DKA, diabetic ketoacidosis.

Appendix 12-2
Sexually Transmitted Infections

STI	Signs and Symptoms	First-Line Treatment
Neisseria gonorrhoeae	Infection can be asymptomatic Mucopurulent discharge—vaginal, penal, rectal Vaginal pruritus Intermenstrual bleeding Symptoms of pelvic inflammatory disease Abdominal/pelvic pain, fever, discharge Dyspareunia UTI symptoms possible Sore throat, exudate, cervical lymphadenopathy Conjunctivitis—neonates	Ceftriaxone
Chlamydia trachomatis	Infection can be asymptomatic Mucopurulent discharge—vaginal Intermenstrual vaginal bleeding UTI symptoms Urethritis in males—watery discharge Epididymitis Anal inflammation, discharge, pain	Doxycycline or azithromycin
Syphilis		
Primary	Localized skin lesion—chancre, painless lesion at point of contact—external genitalia, vagina, anus	Penicillin
Secondary	Systemic illness: fever, headache, muscle/joint pain, sore throat, weight loss, rash, lymphadenopathy, alopecia, condyloma	Penicillin
Tertiary	Neurological and cardiovascular manifestations	Penicillin
Genital herpes simplex virus		
Primary	Painful genital lesions, fever, headache, dysuria, inguinal lymphadenopathy Extragenital manifestations—aseptic meningitis, acute urinary retention Can be transmitted to newborn during vaginal delivery	Antiviral therapy
Recurrence	Expected, more common in immunosuppression Viral shedding can occur without lesion eruption	Breakthrough antiviral therapy versus daily therapy

(continues)

STI	Signs and Symptoms	First-Line Treatment
Chancroid	Papules occur 4–10 days after sexual contact evolving into pustules, then ulcers Lymphadenopathy	Varied antibiotic options
Pubic lice	Pruritus in affected area Lesions in lower abdomen, thighs, buttocks Blood stains on underwear	Topical pediculicides

Data from Workowski, K. A., Bachmann, L. H., Chan, P. A., Johnston, C. M., Muzny, C. A., Park, I., Reno, H., Zenilman, J. M., & Bolan, G. A. (2021). Sexually transmitted infections treatment guidelines, 2021. *Morbidity and Mortality Weekly Report: Recommendations and Reports, 70*(4), 1–187. https://doi.org/10.15585/mmwr.rr7004a1

The Child with a Rash

Kelly Williams, MSN, RN, CEN, CPN, CPEN, NPD-BC, CNE, TCRN

OBJECTIVES

Upon completion of this chapter, the learner will be able to:

1. Describe characteristics and selected causes of pediatric rashes.
2. Apply the Pediatric Nursing Process to a child experiencing a rash.
3. Determine appropriate infection control measures based on the presentation of the child with a rash.
4. Identify pediatric patients with a rash who are at risk for underlying complications.
5. Plan appropriate interventions and treatments for the child presenting with a rash.

Introduction

Rash is a common complaint in the emergency department. A large number of pediatric patients presenting with a rash are diagnosed with a benign cause, with one of the most common being diaper rash. However, a rash can also be an assessment finding indicative of a more serious underlying illness. It is important to consider the patient's history and any other signs and symptoms. Although a well-appearing child with a rash is less likely to have a life-threatening illness, assessment of the rash can serve as a diagnostic tool to narrow the possible etiologies.[28]

Performing a thorough assessment and collecting a complete patient history can help determine the cause of the rash. A rash can signify an allergic or anaphylactic reaction, a viral or bacterial infection, an infestation, or a serious underlying condition. An assessment and history can also determine what precautions should be initiated for a possible infectious disease.[28]

Initial Assessment

Use the Pediatric Nursing Process to ensure that immediate threats to life are identified and addressed in the primary survey. The initial assessment of a pediatric patient presenting with a rash includes a complete history and a thorough assessment. Ask about any other signs and symptoms and when the rash appeared within the timeline of the illness. Assess any other symptoms, such as fever and any gastrointestinal or neurologic complaint. Ask about any recent illness, infection, or medications taken.[28] Ascertain information regarding allergies to food or medication and determine the immunization status of the patient.[79(Ch19)] Review the patient's vital signs and look for any lethargy or distress. Perform an assessment of the rash, noting its characteristics (see **Table 13-1**).

Implement any isolation precautions as indicated based on the findings.[28] **Table 13-2** lists the isolation precautions recommended for specific conditions. In most

TABLE 13-1 Rash Descriptors

Type of Rash	Description	Examples/Causes
Macule	Flat, nonpalpable, < 10 mm diameter	Freckle, flat mole, port-wine stain
Patch	Large macule, > 10 mm diameter	Freckle, flat mole, port-wine stain
Papule	Elevated, < 10 mm diameter	Warts, insect bites, acne, cancer
Plaque	Elevated or depressed, > 10 mm diameter	Psoriasis
Nodule	Firm papules that extend into skin	Cyst, lipoma
Vesicle	Clear, fluid-filled blister, < 10 mm diameter	Herpes, contact dermatitis
Bullae	Clear, fluid-filled blister, > 10 mm diameter	Burns, bites, contact dermatitis
Pustule	Vesicles that contain pus	Bacterial infections, pustular psoriasis
Petechiae	Nonblanchable, pinpoint area of hemorrhage	Straining (coughing, vomiting), coagulopathy, vasculitis
Purpura	Nonblanchable, larger area of hemorrhage than petechiae	Coagulopathy, vasculitis
Targeted/targetoid	Ring-shaped with a dusky center	Erythema multiforme
Urticaria	Elevated, pruritic plaques, varying in size, also known as wheals or hives	Allergic reaction to food, insect bite, or medication

Data from Benedetti, J. (2019). Description of skin lesions. *Merck Manual: Professional version.* https://www.merckmanuals.com/professional/dermatologic-disorders/approach-to-the-dermatologic-patient/description-of-skin-lesions

TABLE 13-2 Infectious Conditions and Isolation Precautions

Infectious Condition	Isolation Precaution
Fifth disease (parvovirus B19, erythema infectiosum)	Droplet
Hand, foot, and mouth	Contact precautions when treating an infant or toddler in diapers
Impetigo	Contact
Lice	Contact until 24 hours after initiation of effective therapy
Meningococcal meningitis	Droplet until 24 hours after initiation of effective therapy
Molluscum contagiosum	Standard
Ringworm	Standard
Roseola infantum	Standard (no longer contagious once symptomatic)
Rubeola (measles)	Airborne until 4 days after onset of rash, for the entire duration of illness in an immunocompromised patient
Scabies	Contact until 24 hours after initiation of effective therapy
Scarlet fever	Droplet
Varicella (chickenpox)	Airborne and contact

Data from Centers for Disease Control and Prevention. (2019, July 22). *Type and duration of precautions recommended for selected infections and conditions.* https://www.cdc.gov/infectioncontrol/guidelines/isolation/appendix/type-duration-precautions.html

cases, the nurse will not know the diagnosis before patient contact begins. Note that infection control recommendations evolve and infectious diseases are always emerging. Err on the side of caution with personal protective equipment (PPE).

> **RED FLAG**
>
> The consideration of safety threats to the team, including infectious disease, takes priority over patient care. Don PPE before approaching the patient.

Assessment Findings of Concern

Any child with a rash who is not well-appearing should raise concerns. Other concerns include respiratory distress with urticaria (anaphylaxis), fever, inconsolability, or diarrhea and abdominal pain. When assessing a rash, concerns include blistering or skin sloughing, mucosal involvement and inflammation, and petechiae or purpura.[28]

> **CLINICAL PEARL**
>
> ### Differentiating Between Rash Types
>
> Many terms are used to differentiate various types of rashes. A quick way to remember the proper term is based on rash size. Some examples include the following:
>
> - A macule becomes a patch once it is larger than 10 mm.
> - A papule becomes a plaque once is it larger than 10 mm.
> - A vesicle becomes a bullae once it is larger than 10 mm.[76]
> - The term "macular–papular" refers to a rash that consists of about a 50–50 ratio of macules and papules.[76] This rash description is used only when macules and papules are both present. The term is often loosely associated with any nonspecific rash, so its use must be specific to the clinical assessment.[10]

Conditions Presenting with a Rash

A rash can be the result of minor irritation, or it can point to a more serious or even life-threatening underlying disease process. Different types of rashes and what they could signify are highlighted in this section.

> **RED FLAG**
>
> A blanching rash is one that fades or turns white when pressure is applied to it. These usually result from a benign cause. A nonblanching rash can signify a more serious illness such as sepsis or meningitis. A patient who presents with a nonblanching rash requires immediate assessment to determine the severity of illness and isolation precautions.[9,41]

Henoch-Schönlein Purpura

Henoch-Schönlein purpura (HSP), also known as immunoglobulin A (IgA) vasculitis, causes IgA to collect in blood vessels, which results in inflammation and the leakage of blood.[55] HSP occurs in young children, usually younger than 10 years of age, and has a higher incidence in males.[1,81] HSP is triggered by an overactive response of the immune system and is usually preceded by an upper respiratory illness.[38,77,81]

The four hallmarks of HSP are arthritis, gastrointestinal complaints (most commonly abdominal pain and gastrointestinal bleeding), kidney inflammation, and a purpuric rash. A macular–petechial rash is commonly found on the lower extremities (**Figure 13-1**) and the buttocks and is described as a raised red or purple spotted rash that is nonblanchable.[77] Petechiae appear as tiny red dots. As bleeding under the skin continues, purpura develops.

There is no definitive test for HSP, and the diagnosis is made clinically through assessment findings. Abdominal imaging and laboratory studies including renal function and urinalysis are performed to rule out other acute causes of abdominal pain.[1]

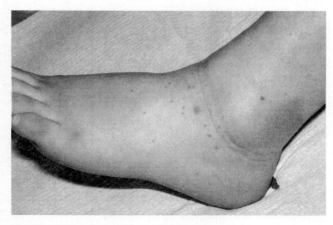

Figure 13-1 *Henoch-Schönlein purpura.*
© Allan Harris/Medical Images.

Treatment includes pain medication and monitoring for hypertension to assess for kidney involvement. The condition is self-resolving within a few weeks, but can reoccur.[77] A small percentage of patients diagnosed with HSP develop bowel or renal disease.[38]

Immune Thrombocytopenic Purpura

Immune thrombocytopenic purpura (ITP; formerly called idiopathic thrombocytopenic purpura and also referred to as immune thrombocytopenia) is one of the most common acquired bleeding disorders, affecting 5 to 10 per 100,000 children every year.[30] ITP occurs in children younger than 10 years of age, with the highest prevalence noted in children aged 1 to 5 years.[34] This disease process is related to autoimmune conditions, and can present as an initial sign of an autoimmune disorder in a child.[43] ITP is an isolated thrombocytopenia that does not involve any bone marrow damage and occurs in response to formation of antiplatelet antibodies.[30,59]

Assessment findings of ITP include petechiae or unexplained bruising; bleeding from the gums, mouth, or gastrointestinal tract; heavy bleeding during the menstrual cycle; and lethargy.[24,60] ITP may be preceded by a viral illness or a recent medication.[37] The petechiae present as a red or purplish rash, with scattered, raised bumps the size of pinpoints.[24] This rash is caused by bleeding under the skin.[54] Most often, petechiae are noted on the lower extremities.[50]

Blood and urine tests, including a platelet count, are required for diagnosis.[37] Diagnosis is determined through assessment findings, low platelet count, and exclusion of other causes of symptoms.

The goal of treatment is to stop and prevent any further bleeding.[30] Education topics include decreased activity to minimize the chance of traumatic injury and the need for immediate medical attention for any injuries sustained to the head or abdomen. Intravenous immunoglobulin (IVIG) may be administered to increase platelet counts, and corticosteroids may be prescribed to decrease the production of antiplatelet antibodies.[37] In ITP, the spleen makes antibodies that destroy platelets rather than fight infections. A splenectomy may be required if the patient does not respond to pharmaceutical treatment.[54]

Kawasaki Disease

Kawasaki disease is an acute inflammatory condition and a common vasculitis found in childhood that can affect the coronary arteries, causing aneurysms, heart failure, myocardial infarction, and arrhythmias. Assessment findings include a rash found on the trunk (**Figure 13-2**) that is described as morbilliform, targeted, or erythematous.[63]

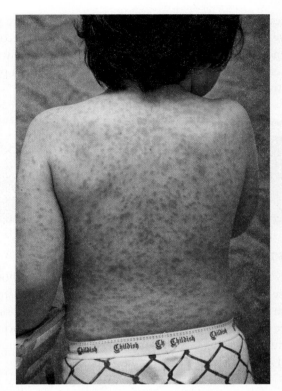

Figure 13-2 *A rash on the trunk from Kawasaki disease.*
Courtesy of Kawasaki Disease Foundation.

Other findings include a fever for at least 5 days; "strawberry tongue" (see Figure 10-1); desquamation, or the shedding of the outer layers of the skin, of the fingers and toes; eye redness; and swollen lymph nodes in the neck.[5,63] See Chapter 10, "The Child with a Fever," for more information on Kawasaki disease.

NOTE

Morbilliform Rash

A morbilliform rash refers to a rash that looks like measles. It consists of macular and papular lesions and is found on the face and the body.[76]

Multisystem Inflammatory Syndrome in Children

Multisystem inflammatory syndrome in children (MIS-C) occurs about 4 weeks after a COVID-19 infection and is diagnosed only in patients younger than the age of 21.[46] Symptoms are similar to those of Kawasaki disease and involve inflammation of a body system. A particular finding is a rash similar to that of Kawasaki disease as well as malar erythema (reddening of the cheeks). This may be an indication, along with a positive history of recent COVID-19 infection, of MIS-C versus Kawasaki disease.[27,65] The patient with more severe MIS-C may present with signs of shock or respiratory failure.[49] See Chapter 10, "The Child with a Fever," for more information on MIS-C.

NOTE

Rash in Kawasaki Versus MIS-C

Both Kawasaki disease and MIS-C present with a morbilliform and erythematous rash found on the trunk. A quick assessment finding that can assist in differentiating these diseases is the presence of erythema of the cheeks, known as malar erythema, on the patient with probable MIS-C.[27,65]

Stevens-Johnson Syndrome/Toxic Epidermal Necrolysis

Stevens-Johnson syndrome (SJS) and toxic epidermal necrolysis (TEN) are hypersensitivity reactions that cause partial- to full-thickness necrosis of the epidermis. Most often SJS or TEN is a drug reaction and will manifest 1 to 3 weeks after the start of a new medication.[8] The medications most commonly associated with SJS or TEN include allopurinol, anticonvulsants, sulfa drugs, nevirapine, and oxicam nonsteroidal anti-inflammatory drugs.[6] These conditions can also present idiopathically or after infection.[8]

Assessment findings include malaise, fever, cough, and sore throat. Painful lesions appear following the flulike symptoms. The rash is erythematous in nature and can present as patches, targetoid, or bullae lesions. Lesions may have a dusky center, signaling necrosis of the epidermis. The rash commonly involves the buccal, genital, or ocular mucosa.[8] A diagnostic finding is a positive Nikolsky sign, a skin finding in which the top layer of skin falls away from the lower layer of skin when rubbed.[47]

Diagnosis relies on patient history and a skin biopsy. All mucous membranes, including the vagina in female patients, should be assessed, as the lesions can present in any mucous membrane of the body.

Initial treatment includes removing the triggering agent. Due to the break in the skin barrier, there is a risk of fluid loss and infection. Fluid loss is treated with fluid resuscitation. Infection is treated with the administration of antibiotics. The patient may require pain medications. The patient is admitted to an intensive care unit (ICU) or a burn unit for continued care.[26]

Rashes Associated with Infectious Disease

Many rashes are associated with an infectious disease. Determining the need for isolation is a priority to protect staff and other patients. When a child presents with a rash, obtain a history to assess for the potential cause for the rash. Gather the following information:

- Does the child have a fever?
- If fever is present, which came first, the rash or the fever?
- Describe the rash.
- Has the child traveled abroad recently?
- What is the child's immunization status?
- Has the child been exposed to anyone actually or potentially ill?

Answers to these questions, the clinical exam, and assessment of the appearance of the rash assist with the determination for infection control measures, appropriate diagnostic testing, and treatment.[63]

Meningococcal Meningitis

Meningococcal meningitis is a bacterial infection of the meninges and/or the blood caused by gram-negative *Neisseria meningitidis*. Infants within the first 3 months of life have the highest risk of contracting bacterial meningitis due to the immaturity of their immune system.[25] Assessment findings include flulike symptoms, fever, headache, a stiff neck, vomiting, altered level of consciousness, and rash. The rash may appear as petechiae, purpura, or ecchymosis. It may initially present as viral in appearance—that is, as splotchy red spots—with the presentation being either sudden or gradual, and either appearing on one section of the body or becoming widespread. As the disease progresses, vesicles and bullae may form and even become gangrenous, leading to possible amputation of limbs. The presence of purpura fulminans (**Figure 13-3**) is a diagnostic sign of a systemic disease.[8]

Meningococcal meningitis is a life-threatening disease, and afflicted children can deteriorate quickly. Upon recognition of the purpuric or petechial rash, immediate intervention is necessary to ensure the optimal outcome for the child.[25] Patients presenting with signs and symptoms of meningococcus are placed on standard and droplet precautions.[16] See Chapter 10, "The Child with a Fever," for information on other types of meningitis.

Definitive diagnosis is determined from the positive identification of *N. meningitidis* in blood cultures or in cerebrospinal fluid via a lumbar puncture. Treatment consists of early administration of antibiotics and symptom support.[8] Patient care includes providing a dark and

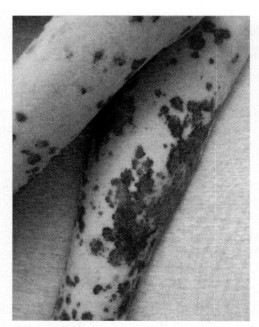

Figure 13-3 *Purpura fulminans.*
Courtesy of DrFO.Jr.Tn.

quiet environment, as patients with meningococcus can be sensitive to light and noise. A side-lying position is best to decrease the discomfort of nuchal rigidity. Continue to reassess for signs and symptoms of increased intracranial pressure (ICP), urine output, and changes in neurologic status.[66] Meningococcal meningitis can quickly lead to septic shock. See Chapter 7, "The Child in Need of Stabilization," for more information on the identification and management of shock.

CLINICAL PEARL

Meningococcal Disease and Vaccines

Meningococcal disease is especially dangerous for young children, though teens and young adults are also at risk. It has a mortality rate of 10% to 15%, with 20% of survivors suffering long-term detriments such as neurologic damage, limb loss, and hearing loss.

Vaccines for meningococcal meningitis are now available. A two-part vaccine is administered to prevent infections with the meningococcal strands A, C, W, and Y. The initial vaccine is administered at age 11, with the booster following at age 16. Although not categorized as a routine recommendation, a B-strand vaccine is also available and is administered to youth between the ages of 16 and 18 for short-term protection. There has been a dramatic decrease in meningococcal infections since the institution of the vaccines.[4]

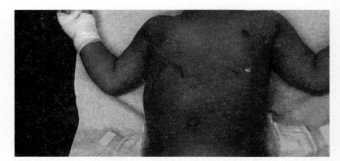

Figure 13-4 *Roseola infantum.*
© Science Source.

Viral Skin Infections

Viral skin infections are primarily due to poor hygiene practices and close contact with other children. Common viral skin infections include roseola infantum, fifth disease, molluscum contagiosum, varicella, and rubeola.

Roseola Infantum

Roseola infantum is caused by a herpesvirus and usually presents in children younger than 3 years of age.[3] The hallmark of roseola infantum is a rash consisting of small, erythematous, blanching papules that begins at the trunk and then spreads distally (**Figure 13-4**). The rash appears 12 to 24 hours after the fever has resolved. The rash typically lasts 1 to 3 days.[63] The child is no longer contagious once symptoms are present.[71]

The diagnosis is determined through clinical findings, which include rhinorrhea, sore throat, conjunctivitis, fever, and rash.[63] Treatment is not required for roseola infantum. Patients are usually discharged, and education includes symptom management.[3,75] Standard precautions are recommended.[16]

Fifth Disease

Fifth disease, also called erythema infectiosum, is a pediatric illness that is caused by parvovirus B19.[18] Assessment findings include fever, runny nose, sore throat, headache, malaise, and rash.[3,18] Some patients will experience joint pain and swelling.

The initial rash appears on the face as bright red cheeks, sometimes called a "slapped cheek" rash, which fades in 5 to 10 days (**Figure 13-5**). Once the initial rash presents, the child is no longer contagious. Following resolution of the initial rash, a lacelike rash can appear on the trunk and extremities, which can fade and reappear for weeks, especially when exposed to heat.[3,18,63,78] Fifth disease is spread through respiratory secretions. Parvovirus B19 can also be spread through blood products; a pregnant woman infected with parvovirus B19 can transmit the infection to her baby.[18,63]

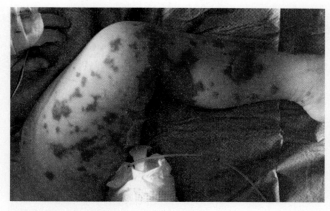

Figure 13-5 *Slapped cheek rash.*
© SPL/Science Source.

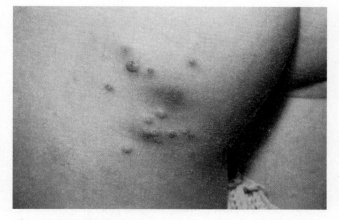

Figure 13-6 *Lesions from molluscum contagiosum.*
© Dr. P. Marazzi/Science Source.

Fifth disease is usually diagnosed by the hallmark "slapped cheek" rash. Treatment is not required, but fever and discomfort can be managed with over-the-counter pain relievers. Discharge teaching includes information about handwashing and refraining from sharing drinks in the home.[3,18,78] Isolation measures include droplet precautions.[16]

Molluscum Contagiosum

Molluscum contagiosum is a highly contagious infection caused by the poxvirus and transmitted through skin-to-skin contact. It is seen most often in children ages 2 through 11 and in sexually active teens.[3] Assessment findings include lesions that measure 2 to 5 mm and are pale or skin colored. The lesions are papular, with central umbilication—an impression in the middle of the lesion that gives the impression of a navel (**Figure 13-6**). The lesions surface on the face, extremities, and the trunk.[2] A child usually presents with 10 to 20 lesions, but there have been cases with hundreds of lesions. When transmitted through sexual activity, lesions will be found in the genital region. A sexually active teenager should also be assessed for other sexually transmitted diseases.

Diagnosis is made based on the characteristics and appearance of the lesions. The illness resolves without treatment, although itching can be treated to prevent further transmission to other body parts. The lesions can last 6 months to years.[3] Children can go to school and participate in sports if lesions that are not protected by clothing are covered with a watertight bandage.[14,36]

Although the lesions will eventually disappear, parents may become anxious and request treatment.[3] Large placebo-controlled trials are lacking, but cryotherapy, curettage, and cantharidin do seem to be effective in removing the lesions. Podophyllotoxin is an option supported by data from a placebo-controlled trial, but its safety in children has not been established.[36] Cantharidin is a fatty substance derived from beetles that is applied to individual lesions, resulting in a blister that irritates the lesion. According to a chart review, cantharidin clears the lesions in 90% of patients and provides overall relief to another 8% of children suffering from molluscum contagiosum.[29,58] Standard precautions are recommended.[16]

Varicella (Chickenpox)

Varicella, commonly known as chickenpox, is caused by a herpesvirus. Assessment findings include a vesicular rash that spreads over the entire body and has been described as looking like a "dewdrop on a rose petal." The rash starts as red or pink bumps on the face, trunk, and extremities (**Figure 13-7**) and transforms into itchy fluid-filled blisters that, after about a week's time, turn into crusted papules.[21,78] History may include fever or malaise 1 or 2 days prior to the development of the rash. However, the rash is usually the first sign of illness in children.[21] The rash may not appear until 10 to 21 days post exposure.[23]

Diagnosis is based on rash presentation, although a swab of the lesion can be performed to detect the presence of varicella.[21] Treatment includes antihistamines and topical calamine lotion to relieve the itching. Discharge instructions should include instructions on good skin care and prevention of scratching, as this can lead to a secondary bacterial infection.[67] Severe complications include encephalitis and pneumonia. Varicella is contagious and requires patients to be placed on standard, contact, and airborne isolation.[21]

A vaccine to prevent varicella is available and is administered in two doses. The first dose is administered between the ages of 12 and 15 months; the second dose is administered between 4 and 6 years of age. Since the start of varicella vaccine administration, cases of positive varicella have decreased from 4 million per year in the United States to 500,000 per year.[21]

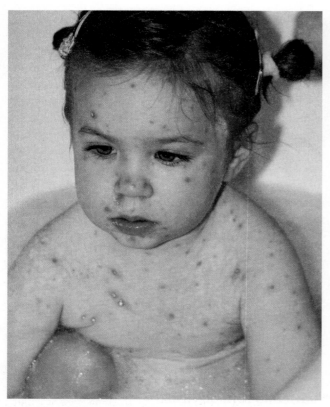

Figure 13-7 *Varicella.*
© Dagfrida/Shutterstock.

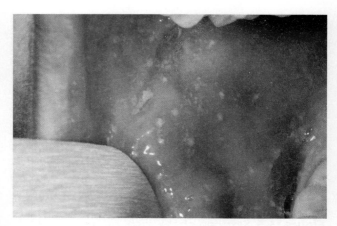

Figure 13-8 *Koplik's spots in the oral mucosa.*
© Dr. P. Marazzi/Science Photo Library.

Rubeola (Measles)

Rubeola, also known as measles, is a highly contagious viral illness. Contagion can occur through exposure to infected persons four days prior to the development of a rash and continues for four days after the rash appears. Transmission occurs primarily through respiratory secretions, although the virus can also be transmitted by blood or urine. Transmission is more common in the winter months.[67] Although the child may complain of malaise, fever, or cough initially, the hallmark sign of rubeola infection is the appearance of Koplik's spots in the oral mucosa (**Figure 13-8**).[23] These small white, gray, or blue spots are surrounded by a reddened ring, and appear along the inner cheek and opposite the molars.[78] A hyperpigmented rash of macules and papules also appears on the head and face, spreading next to the trunk and extremities.[23,78] Unvaccinated children presenting with fever, a maculopapular rash, and a hyperpigmented rash should be suspected to have measles.[35]

Diagnosis is made clinically, although definitive diagnosis can be made through nasopharyngeal swab, urine, or blood test.[23] Treatment includes antipyretics for fever, rest, skin care in a tepid bath, and removing crust from the eyes with a warm, moist cloth.[67] Infection control measures include standard and airborne precautions.[16]

After the rollout of a two-dose vaccine received in childhood, measles was declared as eliminated from the United States in the year 2000. However, measles outbreaks occasionally occur, mostly within the unvaccinated population or due to international travel. In an effort to control the spread of this highly contagious disease, rubeola is reportable by law in many parts of the world.[31,80]

Hand, Foot, and Mouth Disease

Hand, foot, and mouth disease is a viral illness most commonly seen in children younger than 5 years of age, although adolescents and adults can become infected.[19] Transmission commonly occurs via the fecal–oral route but may occur after oral–oral or respiratory droplet contact.

Assessment findings include fever, maculopapular or papulovesicular rash on the hands and the soles of the feet, and ulcers in the oral mucosa. The ulcers in the mouth may cause discomfort, resulting in the child's refusal to eat or drink, which may lead to dehydration. The rash resolves after 7 to 10 days. Treatment consists of system support. Analgesics are administered for pain relief. Intravenous fluids may need to be delivered if the child is dehydrated due to decrease in oral intake. Discharge instructions include hand hygiene and disinfection of contaminated surfaces.[72] Contact precautions are recommended when treating an infant or toddler still wearing diapers.[16]

Bacterial Infections

Bacterial skin infections in children are common. Most pediatric skin infections are caused by gram-positive bacteria, mainly *Staphylococcus aureus* and group A streptococci. Impetigo is a common bacterial skin infection, while scarlet fever presents with a rash after a bacterial illness.[48]

Impetigo

Impetigo, a bacterial infection of the epidermal layer of the skin, is one of the most common bacterial infections to the skin found in children.[64] An outbreak of impetigo is usually limited to the superficial skin surrounding the nose and mouth. Healthy bacteria live on skin and provide a barrier that fights against penetration of harmful bacteria. When there is an area of breakdown, bacteria are able to enter and infect the skin tissue.[62] Impetigo is caused specifically by the invasion of *S. aureus* and group A *Streptococcus*.[3,51,64] Assessment findings include pus-filled vesicles that eventually burst, leaving a layer of thick, yellow crust on the face and extremities (**Figure 13-9**).[3,62,64]

Bullous impetigo presents with fluid-filled bullae. A thin brown crust is evident after the bullae rupture. This form of impetigo is frequently seen on the trunk.[7]

If bacteria continue to invade deeper into the tissue, complications can occur. Cellulitis or an abscess may form. The bacteria may enter the bloodstream, causing more severe infection. Warning signs to watch for include redness, swelling, pain, drainage, fever, or vomiting.[62] A streptococcal impetigo infection can cause rheumatic fever, an illness that affects the heart, joint, skin, and brain.[13]

Diagnosis is based on assessment findings, although a swab of the lesion can determine the causative agent.[64] Treatment includes either oral or topical antibiotics.[3,62] Impetigo can be caused by scratching due to a scabies infestation, so concurrent treatment of scabies can be considered.[70] Discharge teaching includes handwashing and encouraging the child not to scratch or pick at the crusts. Skin care including cleansing and moisturizing is also important.[62] Impetigo is contagious and requires standard and contact precautions until 24 hours after the initiation of effective therapy.[16]

Scarlet Fever

Scarlet fever is a bacterial infection caused by group A *Streptococcus*. The illness begins with a fever and sore

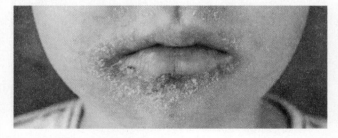

Figure 13-9 *Impetigo.*

Reproduced from Centers for Disease Control and Prevention. (2021, July 15). *Impetigo: All you need to know.* https://www.cdc.gov/groupastrep/diseases-public/impetigo.html

throat, which is followed by a sandpaper-like rash. The rash is seen first on the trunk and spreads outward, but avoids the palms of the hands and the soles of the feet. The rash consists of papules that blanch.[3,15,20,22,78] Red streaks, called Pastia's lines, may appear in body creases, such as the armpit, elbow, or groin.[15,78] Petechiae may be observed on the palate of the mouth, with the skin around the lips paling (circumoral pallor). The tongue may have a yellow-white coating initially. As the coating disappears, papillae coating the tongue create a "strawberry tongue" appearance similar to that noted in Kawasaki disease. The rash lasts about 7 days before desquamation, or peeling of the skin, begins.[3,20,22,78]

Diagnosis is made from a positive strep test or throat culture. First-line treatment of scarlet fever is penicillin or an alternative antibiotic if an allergy exists. Antibiotic therapy shortens the duration and the severity of the illness.[3,20,22,78] Symptom support treatment includes rest, antipyretics for fever, analgesics for sore throat, and antipruritics for itching. Discharge teaching includes reinforcing the importance of completing the antibiotic treatment. The parent is also instructed to discard the child's toothbrush and to not allow sharing of drinks or utensils.

Transmission of the bacteria occur through nasopharyngeal secretions. Standard and droplet precautions are recommended until 24 hours after the initiation of effective therapy.[16]

Allergic Rashes

Because the skin is the largest organ of the body and part of the immune system, rashes are a common symptom of an allergic response.[11]

Urticaria (Hives)

Urticaria, or hives, can be either a benign response to an allergen or an early sign of anaphylaxis. It can also be a response to physical stimuli or stress, signal the presence of an infection, or have an idiopathic origin. Urticaria presents as an acute, edematous rash with wheal and flare–type lesions (**Figure 13-10**). The lesions are itchy and usually fleeting, resolving in 2 to 3 hours.[39,73] Treatment of urticaria involves removing the cause of the allergic response and providing relief for the pruritis (itching) with antihistamines and corticosteroids.[39]

If urticaria is recognized in the presence of anaphylaxis, a severe life-threatening allergic reaction, immediate action must be taken. Administration of intramuscular epinephrine is the priority. Intubation may be required to maintain a patent airway. Crystalloid boluses may be required for anaphylactic shock. Adjunctive treatments include nebulized albuterol,

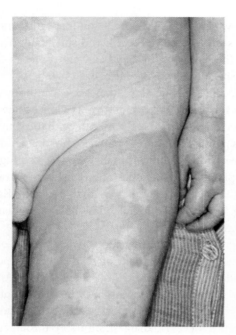

Figure 13-10   *Urticaria.*
© Dr. P. Marazzi/Science Source.

antihistamines, and corticosteroids.[12] See Chapter 7, "The Child in Need of Stabilization," for more information on anaphylaxis.

Atopic Dermatitis

Atopic dermatitis (AD) is the most common form of eczema, a group of conditions that cause an itchy and inflamed rash on the skin.[53] AD usually begins in infancy or childhood, with a higher prevalence found in children with a family history of eczema. AD is classified as an immune-mediated disease and is affected by both genes and external factors. This condition is recurring and can be triggered by an environmental exposure.[52]

Assessment findings include rash, surrounding redness, itchiness, dry or scaly skin, and open, weeping sores. Infants and toddlers may show initial symptoms on the face, elbows, or knees, as these are areas of the body that are often disturbed and irritated while crawling. AD is usually not found in the diaper area, as moisture prevents an outbreak. Older children may present with areas of rash on the elbows, hands, behind the knees, feet, scalp, or behind the ears. If scratched, the affected areas can become infected and form a yellow crust.[52] AD and rhinitis are commonly found together, signifying a possible commonality in pathophysiology.[42] AD is also associated with allergies such as asthma, food allergy, and hay fever.[52]

Diagnosis is based on clinical findings. Treatment includes topical anti-inflammatory agents and hydration of the skin. In some cases, phototherapy or immune-suppressing drugs are used.[52] Discharge teaching includes minimizing

further exacerbation or reoccurrence once the precipitating factor is identified. Baths should be taken in tepid water either with mild soap or without soap. Emulsifying oils can be used to trap moisture in the skin. Affected children are instructed not to scratch the rash to avoid further irritation or secondary bacterial infection.[69]

Rashes Associated with Infestations

A common complaint in the pediatric emergency department is infestation of the skin. Early identification of the infestation decreases the risk of complications and enables prompt treatment and recovery.[57]

Scabies

Scabies is a contagious parasitic skin infestation of mites, in which female mites burrow into the epidermis, depositing eggs and feces there.[57,68] Scabies can be found in any person regardless of age, sex, hygiene practices, or socioeconomic status.[68] Assessment findings include a generalized pruritic rash, which worsens at night.[40] A hallmark sign of scabies is itchy skin lesions on the palms and soles, although the lesions may also be found on other areas of the body.[57] Lesions may present as erythematous papules or vesicular lesions. Upon magnified assessment, burrows—which take the form of gray lines measuring about 5 mm—may be noted (**Figure 13-11**). A classic infestation involves 10 to 15 mites. However, in an immunosuppressed patient, a hyperinfestation may occur, resulting in crusted scabies. In crusted scabies, deep fissures will be seen on the palms and soles.[74]

Scabies is transmitted through skin-to-skin contact; therefore, family members may also become infected.[40,74]

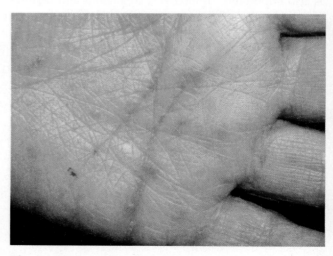

Figure 13-11   *Scabies burrows.*
Reproduced from Gilson, R. L., & Crane, J. S. (2021, July 18). *Scabies.* StatPearls Publishing. https://www.ncbi.nlm.nih.gov/books/NBK544306/figure/article-28727.image.f2/

Mites are resistant to soap and water, and scabies is exacerbated if treated with topical steroids. Scratching can introduce bacteria, resulting in a secondary bacterial infection.[40] Itching is worse at night.

Diagnosis is based on the clinical assessment and physical examination. Occasionally, skin scapings may be obtained. Lab work is usually not required, but eosinophilia—an abundance of disease-fighting white blood cells that can indicate a parasitic infection—has been found in some cases of scabies.

Treatment includes the application of a topical scabicide. Permethrin is the preferred first-line agent for children older than 2 months of age.[40,57] This topical agent is applied over the entire skin surface, including between the finger and toe creases, the cleft of the buttocks, and under the nails.[40] Ivermectin is an oral alternative to permethrin.[68] Discharge education includes hygiene measures, such as washing of all clothes, towels, and linens in hot water. Items that cannot be washed should be placed in a sealed plastic bag for 72 hours. The infestation period before physical symptoms arise is 30 to 60 days, so anyone in close contact with the patient during this time should be treated.[68] Contact precautions are recommended.[16]

Tinea Corporis (Ringworm)

Tinea corporis is a superficial fungal skin infection. It is most common in tropical regions and in postpubertal children and young adults. Ringworm is the most common infection found in wrestlers because of their close and prolonged skin contact.[68] It can be transmitted via person-to-person contact as well as through contact with dogs, cats, soil, or fomites. Ringworm is usually contracted in warmer environments when sharing towels or clothes.

The typical assessment finding is a well-demarcated, sharply circumscribed oval or circular lesion. The lesion presents as a scaly patch or plaque with a raised edge and mild erythema. The center of the lesion is hypopigmented or brown. The border may be irregular (**Figure 13-12**). Ringworm appears primarily on the trunk and can be associated with mild pruritis.[44] It can also be found on the extremities, usually unilaterally, and on the nails.[68]

Diagnosis is clinical, although a fungal culture can be performed for definitive diagnosis. Treatment includes a topical antifungal. Topical treatment is applied for the entire course, as early cessation can result in reoccurrence. The patient is also advised to stay dry and to wear light and loose clothing.[44] Wrestlers are encouraged to shower immediately after wrestling, remove and separate their dirty clothes, treat any cuts on their skin, and clean the mats after use to prevent transmission of ringworm.[56] Standard precautions are normally

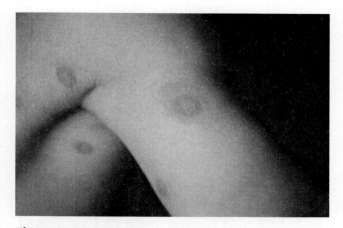

Figure 13-12 *Ringworm.*
© alejandrophotography/iStock/Getty Images Plus/Getty Images.

recommended. However, in the case of an institutional outbreak, contact precautions are also initiated.[16]

Lice

Parasitic insects known as lice (singular: *louse*) can also cause infestations. Lice spread by close person-to-person contact. They do not hop or fly and are not spread by animals. These parasites can be eradicated from clothing, linens, and towels with hot washing and drying.[17,32,33]

Pediculosis corporis, or body lice, live on clothing or bedding and are associated with crowded living conditions and poor hygiene. The louse crawls onto the human body during sleep to feed on blood. Common bite areas include the neck, shoulders, armpits, waist, and groin. A key assessment finding is a pruritic rash. After long exposure to lice, thickening and darkening of the skin can occur. Diagnosis is based on clinical findings. Thorough bathing and hot washing and drying of all clothes, linens, and towels is often the only treatment required. In some cases, a topical pediculicide, either an over-the-counter or prescription agent, is recommended.[32,45]

Pediculosis capitis, or head lice, are common in children and not associated with socioeconomic status. Head lice and their nits (eggs) can be seen on the hair shaft. Wet combing and topical pediculicides are used to eliminate head lice. Advise the child against sharing clothes, a bed, or hair supplies with anyone.[33,68]

Isolation precautions vary depending on the location of the lice. For head lice, contact precautions are recommended until after 24 hours of effective treatment. Standard precautions are advised for body lice with the addition of contact precautions if removing clothes from the patient. Standard precautions are recommended for pubic lice.[16]

Cimex lectularius (Bed Bugs)

Bed bugs are flat, brown insects that infest walls or the structure of a bed. They emerge at night to feed on

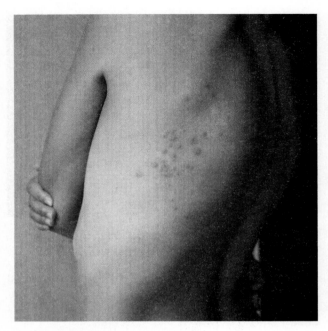

Figure 13-13 *Bed bug bites.*
© Joel Carillet/iStock/Getty.

human blood. These organisms are 1 to 7 mm in length and emit an almond or berry-like smell. Evidence of a bed bug infestation is discarded exoskeletons found in bedding.[45,61]

Assessment findings include bites or painless skin lesions, which are usually found on exposed parts of the body such as arms, legs, feet, face, and neck. The lesions are 2 to 5 mm in diameter and present in clusters of three or more bites (**Figure 13-13**). This is remembered by labeling the cluster of bites "breakfast, lunch, and dinner."[61] Often the bites follow a linear pattern and are found when the patient wakes up.

Diagnosis is based on clinical findings. Symptomatic treatment for pruritis includes topical steroids or antihistamines. Discharge instructions include maintaining good hygiene and avoiding scratching to prevent infection. All clothes, linens, and towels must be hot washed and dried. Thorough vacuuming of the living area and furniture is required. Professional pest control may be necessary to eradicate the infestation.[45,61]

Summary

A rash can indicate a significant systemic condition or a benign localized reaction. It may be a sign of an infectious disease, a parasitic infestation, or an allergic response. Recognizing the signs of an infectious process is key to initiating the appropriate infection control measures. It is important to assess whether the child is sick or well-appearing to determine the significance of the rash itself. Accurate assessment and description of the rash and patient history aids in determining the etiology. Although most rashes are benign and easily managed, some can be a sign of a life-threatening illness that requires immediate recognition and intervention. Astute assessment and awareness of concerning presentations facilitates early identification and interventions.

References

1. Adrogue, H., & Hayde, N. (2021). Henoch-Schönlein purpura. In T. K. McInerny, H. Adam, D. Campbell, T. DeWitt, J. Foy, & D. Kamat (Eds.), *Textbook of pediatric care* (2nd ed., Chapter 264). American Academy of Pediatrics. https://pediatriccare.solutions.aap.org/chapter.aspx?sectionId=124509885&bookId=1626&resultClick=1

2. Aggarwal, P. (2019, August 19). Emergent itchy rash in a 5-year-old boy. *Contemporary Pediatrics.* https://www.contemporarypediatrics.com/view/emergent-itchy-rash-5-year-old-boy

3. Allmon, A., Deane, K., & Martin, K. (2015). Common skin rashes in children. *American Family Physician, 92*(3). https://www.aafp.org/afp/2015/0801/p211.html

4. American Academy of Family Physicians. (2021). *Meningococcal disease vaccine.* https://www.aafp.org/family-physician/patient-care/prevention-wellness/immunizations-vaccines/disease-pop-immunization/meningococcal-disease-vaccine.html

5. American Heart Association. (2019, November 19). *Kawasaki disease.* https://www.heart.org/en/health-topics/kawasaki-disease

6. Amrol, D. (2020, February). What are the most common causes of Stevens-Johnson syndrome? *NEJM Journal Watch.* https://www.jwatch.org/na50905/2020/02/18/what-are-most-common-causes-stevens-johnson-syndrome

7. Baddour, L. M., (2020). Impetigo. *UpToDate.* Retrieved February 5, 2022, from https://www.uptodate.com/contents/impetigo

8. Barnes, B. (2020). *Deadly pediatric rashes.* Relias Media. https://www.reliasmedia.com/articles/145643-deadly-pediatric-rashes

9. Barrell, A. (2021, January 27). Causes for a non-blanching rash in adults and children. *Medical News Today.* https://www.medicalnewstoday.com/articles/non-blanching-rash

10. Benedetti, J. (2019). Description of skin lesions. *Merck Manual: Professional version.* https://www.merckmanuals.com/professional/dermatologic-disorders/approach-to-the-dermatologic-patient/description-of-skin-lesions

11. Blank Children's Hospital. (2019, January 1). *Watch out for the most common allergies in children.* Unity Point Health. https://www.unitypoint.org/livewell/article.aspx?id=5dbd67a7-f210-405d-ba37-47471b898dbd

12. Campbell, R. L. (2021). Anaphylaxis: Emergency treatment. *UpToDate.* Retrieved February 5, 2022, from https://www.uptodate.com/contents/anaphylaxis-emergency-treatment

13. Cedars Sinai. (2021). *Impetigo.* https://www.cedars-sinai.org/health-library/diseases-and-conditions/i/impetigo.html

14. Centers for Disease Control and Prevention. (2015, May 11). *Molluscum contagiosum: Day care centers and schools.* https://www.cdc.gov/poxvirus/molluscum-contagiosum/day_care.html

15. Centers for Disease Control and Prevention. (2018, November 1). *Group A streptococcal (GAS) disease: Scarlet fever.* https://cdc.gov/groupastrep/diseases-hcp/scarlet-fever.html

16. Centers for Disease Control and Prevention. (2019, July 22). *Type and duration of precautions recommended for selected infections and conditions.* https://www.cdc.gov/infectioncontrol/guidelines/isolation/appendix/type-duration-precautions.html

17. Centers for Disease Control and Prevention. (2019, September 11). *Parasites: Lice.* https://www.cdc.gov/parasites/lice/index.html

18. Centers for Disease Control and Prevention. (2019, November 26). *Fifth disease.* https://www.cdc.gov/parvovirusb19/fifth-disease.html

19. Centers for Disease Control and Prevention. (2021, February 2). *Hand, foot, and mouth disease.* https://www.cdc.gov/hand-foot-mouth/index.html

20. Centers for Disease Control and Prevention. (2021, March 22). *Scarlet fever: All you need to know.* https://www.cdc.gov/groupastrep/diseases-public/scarlet-fever.html

21. Centers for Disease Control and Prevention. (2021, April 28). *Chickenpox (varicella): For healthcare professionals.* https://www.cdc.gov/chickenpox/hcp/index.html

22. Centre for Health Protection. (2019, August 28). *Scarlet fever.* https://www.chp.gov.hk/en/healthtopics/content/24/41.html

23. Chen, C., & Whitehead, A. (2021). Emerging and re-emerging infections in children: COVID/ MIS-C, Zika, Ebola, measles, varicella, pertussis: Immunizations. *Emergency Medicine Clinics of North America, 39*(3), 153–465. https://doi.org/10.1016/j.emc.2021.04.002

24. Cherney, K. (2018, February 14). *Immune thrombocytopenic purpura symptoms.* Healthline. https://www.healthline.com/health/understanding-itp/strange-symptoms-itp

25. Chiumento, S., & Owusu-Ansah, S. (2021). Medical emergencies. In S. Fuchs & M. McEvoy (Eds.), *Pediatric education for prehospital providers* (4th ed., pp. 111–136). American Academy of Pediatrics.

26. Cleveland Clinic. (2020, December 18). *Stevens-Johnson syndrome.* https://my.clevelandclinic.org/health/diseases/17656-stevens-johnson-syndrome

27. Cleveland Clinic. (2020, December 20). *Skin symptoms in most children with multi-system inflammatory syndrome related to COVID-19.* Consult QD. https://consultqd.clevelandclinic.org/skin-symptoms-in-most-children-with-multi-system-inflammatory-syndrome-related-to-covid-19/

28. Consolini, D. M. (2020, June). Rash in infants and young children. *Merck Manual: Professional version.* https://www.merckmanuals.com/professional/pediatrics/symptoms-in-infants-and-children/rash-in-infants-and-young-children

29. Coyner, T. (2020). Molluscum contagiosum. *Journal of the Dermatology Nurses' Association, 12*(3), 115–120. https://doi.org/10.1097/JDN.0000000000000534

30. Despotovic, J., & Grimes, A. (2018). Pediatric ITP: Is it different from adult ITP? *American Society of Hematology, 2018*(1), 405–411. https://doi.org/10.1182/asheducation-2018.1.405

31. Gastanaduy, P. A., Redd, S. B., Clemmons, N. S., Lee, A. D., Hickman, C. J., Rota, P. A., & Patel, M. (2019, May 13). Measles. In S. W. Roush, L. M. Baldy, & M. A. Kirconnel Hall (Eds.), *Manual for the surveillance of vaccine-preventable diseases* (Chapter 7). Centers for Disease Control and Prevention. https://www.cdc.gov/vaccines/pubs/surv-manual/chpt07-measles.html

32. Goldstein, A. O., & Goldstein, B. G. (2020). Pediculosis corporis. *UpToDate.* Retrieved February 5, 2022, from https://www.uptodate.com/contents/pediculosis-corporis

33. Goldstein, A. O., & Goldstein, B. G. (2021). Pediculosis capitis. *UpToDate.* Retrieved February 5, 2022, from https://www.uptodate.com/contents/pediculosis-capitis

34. Hockenberry, M. F. (2018). The child with hematologic or immunologic dysfunction. In S. E. Perry, M. J. Hockenberry, D. L. Lowdermilk, D. Wilson, K. Cashion, C. C Rodgers, & K. R. Alden (Eds.), *Maternal child nursing care* (6th ed., pp. 1271–1298). Elsevier.

35. Husada, D., Kusdwijono, Puspitasari, D., Kartina, L., Basuki, P. S., & Ismoedijanto. (2020). An evaluation of the clinical features of measles virus infection for diagnosis in children within a limited resources setting. *BMC Pediatrics, 20*(5). https://doi.org/10.1186/s12887-020-1908-6

36. Isaacs, S. N. (2020). Molluscum contagiosum. *UpToDate.* Retrieved February 5, 2022, from https://www.uptodate.com/contents/molluscum-contagiosum

37. Johns Hopkins Medicine. (n.d.). *Idiopathic thrombocytopenia purpura.* https://www.hopkinsmedicine.org/health/conditions-and-diseases/idiopathic-thrombocytopenic-purpura

38. Johns Hopkins Vasculitis Center. (n.d.). *Henoch-Schönlein purpura.* https://www.hopkinsvasculitis.org/types-vasculitis/henochschnlein-purpura/

39. Kayiran, M. A., & Akdeniz, N. (2019). Diagnosis and treatment of urticaria in primary care. *Northern Clinics of Istanbul, 6*(1), 93–99. https://doi.org/10.14744/nci.2018.75010

40. Kazeminejad, A., Hajheydari, Z., & Ghahari, M. J. (2019). Scabies treatment in children: A narrative review. *Journal of Pediatrics Review, 7*(2), 105–112. https://doi.org/10.32598/jpr.7.2.105

41. Kingston Hospital. (n.d.). *Non blanching rashes in children.* https://kingstonhospital.nhs.uk/healthcare-professionals/paediatrics-referrals/non-blanching-rashes-in-children/

42. Knudgaard, M. H., Andreasen, T. H., Ravnborg, N., Bieber, T., Silverberg, J., Egeberg, A., Halling, A., & Thyssen, J. (2021). Rhinitis prevalence and association with atopic dermatitis: A systematic review and meta-analysis. *Annals of Allergy, Asthma, & Immunology, 127*(1), 49–56. https://doi.org/10.1016/j.anai.2021.02.026

43. Konda, M., Fletcher, M., & Warrier, R. (2021). ITP is neither idiopathic nor always benign. *Clinical Pediatrics, 60*(3), 193–194.

44. Leung, A. K., Lam, J. M., Leong, K. F., & Hon, K. L. (2020). Tinea corporis: An updated review. *Drugs in Context, 9*, 5–6. https://doi.org/10.7573/dic.2020-5-6

45. Lillis, C. (2018, August 7). How to identify lice bites. *Medical News Today*. https://www.medicalnewstoday.com/articles/322691

46. Louie, M., Mikesell, C., & Chang, Y. K. (2020). *MIS-C: Multisystem inflammatory syndrome in children*. C. S. Mott Children's Hospital. http://med.umich.edu/mott/pdf/mis/MIS-C-ED-Inpt-Overview.pdf

47. Maity, S., Banerjee, I., Sinha, R., Jha, H., Ghosh, P., & Mustafi, S. (2020). Nikolsky's sign: A pathognomic boon. *Journal of Family Medicine and Primary Care, 9*(2), 526–530. https://doi.org/10.4103/jfmpc.jfmpc_889_19

48. Marathe, K., & Williams, J. (2017). Bacterial skin infections. In H. Adam, D. Campbell, T. DeWitt, J. Foy, & D. Kamat (Eds.), *Textbook of pediatric care* (2nd ed., Chapter 222). American Academy of Pediatrics. https://pediatriccare.solutions.aap.org/chapter.aspx?sectionId=135604823&bookId=1626

49. Mayo Clinic. (2021). *Multisystem inflammatory syndrome in children (MIS-C) and COVID-19*. https://www.mayoclinic.org/diseases-conditions/mis-c-in-kids-covid-19/diagnosis-treatment/drc-20502561

50. Mayo Foundation for Medical Education and Research. (2021). *Immune thrombocytopenia (ITP)*. https://www.mayoclinic.org/diseases-conditions/idiopathic-thrombocytopenic-purpura/symptoms-causes/syc-20352325

51. Murren-Boezem, J. (2018). *Impetigo*. Nemours KidsHealth. https://kidshealth.org/en/kids/impetigo.html#:~:text=Impetigo%20is%20contagious%2C%20which%20means,sores%20should%20begin%20to%20heal

52. National Eczema Association. (n.d.). *Atopic dermatitis in children*. https://nationaleczema.org/eczema/children/atopic-dermatitis/

53. National Eczema Association. (n.d.). *What is eczema?* https://nationaleczema.org/eczema/

54. National Heart, Lung, and Blood Institute. (n.d.). *Immune thrombocytopenia*. https://www.nhlbi.nih.gov/health-topics/immune-thrombocytopenia

55. National Institute of Diabetes, Digestive, and Kidney Diseases. (2020, April). *IgA Vasculitis*. https://www.niddk.nih.gov/health-information/kidney-disease/iga-vasculitis

56. Neidecker, J. (n.d.). *Preventing skin problems in wrestling*. https://orthonc.com/uploads/Wrestling-Skin.pdf

57. Ogbuefi, N., & Kenner-Bell, B. (2021). Common pediatric infestations: Update on diagnosis and treatment of scabies, head lice, and bed bugs. *Current Opinion in Pediatrics, 33*(4), 410–415. https://doi.org/10.1097/MOP.0000000000001031

58. Ogilvie-Turner, K., & Goldman, R. D. (2020). Cantharidin for molluscum contagiosum. *Canadian Family Physician, 66*(6), 419–420. https://www.cfp.ca/content/66/6/419.long

59. Onisai, M., Vladareanu., A., Spinu, A., Gaman, M., & Bumbea, H. (2019). Idiopathic thrombocytopenic purpura (ITP): New era for an old disease. *Romanian Journal of Internal Medicine, 57*(4), 273–283. https://doi.org/10.2478/rjim-2019-0014

60. Oved, J. H., Lee, C. S. Y., & Bussel, J. B. (2017). Treatment of children with persistent and chronic idiopathic thrombocytopenic purpura: 4 infusions of rituximab and three 4-day cycles of dexamethasone. *Journal of Pediatrics, 191*, 225–231. https://doi.org/10.1016/j.jpeds.2017.08.036

61. Parola, P., & Izri, A. (2020). Bedbugs. *New England Journal of Medicine, 382*, 2230–2237. https://doi.org/10.1056/NEJMcp1905840

62. Patrick, M. (2021, January 13). *Impetigo: What you need to know*. Nationwide Children's. https://www.nationwidechildrens.org/family-resources-education/700childrens/2021/01/impetigo

63. Philopena, R., Hanley, E., & Dueland-Kuhn, K. (2020). Emergency department management of rash and fever in the pediatric patient. *EB Medicine, 17*(1). https://www.ebmedicine.net/topics/infectious-disease/pediatric-rash-fever

64. Preda-Naumescu, A., Elewski, B., & Mayo, T. (2021). Common cutaneous infections: Patient presentation, clinical course, and treatment options. *Medical Clinics of North America, 105*(4), 783–797. https://doi.org/10.1016/j.mcna.2021.04.012

65. Rekhtman, S., Tannenbaum, R., Strunk, A., Birabaharan, M., Wright, S., & Garg, A. (2021). Mucocutaneous disease and related clinical characteristics in hospitalized children and adolescents with COVID-19 and multisystem inflammatory syndrome in children. *Journal of the American Academy of Dermatology, 84*(2), 408–414. https://doi.org/10.1016/j.jaad.2020.10.060

66. Rodgers, C. (2018). The child with cerebral dysfunction. In E. F. Olshansky (Ed.), *Maternal child nursing care* (6th ed., pp. 1355–1392). Elsevier.

67. Rodgers, C. (2018). The preschooler and family. In E. F. Olshansky (Ed.), *Maternal child nursing care* (6th ed., pp. 904–935). Elsevier.

68. Rodgers, C. (2018). The school-age child and family. In E. F. Olshansky (Ed.), *Maternal child nursing care* (6th ed., pp. 937–960). Elsevier.

69. Rodgers, C. (2018). The toddler and family. In E. F. Olshansky (Ed.), *Maternal child nursing care* (6th ed., pp. 867–903). Elsevier.

70. Romani, L., Whitfield, M. J., Koroivueta, J., Kama, M., Wand, H., Tikoduadua, L., Tuicakau, M., Koroi, A., Ritoya, R., Andrews, R., Kaldor, J. M., & Steer, A. C. (2017). The epidemiology of scabies and impetigo in relation to demographic and residential characteristics: Baseline findings from the skin health intervention Fiji trial. *American Journal of Tropical Medicine and Hygiene, 97*(3), 845–850. https://doi.org/10.4269/ajtmh.1-073

71. Royal Children's Hospital Melbourne. (2020). *Roseola infantum*. https://www.rch.org.au/kidsinfo/fact_sheets/Roseola_infantum/

72. Saguil, A., Kane, S. F., Lauters, R., & Mercado, M. G. (2019). Hand-foot-and-mouth disease: Rapid evidence review. *American Family Physician, 100*(7), 408–414. https://www.aafp.org/afp/2019/1001/p408.html

73. Techasatian, L., Phungoen, P., Chaiyarit, J., & Uppala, R. (2021). Etiological and predictive factors of pediatric urticaria in an emergency context. *BMC Pediatrics, 21*(92), 408–414. https://doi.org/10.1186/12887-021-02553-y

74. Thadchanamoorthy, V., & Dayasiri, K. (2020). Diagnosis and management of scabies in children. *Sri Lanka Journal of Child Health, 49*(4), 383–389. http://doi.org/10.4038/sljch.v49i4.9273

75. Tremblay, C., & Brady, M. T. (2021). Roseola infantum (exanthem subitem). *UpToDate*. Retrieved February 5, 2022, from https://www.uptodate.com/contents/roseola-infantum-exanthem-subitum

76. Van Durme, D. (2018). *Fundamentals of dermatology: Describing rashes and lesions* [Fact sheet]. https://camls-us

.org/wp-content/uploads/2018/05/Handout-Fundamentals -of-Dermatology.pdf

77. Watson, S. (2018, November 12). *Henoch-Schönlein purpura.* Healthline. https://www.healthline.com/health/henoch-schonlein -purpura

78. Williams, S. E. (2020, November 5). *Fifth disease (parvovirus B19).* American Academy of Pediatrics. https://www.healthy children.org/English/health-issues/conditions/skin/Pages/Fifth -Disease-Parvovirus-B19.aspx

79. Wilson, S. F., & Giddens, J. F. (2017). *Health assessment for nursing practice* (6th ed.). Elsevier.

80. World Health Organization. (2021). *Global progress against measles threatened amidst COVID-19 pandemic.* https:// www.who.int/news/item/10-11-2021-global-progress-against -measles-threatened-amidst-covid-19-pandemic

81. Wu, Y. F., Wang, J. J., Liu, H. H., Chen, W. X., & Hu, P. (2021). Scabies, incomplete lupus erythematosus and Henoch-Schonlein purpura. *Archives of Medical Science, 17*(2), 564–568. https://doi.org/10.5114/aoms/131542

The Child with an Altered Mental Status

Geraldine Siebenga St Jean, RN, BScN, ENC(C)

OBJECTIVES

Upon completion of this chapter, the learner will be able to:

1. Describe characteristics and selected causes of pediatric altered mental status, including toxicologic, metabolic, and neurologic emergencies.
2. Apply the Pediatric Nursing Process to a child with an altered mental status.

Introduction

Presentation of a child with an altered mental status can be challenging. There are many potential causes of this condition, whose severity ranges from relatively benign to life-threatening. Symptoms may include hypoxia, an electrolyte or metabolic imbalance, exposure or ingestion of toxins, or a condition related to brain structure or function.[28] Altered mental status in children is characterized by the failure to respond to a verbal or physical stimulus that is appropriate for the child's developmental level. Pediatric patients can present to the emergency department (ED) for as simple a reason as "they are not acting right." Parents may or may not know the reason for the child's altered mental status, but they do know they need to seek a higher level of care to determine the cause. Initial treatment of the underlying cause starts in the emergency department.

General Approach

Hypoxia and hypoglycemia are common and reversible causes of altered mental status. Several other specific conditions, such as drug, toxin, or substance exposure (intentional or unintentional) and specific disease processes, can present similarly, but the interventions vary, depending on the cause. To determine the cause of the child's altered mental state, nurses can anticipate some or all of the following diagnostic tests:

- Glucose
- Blood gas
- Electrolytes
- Complete blood count
- Blood cultures
- Toxicology screen including ethanol level
- Metabolic panel
- Coagulation studies

- Advanced metabolic studies (serum amino acids, carnitine level, and urine organic acids)
- Urinalysis and culture
- Serum ammonia level
- Computed tomography (CT) of the head for suspected trauma, status epilepticus, a severely obtunded state, or unremarkable diagnostic findings with persistent symptoms
- Lumbar puncture and collection of cerebral spinal fluid[102] following a CT scan if an infectious source is thought to be the cause[114]

Altered mental status is a symptom—not a diagnosis—that is caused by an underlying illness or trauma. Signs and symptoms of altered mental status can be observed upon presentation and determine the immediacy of care using the Pediatric Assessment Triangle. Look for age-specific behaviors. Assess the child's interactions and behavior. How does the child appear? How alert is the child? What are their speech, mood, and affect? Changes are often subtle.[28] Look for signs and symptoms of poor responsiveness to the family or the environment, weak or absent cry, eye deviation or changes in pupil reaction, abnormal respiratory assessment, abnormal motor movements, and decreased response to painful stimuli.[102] A mnemonic that can be used to remember possibilities for altered mental status in children is AEIOU TIPS (**Box 14-1**).

Hypoglycemic or Hypoxic—Until Proven Otherwise

There are many causes of altered mental status, but the two most common reasons for this symptom to appear in children are hypoglycemia and hypoxia.

Hypoglycemia

A very common reason for children to present with an altered mental status is hypoglycemia.[100] The human body requires glucose for energy production. Children, especially infants, have smaller glycogen stores and increased metabolism compared to adults, putting them at greater risk for hypoglycemia.

Hypoglycemia is considered a glucose value less than 70 mg/dL (3.9 mmol/L). Values less than 54 mg/dL (3 mmol/L) require immediate intervention.[2] Decreased levels of glucose to the brain cause signs and symptoms of altered mental behavior such as confusion, irritability, seizures or seizure-like activity, and focal symptoms that can mimic a stroke. Risk factors for hypoglycemia include the following[46,103]:

- First 48 hours of life
- Birth to a mother with diabetes or gestational diabetes

BOX 14-1 Mnemonic for Altered Mental Status (AEIOU TIPS)

Those concepts in bold are covered in this chapter.[28,102]

- **A** Abuse, **alcohol**, arrhythmia
- **E** **Electrolyte imbalances**, epilepsy, encephalopathy, **electrolyte abnormalities**, **endocrine**
- **I** Insulin-related issues **(hyperglycemia/hypoglycemia and diabetic ketoacidosis [DKA])**, infection, intussusception, inborn errors of metabolism, **ingestions**
- **O** **Overdose/ingestion**, **oxygen deprivation (hypoxia)**
- **U** Uremia
- **T** Trauma, temperature (hypothermia/hyperthermia), tumor
- **I** Infection
- **P** **Poisonings**, psychiatric, **postictal**
- **S** Shock, **seizures**, **stroke**, **shunt malfunction**

Data from Forti, R., & Avner, J. (2017). Altered mental status. In T. K. McInerny, H. M. Adam, D. E. Campbell, T. G. DeWitt, J. M. Foy, & D. M. Kamat (Eds.), *American Academy of Pediatrics textbook of pediatric care* (2nd ed., pp. 2786–2791). American Academy of Pediatrics; Swan, T. (2018). Pediatric altered mental status. In C. M. Zeretzke-Bien, T. B. Swan, & B. R. Allen (Eds.), *Quick hits for pediatric emergency medicine* (pp. 89–91). Springer International Publishing. https://doi.org/10.1007/978-3-319-93830-1_18

- Poor feeding
- Known history of diabetes
- History of hypoglycemic events
- Ingestion of a known oral hypoglycemic medication
- Side effect of many medications
  - Beta blockers, ethanol, salicylates, nonsteroidal anti-inflammatory drugs, and phenytoin
- Inborn errors of metabolism (congenital or genetic) such as glycogen storage disease
- Hormone deficiency such as panhypopituitarism (though often not diagnosed in the ED)
- Neuroblastoma, fibrosarcoma, and Wilms' tumor

Healthy neonates experience a drop in blood glucose as part of the normal physiological transition to extrauterine life. Infants are at higher risk for developing hypoglycemia due to insufficient glucose supplies, low glycogen or fat stores, or increased glucose utilization.[18] Stressors from illness and injury increase the child's demand for glucose, and may cause this demand to exceed the supply.[47]

Assessment Findings and Interventions

Signs and symptoms of hypoglycemia may include the following[20]:

- Lethargy
- Irritability
- Poor feeding
- Cyanosis
- Tremor
- Seizure
- Coma
- Death

Infants and toddlers often display nonspecific symptoms. The only symptom in an infant may be a hypoglycemic seizure. Additional findings for a neonate may include hypothermia, respiratory distress, apnea, and bradycardia. Older children may have complaints of dizziness, sweating, or hunger, and may appear anxious or confused. Confirm hypoglycemia with a bedside glucose measurement. Obtain a blood sample for laboratory analysis. Do not delay glucose supplementation if bedside glucose testing is not immediately available, and do not wait for venipuncture and laboratory confirmation. If the child has an insulin pump, immediately turn it off.[20,47]

For children who can safely swallow, interventions include the following[20]:

- Administer 0.3 g/kg (10–20 g) of oral simple carbohydrates. Examples include the following:
  - 5 ounces (150 mL) of fruit juice or regular soft drink (15 g)
  - 3 teaspoons (15 mL or 3 packages) of sugar— may dissolve in water (12.5 g)
  - 1 tablespoon (15 mL) honey (17 g)
  - 4 ounces (120 mL) unsweetened applesauce (15 g)
  - 1 pouch of squeezable applesauce/fruit puree (15 g)
    - Pouches that also contain protein or fat will not raise glucose levels as rapidly.
  - Glucose gel (see the label; usually15 g per tube; must be swallowed)
  - Glucose tablet (see the label; usually 5 g per tablet)
- Follow with a protein and starch snack such as peanut butter or cheese and crackers.
- More rapidly absorbed carbohydrates may be repeated in 10 to 15 minutes if the blood glucose level remains less than 70 mg/dL (3.89 mmol/L) and the child is still alert and able to safely swallow.

For children with altered mental status or who are unable to safely swallow and have severe symptoms (blood glucose usually less than 54 mg/dL [2.8 mmol/L]), interventions include the following[20,23]:

- Intramuscular or subcutaneous glucagon if intravenous (IV) access is not immediately available
  - 0.5 mg if patient weight < 25 kg
  - 1 mg if patient weight ≥ 25 kg
- IV dextrose
  - 2.5 to 5 mL/kg of 10% dextrose ($D_{10}W$)
  - 1 to 2 mL/kg of 25% dextrose for children > 5 years of age
    - 25% dextrose is an inappropriate concentration for infants and small children due to potential for vein damage

Reassessment should include the following steps[20,23]:

- Evaluate the child's response to the initial treatment, paying close attention to mental status and respiratory effort.
- Repeat a bedside glucose test 15 minutes after the initial treatment is given.
- Repeat treatment as indicated for a glucose level less than 70 mg/dL (3.9 mmol/L).
- Consider the need to administer IV dextrose infusions for recurrent hypoglycemia if oral intake is not possible or sufficient.

Hypoxia

Another common cause of altered mental status is hypoxia.

Assessment Findings and Interventions

Children with hypoxia can present in much the same way as children with hypoglycemia, albeit with a progression of respiratory distress or depression leading to a hypoxic event. If appropriate interventions are not taken, the child may follow the continuum to respiratory failure and possibly cardiac arrest.[108]

Early signs and symptoms of hypoxia include the following[3]:

- Tachypnea
- Increased respiratory effort
- Tachycardia
- Pallor, mottling, and cyanosis
- Agitation, anxiety, and irritability

Later signs and symptoms of hypoxia include the following[3]:

- Decreasing level of consciousness
- Signs of increased respiratory effort such as head bobbing, seesaw breathing, and grunting

- Bradypnea, inadequate respiratory effort, and apnea
- Bradycardia

Initial treatment is to provide supplemental oxygen and to optimize positioning (e.g., elevate the head of the bed or sit upright if possible, place a towel under the upper torso). Work with the physician or advanced practice provider to determine the cause of hypoxia and intervene as indicated (e.g., albuterol [salbutamol], antibiotics, relief of pneumothorax). Oxygen therapy can start with low-flow systems, including a nasal cannula and simple face mask, progressing to the use of high-flow systems such as a high-flow nasal cannula, noninvasive positive-pressure ventilation, and, if needed, manual positioning or use of artificial methods such as an oral pharyngeal airway, nasal pharyngeal airway, or intubation and mechanical ventilation.[28] See Chapter 7, "The Child in Need of Stabilization," and Chapter 8, "The Child with a Cough," for more information.

Toxicology

Toxicology encompasses both poisonings and overdoses. Paracelsus (1493–1541) stated, "All substances are poisons; there is none that is not a poison. The right dose differentiates a poison from a remedy."[111] This is still true today. A once-a-day medication that is therapeutic for an adult disease process can kill a child.[60] Medicine organizers such as blister packs and pill boxes that are meant to improve compliance among adults are a potential source of pediatric medication exposure due to lack of child-protective packaging.[26]

Children can present to the ED after ingestion, inhalation, or injection of a toxic substance or following ocular or dermal exposure. The toxic substances involved may not always be identifiable at the time of presentation and can lead to systemic or specific organ system damage. Suspect a toxicologic etiology when the pediatric patient has a sudden onset of symptoms.[62]

Assessment Findings and Interventions

The Pediatric Nursing Process is a valuable tool to prioritize assessments and interventions for a child experiencing a toxicologic emergency. Adding a few additional Ds for "donning and decontamination," an additional F for "find the antidote," and I for "identify the toxin or antidote" incorporates a few toxicologic considerations into the A–J mnemonic. Donning personal protective equipment always takes precedence over patient care. If a topical substance is causing significant patient harm, immediate patient decontamination may be the next priority intervention. Then, focus on the ABCDEs. Often,

supportive care and monitoring until the toxin is no longer active are the only interventions available. When toxic-specific antidotes or therapies are available, pediatric data on their use are frequently limited. Note the additional assessments and interventions that may be indicated for toxicologic presentations[34,81]:

A: Assess for airway patency.
- Look for any pills, packets, powder, or other substances in the oropharynx.
- Be aware of aspiration risk.
- Observe for airway swelling and obstruction.
- Be prepared to protect the airway with positioning, suctioning, or intubation.

B: Assess breathing rate, rhythm, depth, and breath sounds.
- Use supplemental oxygen as needed.
- Be prepared to assist ventilations for ineffective respirations or apnea.
  - Naloxone may be required if the patient is apneic.

C: Apply a cardiac monitor early.
- Dysrhythmias and other electrocardiogram changes are associated with a variety of toxins.

D: Assess disability (neurologic status), including pupils and presence of cough or gag reflex.
- Look for an altered level of consciousness.
  - Obtain a blood glucose level and manage hypoglycemia.
  - Consider naloxone administration if the patient's pupils are very small/pinpoint.
  - Consider stimulant exposure if the patient's pupils are large.
- Be alert for and manage seizure activity.

E: Expose and environment.
- Maintain patient and staff safety.
  - Inspect for needles, medication patches, other drug paraphernalia, tablets, or containers.
  - Odors may be a clue to identify the toxin but can also be an inhalation hazard.
- Decontaminate the patient, if not done earlier.
  - Dermal
    □ Remove clothing; brush off dry substances.
    □ Rinse with copious amounts of water.
    □ Corrosive agents injure the skin and have systemic effects.
  - Ocular
    □ Remove contact lens.
    □ Irrigate with copious amounts of fluid until pH is in target range.
    □ The target level of pH post chemical exposure to the eye(s) is 6.5 to 7.5.[53,90]
    □ Do not irrigate if there is also an ocular foreign body or globe rupture.

F: Obtain a full set of vital signs and family presence.

- Hypotension: Vasopressors may be required if IV fluid resuscitation is ineffective.
- Hypertension is often short-lived.
    - Benzodiazepines are the most common treatment, if indicated.
    - Antihypertensives may be considered if hypertension is severe.
        - Short-acting hypertensives are recommended.
            - Medications may be short or long acting.
            - Blood pressures can be labile with many toxins.
- Passive and/or active measures as required for hypothermia or hyperthermia.
- Find the antidote (**Table 14-1**).[7,8,11,14,31]
    - Recruit the family to help identify the toxin.
    - Identification of the toxin may not be possible; treat the patient based on symptoms and toxidrome (**Figure 14-1**).

G: Get adjuncts to the primary survey.

- Labs: These are all dependent on the substance or suspected substance.
    - Serum electrolytes—may include renal and hepatic function
    - Blood gas
    - Blood and urine toxicology screen
    - Serum drug levels
- Monitor: Obtain a 12-lead electrocardiogram, trend vital signs, and be alert for electrocardiogram changes.
- Nasogastric or orogastric tubes
    - May increase aspiration risk if used to administer charcoal[81]
    - Can be used to administer polyethylene glycol electrolyte (PEG) solution
- Oxygenation: Perform continuous pulse oximetry, capnography, and co-oximetry (if available).
- Decontaminate as indicated.
    - Gastrointestinal decontamination: Risk versus benefit should always be considered.
        - Activated charcoal: Limits absorption of some specific toxins in the gastrointestinal tract and should not be routinely administered to all patients with poisoning.
            - Risks include vomiting, aspiration, and lung injury.
            - Those at highest risk are patients with altered mental status, poor airway control, seizures, or bowel obstruction or perforation.

TABLE 14-1 Toxins and Antidotes*	
Toxicity	**Antidote**
Acetaminophen	Acetylcysteine
Anticholinergics	Physostigmine
Anticoagulants (drug-specific antidotes)	Andexanet alfa, idarucizumab, phytonadione (vitamin K), plasma, protamine, prothrombin complex concentrate, recombinant factor VIIa
Benzodiazepines	Flumazenil (Caution: May cause status epilepticus in benzodiazepine-dependent patients and others.)
Beta blockers and calcium channel blockers	Calcium, glucagon, high-dose insulin/glucose/potassium, lipid emulsion, vasopressors
Botulism	Botulinum antitoxin, botulism immune globulin
Cholinergics	Atropine, pralidoxime (organophosphate poisoning)
Carbon monoxide	100% O_2, hyperbaric chamber
Cyanide	Hydroxocobalamin
Digoxin	Digoxin immune FAB
Heparin	Protamine
Iron	Deferoxamine

(continues)

TABLE 14-1 Toxins and Antidotes* (*continued*)

Toxicity	Antidote
Isoniazid (antibiotic for tuberculosis)	Pyridoxine
Methemoglobinemia	Methylene blue
Opioids	Naloxone
Organophosphates	Atropine, pralidoxime
Salicylates	Sodium bicarbonate
Selective serotonin reuptake inhibitors	Cyproheptadine
Sulfonylureas (oral hypoglycemic)	Dextrose, octreotide
Toxic alcohols (ethylene glycol, methanol)	Fomepizole, ethanol (oral or intravenous), dialysis
Tricyclic antidepressants	Sodium bicarbonate, lipids

* Not a comprehensive list. Not all toxins and antidotes listed in this table are discussed in this chapter. Pediatric data are often limited.

Data from Barrueto, F. (2020). Beta blocker poisoning. *UpToDate*. Retrieved March 19, 2022, from https://www.uptodate.com/contents/beta-blocker-poisoning; Barrueto, F. (2021). Calcium channel blocker poisoning. *UpToDate*. Retrieved March 19, 2022, from https://www.uptodate.com/contents/calcium-channel-blocker-poisoning; Boyer, E. W. (2021). Serotonin syndrome (serotonin toxicity). *UpToDate*. Retrieved March 10, 2022, from https://www.uptodate.com/contents/serotonin-syndrome-serotonin-toxicity; Canadian Association of Poison Control Centres. (2021). *Canadian antidote guide for acute care toxicology*. https://www.ciusss-capitalenationale.gouv.qc.ca/antidotes?lang=en; Garcia, D. A., & Crowther, M. (2021). Management of bleeding in patients receiving director oral anticogulants. *UpToDate*. Retrieved March 19, 2022, from https://www.uptodate.com/contents/management-of-bleeding-in-patients-receiving-direct-oral-anticoagulants

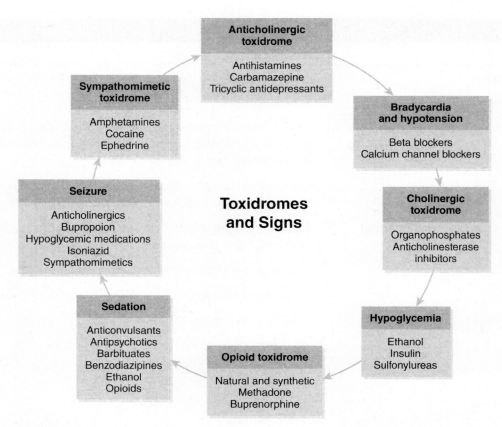

Figure 14-1 *Toxidromes and signs with potential causative agents.*

ACTIVATED CHARCOAL

The risks associated with using activated charcoal for gastric decontamination often outweigh the benefits. The potential for aspiration and lung injury is high in anyone with an altered mental status. Other contraindications include bowel obstruction, ileus, or perforation. Even when the patient is currently alert, many toxins will gradually cause an altered mental status, increasing aspiration risk.[44]

□ Whole-bowel irrigation: PEG solution is indicated for ingestions of life-threatening amounts of sustained-release medications, iron supplements, lead-containing foreign bodies, lithium, and illicit drug packs (no sign of leakage).
  ○ Contraindicated in a patient with unprotected airway, bowel obstruction, frequent vomiting, and unstable vital signs
- Enhanced elimination
  □ Urinary: Diuresis and alkalization
  □ Hemodialysis
  □ Peritoneal dialysis
  □ Repeat dose of activated charcoal for large ingestions or sustained preparations.

H: History may be inaccurate or unknown. Continue to enlist family and friends to determine the events related to the patient's condition.

I: Inspect all body surfaces and clothing for medication patches, tablets, and containers if not done already.
- Identify the substance with any new information obtained.
- Count the remaining tablets in a container and compare this number to the prescribed quantity and date.
- Use tablet shape, size, color, and imprint with online software to identify the medication.

J: Just keep evaluating.
- Consider the duration of action for any identified toxin.
- Call the poison control center or consult toxicology information sources for recommended management and ongoing monitoring.

Toxidromes

To help with the identification of potential poisonings or overdoses, toxins can be grouped based on their common physical findings. Assessment and treatment may then be based on the symptoms or toxidrome. A variety of toxidrome classifications exist. Figure 14-1 shows one depiction of various causative agents, toxidromes, and presenting signs.

The signs and symptoms of the various toxidromes are presented in **Table 14-2**.[12,60,112]

Medication Toxicity

Poisonings in children are often the result of a child getting access to adult medications or taking too much of a pediatric medication. The substances taken may be simple, over-the-counter medications, but when consumed by the child in quantity they can become deadly. One adult dose of commonly prescribed medications may be life-threatening for children.

Acetaminophen

Pediatric acetaminophen overdose is a significant problem worldwide. This product is available in multiple formulations, both as an individual product and in combination forms. Because acetaminophen is so readily accessible, it is a common cause of intentional and unintentional overdose.[69] A toxic ingestion in children is more than 150 mg/kg.[72] Peak serum levels are reached at 4 hours after ingestion.[72] The initial toxicity can produce mild effects but result in life-threatening hepatotoxicity. A complicating factor, especially for parents, is the large number of over-the-counter medications that contain acetaminophen. Parents may inadvertently overdose their child if they do not read labels carefully or note the amount of acetaminophen in the medication.[72]

Stages of acetaminophen toxicity are as follows[85]:

- Stage I (0–24 hours): Nausea and vomiting, but most patients are asymptomatic.
- Stage II (24–72 hours): Right upper quadrant (RUQ) tenderness, tachycardia, and hypotension. May have decreased urine output, elevated liver enzymes, and abnormal coagulation studies.
- Stage III (72–96 hours): Liver failure, RUQ pain, vomiting, jaundice, coagulopathy, hypoglycemia, renal failure, metabolic acidosis, multi-organ failure.
- Stage IV (4 days–2 weeks): Resolution of hepatic dysfunction.

The history should include which product was ingested or the name of the drug, with special consideration given to combination drugs. Baseline diagnostic studies include the following:

- Serum acetaminophen level
- Aminotransferases (alanine transaminase [ALT] with or without aspartate transaminase [AST])

TABLE 14-2 Common Toxidromes

Toxidrome	Vital Signs	Pupils	Skin	Mental Status
Anticholinergic	↑HR ↑BP ↑T	Dilated (mydriasis)	Dry Flushed Warm or hot	Agitation Delirium Hallucinations Seizures Coma
Cholinergic	↓HR	Constricted (miosis)	Diaphoretic Drooling Tearing	Depressed Confused Seizures
Hallucinogenic	↑HR	Normal Dilated	Normal	Confused Hallucinations
Opioid	↓RR ↓BP	Constricted	Normal	Depressed
Sedative/hypnotic	Normal	Varies	Normal	Depressed
Sympathomimetic	↑HR ↑BP ↑RR	Dilated	Warm or hot Diaphoretic	Alert Agitated Seizures

Abbreviations: BP, blood pressure; HR, heart rate; RR, respiratory rate; T, temperature.

Data from Brocato, C., & Paley, R. (2021). Toxidromes: Common poisoning syndromes to know. *Journal of Emergency Medical Services, 46*(2). https://www.jems.com/patient-care/common-poisoning-syndromes-to-know/; Lucas, J. (2018). Pediatric toxicology. In C. Zeretzke-Bienm, T. Swan, & B. Allen (Eds.), *Quick hits for pediatric emergency medicine* (pp. 133–145). Springer International Publishing. https://doi.org/10.1007/978-3-319-93830-1_18; Velez, L. I., Shepher, J. G., & Goto, C. S. (2020). Approach to the child with occult toxic exposure. *UpToDate*. Retrieved March 21, 2022, from https://www.uptodate.com/contents/approach-to-the-child-with-occult-toxic-exposure

- Coagulation studies including international normalized ratio (INR)
- Serum creatinine

Decontamination is also a possibility. If the child presents within the first hour of ingestion, consideration is given to a single dose of activated charcoal orally unless contraindicated due to the patient's altered mental status with associated risk of aspiration. Charcoal may benefit the pediatric patient when administered up to 4 hours post ingestion, especially with acetaminophen ingestions of more than 500 mg/kg.[61]

For single acute ingestions, compare the 4-hour acetaminophen level to the Romack-Matthews nomogram. If the child's serum level falls in the possible or probable range, prepare to administer *N*-acetylcysteine (NAC) within 8 hours of ingestion or as soon as possible according to your local protocols.[61]

Intravenous NAC administration is recommended. Many clinicians are now using a two-step approach. With this regimen, the child receives a bolus infusion at 150 mg/kg over the first hour. After the first hour, the infusion is decreased to a dose of 12.5 to 25 mg/kg/hr for a minimum of 20 hours, based on local dosing protocols.[49,61] Near the end of the 21-hour infusion, the initial blood tests are repeated, and the infusion can be terminated if the child meets the following criteria:

- Serum acetaminophen concentration is undetectable (i.e., below the lower limit of quantification measured by the local laboratory).
- Aminotransferases (ALT with or without AST) are normal or declining on at least one measurement.
- INR is less than 1.5.
- Serum creatinine is normal or declining.
- The patient is clinically well (no evidence of encephalopathy).

If the child does not meet these criteria, the NAC infusion can be continued until the criteria are met.[61]

Antidepressants

Multiple classifications of antidepressants exist, but selective serotonin reuptake inhibitors (SSRIs) and tricyclic antidepressants (TCAs) are of particular concern when considering pediatric overdose. An overdose of either of these types of medications can be lethal if not recognized early. Antidepressant prescriptions of both SSRIs and TCAs are on the rise, and healthcare providers need to be aware that they are often prescribed in combination with other medications.[56]

Selective Serotonin Reuptake Inhibitors

SSRIs are more widely used than other antidepressants, in part because they have fewer dangerous side effects in the event of an overdose. Fluoxetine (Prozac), paroxetine (Paxil), and sertraline (Zoloft) are just a few of the SSRIs that are more commonly prescribed. When taken in excessive amounts, they can lead to life-threatening serotonin syndrome. SSRI overdoses typically produce central nervous system (CNS) depression and seizures. Serotonin syndrome causes hyperthermia, hypertension, tachycardia, and muscular rigidity and may be treated with benzodiazepines and cyproheptadine. Short-acting antihypertensives are used to treat the blood pressure lability.[11,81]

Tricyclic Antidepressants

An overdose of a TCA can cause cardiovascular dysrhythmias and cardiovascular collapse. As little as one tablet can kill a child. TCA prescriptions appear to be on the rise again despite warnings about their dangers.[56] In particular, they are often prescribed in combination with other psychotropic drugs. Amitriptyline (Elavil) and doxepin (Sinequan) are examples of TCAs. Symptomology in case of an overdose falls into the anticholinergic category.[104]

Children with TCA overdose can present with the anticholinergic toxidrome: dry mucous membranes (dry as a bone), mental status changes (mad as a hatter), mydriasis (blind as a bat), flushed skin (red as a beet), hyperthermia (hot as a hare/pistol), tachycardia, prolonged QRS interval, heart block or ventricular dysrhythmias, hypertension, decreased bowel sounds, urinary retention, ataxia, and even seizures.[55]

Activated charcoal may be administered for gastric decontamination if the patient presents within 2 hours of ingestion and there are no contraindications such as bowel obstruction or altered mental status. Intravenous sodium bicarbonate is the first-line therapy for hypotension or dysrhythmias. Lipid emulsion therapy, lidocaine, magnesium, and benzodiazepines are other treatment considerations.[88]

Benzodiazepines

Whether they are prescribed as an anticonvulsant, antispasmodic, anxiolytic, or sleep aid, benzodiazepines can be abused or inadvertently ingested. Toxicity is significantly increased if these medications are taken in combination with alcohol or other CNS depressant drugs. Examples include alprazolam (Xanax), clonazepam (Klonopin, Rivotril), diazepam (Valium), lorazepam (Ativan), midazolam (Versed), and temazepam (Restoril).

Symptoms of benzodiazepine overdose include respiratory and CNS depression. Treatment is primarily supportive care. Caution should be used when reversing benzodiazepine overdose with the antidote flumazenil. Flumazenil can cause status epilepticus in patients who routinely take benzodiazepines or who have epilepsy.[62]

Beta Blockers and Calcium Channel Blockers

Ingestion of a cardiac medication can be life-threatening for children. The effects of such medications that are desired in an adult are amplified in children, leading to hypotension, bradycardia, and conduction defects. Hypoglycemia is associated with beta blocker overdose, while hyperglycemia is associated with calcium channel blocker overdose. Treatment options for are based on symptom severity and include the following[7,8,46]:

- IV fluids for hypotension: 5–10 mL/kg repeated as necessary to decrease the chance of fluid overload due to myocardial depression.[4]
- Atropine and pacing may be attempted but are often ineffective.
- Glucagon (may cause vomiting, be prepared with suction)
- Calcium
- Dextrose infusion and high-dose insulin
- Monitor blood glucose every 30 minutes.
- Monitor potassium every hour; insulin will lower potassium levels.
- Vasopressors for persistent hypotension
- Lipid emulsion
- Activated charcoal if not contraindicated, as there is a high risk for aspiration with altered mental status
- Venous arterial extracorporeal membrane oxygenation (ECMO)[9]

Iron

Iron is found in many vitamin formulations, with the greatest lethality occurring from ingestion of prenatal vitamins. Iron is toxic to the gastrointestinal, cardiovascular, and central nervous systems, though the underlying mechanism is unclear. Doses between 20 and 60 mg/kg produce a mild to moderate toxicity, while doses greater than 60 mg/kg can cause severe symptoms, even death.[74]

Initial presentation of iron poisoning may include vomiting, diarrhea, and gastrointestinal bleeding. Late stages of iron ingestion may present as acidosis, coagulopathy, and organ failure. Gastrointestinal scarring and obstruction can occur as long as 1 month after the ingestion.[105]

Serum iron levels 4–6 hours post ingestion are useful in predicting the clinical course of treatment. An abdominal radiograph may be helpful in determining the number of tablets that were ingested, as the iron may be visible on the image. Options for treatment include chelation therapy with deferoxamine or whole-bowel irrigation if a large volume was ingested.[21]

Opioids

Opioid overdose–related hospitalizations are rapidly increasing among youth and adolescents.[46] Addiction is a disease that often starts in adolescence. The parts of the brain that are most involved in attention regulation, inhibition of impulses, and appreciation of the consequences of actions are not fully formed until individuals reach their mid to late twenties. Consequently, many adolescents underestimate the risks associated with dangerous behaviors and overvalue the rewards. Adolescents may also discount parental advice, giving in to peer pressure to engage in risky behaviors. All of these attributes predispose the adolescent to substance abuse.[115]

Opioids are available in many formulations and can be administered by almost any route. Fentanyl, carfentanyl, and other potent synthetic drugs not only pose a risk to those who use, abuse, or are accidentally exposed to them, but may also pose a risk to healthcare workers who come in contact with them.[25]

The most common presentation with opioid overdose is respiratory depression with constricted pupils (miosis). Oxygenation and ventilation are the priority treatments in such a case, along with initiation of naloxone. Be aware that naloxone has a short half-life and may need to be repeated; alternatively, the child may need to be placed on a naloxone infusion.[46] This medication can be administered intranasally, intramuscularly, subcutaneously, or intravenously.[76]

A unique type of opioid overdose that has markedly increased in recent years is tramadol overdose. Tramadol works on both opioidergic and nonopioidergic pathways, resulting in CNS depression from the opioid properties and seizures from the nonopioid pathways. In laboratory studies, naloxone alone has been shown to reduce respiratory depression but causes an increase in seizures when used in isolation.[58] More studies are needed to obtain evidence that would support best practices with this type of presentation. Until future studies and data

can be collected, there are no clear recommendations for treating patients with tramadol overdose. The literature suggests considering benzodiazepines as the first line of treatment in combination with naloxone to reverse tramadol's CNS-related toxicity.[13]

Oral Hypoglycemics

Ingestion of oral hypoglycemics in a child can cause significant hypoglycemia. Correction of the low blood sugar takes priority. Even small amounts of sulfonylureas can cause significant hypoglycemia.[60] Interventions include the following[109]:

- Initiate IV access for dextrose administration. This treatment will quickly resolve the effects of hypoglycemia, and the onset of action is much quicker than with oral sugar. It is also safer for children who present with an altered mental status and lowers the risk of aspiration.
- Glucagon may be ineffective due to the lower glycogen stores in children.
- Octreotide or diazoxide may be given to inhibit pancreatic insulin release.
- If the patient is alert, able to maintain an airway, and able to swallow, oral supplementation may be used to treat hypoglycemia.

Salicylates

The majority of salicylate exposures are from oil of wintergreen (1 mL is equivalent to 1400 mg of aspirin), herbal oils, and topical analgesic rubs. Early presentation includes tinnitus, fever, tachypnea, diaphoresis, and abdominal distress. The respiratory center in the brainstem is directly stimulated, causing hyperventilation, respiratory alkalosis, and metabolic acidosis with an increased anion gap. Seizures, coma, and hemodynamic instability are seen in severe toxicity.[46]

Early gastric decontamination and aggressive fluid resuscitation may help maintain tissue perfusion and renal function. The use of sodium bicarbonate to alkalinize the urine has been shown to increase the elimination of salicylates and help correct acidemia. Potassium supplementation is important to consider whenever sodium bicarbonate is administered. Severe toxicity may require hemodialysis to decrease salicylate levels and correct electrolyte abnormalities.[46]

Other Toxins

Pediatric poisonings also result from a variety of other toxic substances, some of which may be used recreationally or be prescribed. For example, sympathomimetics are found in medications used for attention deficit or hyperactivity, and cannabis-based medications are used for conditions such as seizures, nausea, and anxiety. Opioids, mentioned in the previous section, are also used both therapeutically and illicitly.

Alcohol

Ethanol is the alcohol found in beer, wine, and liquor, but is also present in some antiseptics and solvents. Ethanol ingestion may present with similar symptoms in people of all ages, but the root cause of the ingestion often differs based on age. Young children are naturally curious and mimic adult behaviors. Glasses of wine or a bottle of beer left on a low table are easily accessed by small children. More recently, with the increased use of alcohol-based sanitizers, children are being exposed to alcohol through dermal absorption and licking or eating hand sanitizer. Even small amounts of alcohol are dangerous for young children.[48,86]

Adolescents may present with intentional poisoning as part of a suicide attempt or experimenting with drugs and alcohol. In such situations, alcohol is often consumed with various other drugs, which compounds their effects and the resulting presentation.[48] The rate of consumption is a significant issue with adolescents, with two-thirds of high school students reporting using alcohol and 20% reporting binge drinking in the past 2 weeks.[15]

Young children are prone to profound hypoglycemia, coma, and hypothermia when they ingest even small amounts of ethanol. The significance of symptoms is positively correlated with blood alcohol levels.[27] Ethanol exposures are treated with IV fluids. Closely monitor and support oxygenation, ventilation, and blood glucose as needed. Hemodialysis is effective but rarely necessary.[81]

Toxic Alcohols

Methanol, isopropyl alcohol, and ethylene glycol are other alcohols that children may be exposed to in household products such as antifreeze and solvent as well as homemade alcoholic beverages. Young children can ingest alcohols due to fluids being poured into smaller containers rather than being kept in their original packaging.[86] Signs and symptoms of such poisonings include nausea, vomiting, ataxia, slurred speech, nystagmus, visual changes, hypotension, seizures, tachycardia, tachypnea, and hypoglycemia.[43]

Fomepizole and ethanol are antidotes for methanol and ethylene glycol poisoning. Fomepizole is the antidote of choice for children, as it does not cause inebriation or have the potential for worsening hypoglycemia. Folic acid enhances methanol elimination and may prevent retinal

toxicity. Hemodialysis is indicated for those patients with end-organ injury and severe metabolic acidosis.[81]

Cannabis

With the increasing legalization of marijuana, more children are presenting with adverse reactions to cannabis products from intentional and unintentional exposures.[22] The widespread availability of enticing marijuana edibles increases the risk for children's inadvertent ingestion of cannabis. The ease of obtaining look-alike products online, whose packaging mimics common candy and food brands (**Figure 14-2**), is a concern for child safety.[1,65]

The most common presentations with cannabis exposures are neurologic in nature, such as a mild tremor, irritability, ataxia, extreme lethargy, stupor, and coma. These symptoms can mimic those of a postictal state, encephalitis, or sepsis, leading to unnecessary diagnostic testing and interventions. Sinus tachycardia and hypertension with respiratory depression necessitating the need for mechanical ventilation have been noted.[122] Vomiting and seizures have also been reported, as well as paradoxical hyperactivity and irritability.[22] Treatment is supportive, including respiratory support, IV fluids, and benzodiazepines for agitation. A urine toxicology screen may be ordered to confirm the presence of tetrahydrocannabinol.[122]

Sympathomimetics

Sympathomimetics encompass agents such as cocaine, amphetamine, methamphetamine, 3,4-methylenedioxymethamphetamine (MDMA, ecstasy), and bath salts. They stimulate the CNS and cause a cascade of adrenergic symptoms. Toxicity can be life-threatening. Although the various amphetamines do have some unique clinical features, there is substantial overlap among this class as a

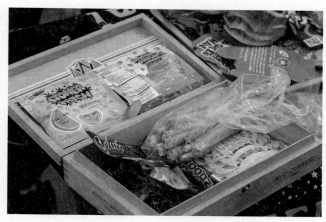

Figure 14-2 *Medicated look-alike candies.*
© Alexi Rosenfeld/Getty Images News/Getty Images.

whole. Treatment is first directed at the patient; identifying the toxin is a secondary consideration.[77]

Amphetamine derivatives such as MDMA, as well as paramethoxyamphetamine and paramethoxymethamphetamine (PMA and PMMA, slang name "death"), tend to be distributed in colorful, branded tablets taken orally. Some of the most widely abused drugs by both university students and teenagers, they are popular with participants in the rave and party scene. PMA/PMMA are more toxic than MDMA. Unfortunately, the initial effects of PMA/PMMA are often delayed and less euphoric than MDMA. This may lead users to believe they have taken a weak MDMA product, resulting in repeated dosing in an effort to obtain the desired effect.[67]

Cocaine is a naturally occurring plant derivative with sympathomimetic properties. It can be used intranasally, injected, or inhaled. Sometimes presentations of cocaine overdose may take the form of a body packer or body stuffer (an individual attempting to smuggle or hide drugs by inserting them into the body cavity or ingesting them). If these individuals present with symptoms related to overdose, emergent removal is needed, as each hidden package contains a significant amount of drug.[77]

Signs and symptoms associated with sympathomimetic use include the following[77,112]:

- Altered mental status (agitation, delirium, coma, visual hallucinations)
- Tachycardia, hypertension, tachypnea, diaphoresis
- Neuromuscular rigidity, tremors, hyperreflexia, nystagmus, seizures
- Dysrhythmias, electrocardiogram abnormalities (QRS prolongation)
- Electrolyte abnormalities (hypoglycemia, hyponatremia, hyperkalemia)

Hyperthermia is an ominous finding and should prompt immediate initiation of treatment, particularly if the patient's body temperature is greater than 106°F (41°C). If such temperatures are sustained for more than 20 minutes, they are likely to lead to fatal multi-system failure. Prolonged hyperthermia may be associated with rhabdomyolysis, seizures, multiple-organ dysfunction, significant metabolic acidosis, and disseminated intravascular coagulation (DIC).[77]

Interventions and treatment include the following:

- In severe presentations (e.g., altered mental status, hyperthermia), laboratory tests should include electrolytes, blood gases, lactate, creatine kinase, partial thromboplastin time (PTT), prothrombin time (PT), international normalized ratio (INR), troponin, and renal/hepatic panel.

- Obtain an electrocardiogram (ECG).
- Treat agitation with aggressive use of benzodiazepines (midazolam, diazepam [more rapid onset], or lorazepam).
- Perform continuous temperature monitoring.
  - In a patient with hyperthermia, body temperature should be brought to less than 102°F (38.8°C) within 20 minutes or less.[77]
  - Completely undress the patient and use ice over water-soaked sheets, ice packs, cooling blankets, cold saline infusions, or cool air to maintain the patient temperature within the normal range.[67] If the patient remains hyperthermic and agitated despite aggressive treatment measures, intubation and paralysis using a nondepolarizing neuromuscular blocker (e.g., rocuronium) is appropriate. Succinylcholine is relatively contraindicated because of the risk of precipitating or worsening hyperkalemia in patients with rhabdomyolysis. Ongoing sedation can be achieved using either propofol or benzodiazepine infusions.
  - If there is persistent muscle rigidity, dantrolene can be used.[36]
  - Physical restraints should be used sparingly, as they may increase injury and the risk of rhabdomyolysis.
- Treat cocaine-associated dysrhythmias.
  - Sinus tachycardia usually resolves after sedation, cooling, and rehydration.
  - Cocaine has sodium channel–blocking effects, which may be reflected on a 12-lead ECG as a widened QRS. Sodium channel blockade should be treated with sodium bicarbonate, 1 to 2 mEq/kg IV push followed by an infusion if the initial bolus is effective. If no effect is seen, lidocaine is recommended.[97]
  - Cocaine use can also result in seizures and hypotension.
- Treat seizures aggressively by administering benzodiazepines (midazolam, diazepam, or lorazepam). If seizures continue despite benzodiazepine therapy, either a barbiturate (e.g., phenobarbital) or propofol may be administered to terminate the seizures. Phenytoin should be avoided in toxin-induced seizures.[67]

Carbon Monoxide Poisoning

Carbon monoxide is formed during incomplete combustion of almost any substance that has a carbon-containing compound. It is an odorless, colorless, and tasteless gas.[57] Presentations of carbon monoxide poisoning can occur from children being involved in a house fire; exposure through the use of combustion of charcoal, wood, or natural gas (especially when the flue is blocked) for heating or cooking in an enclosed space; the use of gasoline-powered generators within an enclosed space; and exhaust fumes from motor vehicles. Symptoms associated with carbon monoxide poisoning are often nonspecific and can be confused with a viral infection. The most common symptoms are headache, nausea, or vomiting, so that this poisoning is often misdiagnosed as influenza, gastroenteritis, or food poisoning, especially in infants and small children.[17]

The brain and the heart are the most sensitive to carbon monoxide poisoning. Carbon monoxide binds to hemoglobin, decreasing the delivery of oxygen to cells, which leads to hypoxia. Carbon monoxide also interferes with cellular respiration by binding to mitochondrial cytochrome oxidase. Patients develop a respiratory alkalosis as the body attempts to compensate for the reduced oxygen-carrying capacity. Carbon monoxide poisoning is associated with neurological sequelae and morbidity even after acute treatment.[17]

Compared to adults, children are more sensitive to the effects of carbon monoxide due to their increased metabolic and respiratory rates. Children become symptomatic at much lower concentrations of carbon monoxide than do adults. The severity of symptoms does not correlate well with serum carboxyhemoglobin levels in younger children due to factors such as air density at the time of occurrence and the child's physiologic characteristics.[91] Be aware that pulse oximeters cannot differentiate oxygenated hemoglobin from carboxyhemoglobin, making pulse oximetry readings unreliable in case of carbon monoxide poisoning. Noninvasive co-oximetry is available, but accuracy of the data obtained from such devices has been questioned.[17] An alternative clinical marker is lactate: Elevated lactate is a significant marker for worse outcomes.[107]

Management includes administering high-flow oxygen via nonrebreathing mask or endotracheal tube. The effect of the oxygen is to enhance dissociation of the carbon monoxide. Hyperbaric oxygen therapy reduces the half-life of carbon monoxide and increases the amount of dissolved oxygen available to cells. When hyperbaric oxygen therapy is used, early treatment provides greater benefit.[17,106]

Cyanide Poisoning

In children, cyanide poisoning is most often associated with smoke inhalation, suicide attempts, and criminal activity. Sources of unintentional exposure include jewelry cleaning and electroplating in jewelry production, ingestion of artificial nail remover, and ingestion of seeds or pits from the *Prunus* species (e.g., almonds, apricots, cherries, peaches, plums). Absorption of cyanide can occur through oral, dermal, inhalational, and parenteral routes.[45]

Cyanide prevents the tissues from extracting oxygen from the blood. Assessment findings include tachypnea, bradypnea, or apnea; tachycardia; altered mental status; seizures; hypotension; dysrhythmias; and cardiovascular collapse. The most notable clinical features are metabolic acidosis with an elevated lactate level.[70] Children who are unresponsive and suspected to have carbon monoxide poisoning from fire exposure are considered to have cyanide poisoning as well.[107]

Antidotes for cyanide poisoning are available. The preferred antidote is hydroxocobalamin, as it has a safer profile and fewer side effects than the cyanide antidote kits used in the past. An alternative antidote is a combination of amyl nitrate, sodium nitrite, or sodium thiosulfate. These latter antidotes have many undesired side effects, and can induce methemoglobinemia, vasodilation, and, subsequently, hypotension.[70]

Detergent Pods

Detergent pods were introduced as degradable, single-use detergent containers in the last 10 years. They have since become a health hazard, especially for children younger than 5 years of age. These brightly colored pods closely resemble candy (**Figure 14-3**),[39] which is very appealing to the younger child.[95] Younger children have a tendency to explore their environment tactilely and often put items they find in their mouth, especially ones that look like candy. Often items are removed from their original container, leading to ingestion as well as ocular and dermal exposure.[19] Among adolescents, a key concern is

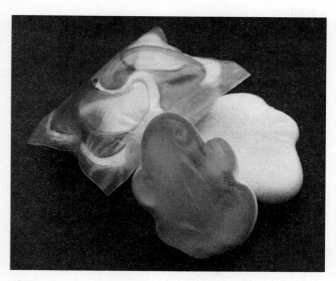

Figure 14-3 *Detergent pod and candy similarity.*
Courtesy of Sarah Zahn.

the dangerous game of intentionally biting or swallowing detergent pods.[37] Detergent pods are pressurized packages; when bitten, the contents are released in an explosive manner that can lead to aspiration, ingestion, and dermal and ocular exposures. The pH of detergent ranges from 7.5 to 8.9; when mixed with water, the pH of detergent pod contents has been recorded as high as 11.[95]

Following the ingestion of single-use detergent pods, children present with emesis, significant mucosal damage, respiratory symptoms, throat pain, drooling, and foaming at the mouth.[96] Assess the child for oral mucosal edema, respiratory distress, apnea, and, in severe cases, respiratory failure. The respiratory distress failure continuum symptoms may include increased bronchial secretions, coughing, wheezing, dyspnea, stertor (lower-pitched airway sound similar to snoring), and stridor. Other symptoms may include CNS depression, drowsiness, and lethargy,.[19] Management depends on the severity of the symptoms.[96]

Interventions include symptomatic and supportive care. Provide supplemental oxygen for hypoxemia, and bronchodilators for laryngeal spasm and bronchospasm. Severe airway edema and chemical burns may require endoscopy and possible intubation and mechanical ventilation.

Ocular exposure causes eye irritation, pain, and conjunctivitis. Flush the eyes with copious amounts of 0.9% sodium chloride. Typical recovery takes about 1 week.

Dermal exposure causes rash, erythema, and skin irritation. On occasion, burns have also developed. Clothing saturated in detergent should be removed immediately and the skin irrigated with soap and water. If burns do develop, they are treated as thermal burns.[19]

Lead

Lead poisoning causes adverse cognitive and behavioral effects in children, most notably developmental delays.[41] Despite awareness and prevention efforts, children continue to be exposed to lead through inhalation, ingestion, or skin contact. Ongoing lead exposure sources include maternal transmission prenatally or while nursing, old paint chips or dust, soil, water (leaching from lead pipes), toys, costume jewelry, pottery, and artificial athletic field turf.[89]

The clinical presentation of lead poisoning includes neurologic changes, fatigue, anorexia and weight loss, vomiting, constipation, and abdominal pain. If lead poisoning is suspected, ask whether there are any walls with paint chips flaking off, as this could be the source of ingestion with young children, who are orally fixated. An abdominal radiograph may be of use if a lead-containing object was ingested.

Though the treatment for lead poisoning may not be initiated in the ED, the diagnosis may be determined due to repeat visits for reoccurring symptoms. Treatment consists of chelation with agents that remove lead from the blood and soft tissues. Close monitoring and follow-up are required during and after treatment.[66]

Organophosphates

Organophosphates are used in industry, agriculture, and home gardens, and as a weapon. They are easily absorbed through skin, via inhalation, or by ingestion.

Once absorbed, the organophosphate molecules bind to the acetylcholinesterase molecules in red blood cells, making the acetylcholine enzyme inactive. The result is an overabundance of acetylcholine within synapses and neuromuscular junctions. Overstimulation of nicotinic receptors found at neuromuscular junctions can lead to fasciculations and myoclonic jerks. These effects are more prominent in children. The resulting depolarizing block will cause flaccid paralysis. Nicotinic receptors also are found in the adrenal glands, so their overstimulation may cause hypertension, sweating, tachycardia, and leukocytosis.[84]

The inhibition of acetylcholinesterase causes a cholinergic toxidrome. There are a few mnemonics to help recall the symptoms. The components of these toxidromes are indicated by the mnemonics SLUDGEBBB and/or DUMBBELLS (**Box 14-2**). In children, the nicotinic effects are especially prominent; a memory aid for these symptoms is based on the days of the week (**Box 14-3**).

Management starts with decontamination. The person affected should be completely undressed and then washed with soap and water. Airway management is a high priority due to bronchospasm and bronchorrhea. Antidotes for organophosphate poisoning include atropine (an anticholinergic drug) and pralidoxime. If atropine administration is aggressive enough, the patient may not require intubation. Larger than usual doses of atropine, as well as repeated doses, may be needed. Pralidoxime works on the nicotinic receptors but must be administered within 48 hours of exposure. The mortality rate from organophosphate exposures is often related to a delay in diagnosis, as symptoms can develop slowly.[84,116]

Injury Prevention and Health Promotion

Every presentation to the ED is an opportunity for injury prevention and health promotion. Have pamphlets or QR codes that link to specific topics available to help parents child-proof their homes and prevent poisonings. Help them understand which substances and solutions are

BOX 14-2 SLUDGE and DUMBBELLS Mnemonics for Cholinergic Toxidromes

SLUDGE mnemonic:

- **S**alivation
- **L**acrimation
- **U**rination
- **D**efecation (diarrhea)
- **G**astrointestinal upset
- **E**mesis

DUMBBELLS mnemonic:

- **D**iarrhea, **d**iaphoresis
- **U**rination
- **M**iosis
- **B**radycardia
- **B**ronchorrhea (watery sputum)
- **E**mesis
- **L**acrimation
- **L**ethargic
- **S**alivation

The killers are the Bs: bradycardia, bronchorrhea, and bronchospasm.

Data from Robb, E. L., & Baker, M. B. (2021, July 26). *Organophosphate toxicity.* StatPearls Publishing. https://www.ncbi.nlm.nih.gov/books/NBK470430/; Welker, K., & Thompson, T. (2018). Pesticides. In R. M. Walls, R. S. Hockberger, & M. Gausche-Hill (Eds.), *Rosen's emergency medicine: Concepts and clinical practice* (9th ed., pp. 1947–1956). Elsevier.

BOX 14-3 Memory Device for Nicotinic Signs of Acetylcholinesterase Inhibitor Toxicity Seen More Prominently in Children

The memory device is simply the days of the week:

Monday = Mydriasis
Tuesday = Tachycardia
Wednesday = Weakness
Thursday = Hypertension
Friday = Fasciculations

Reproduced from Robb, E. L., & Baker, M. B. (2021, July 26). *Organophosphate toxicity.* StatPearls Publishing. https://www.ncbi.nlm.nih.gov/books/NBK470430/

poisonous and how to best store these items to safeguard their own children and any other children who visit their homes. Provide parents with the phone number for the local poison control center.[86]

Many overdoses and poisonings may be unintentional, but others are intentional, especially in the adolescent population. Screen pediatric patients presenting with toxicities for suicide risk and the need for subsequent interventions.[6,30]

Discharge teaching post opioid overdose includes how to use naloxone, how to reduce the risk associated with opioid use disorders, and how to mitigate harm associated with opioid misuse.[120] Discharge discussions may also include the option of medication-assisted treatment for opioid use disorders. Despite the proven efficacy of these programs, they often are not utilized.[73] Another promising development is programs in which individuals with a history of substance use disorder are trained as recovery coaches.[63]

Seizure

Pediatric seizures are a common chief complaint in the ED, with approximately 5% of all children having a seizure by the time they are 16 years old.[42] Seizure presentations may have any of several causes. The most commonly encountered is febrile seizures, discussed in Chapter 10, "The Child with a Fever." Other causes may include trauma (discussed in Chapter 9, "The Child with an Injury"), toxins, hypoglycemia, electrolyte imbalances, improper formula dilution, tumors, and issues that may arise with anticonvulsant medications. Seizures can be classified as generalized or focal (partial), and pediatric seizures may present differently than adult seizures. Not all seizures cause unresponsiveness—that is, patients may maintain their awareness during a focal seizure.[119]

Epilepsy is a seizure disorder that is characterized by two or more seizures without provocation. A provoked seizure has a known cause, such as trauma, hyponatremia, or fever.[119] Diagnosing epilepsy can be difficult, as seizures present in many different forms. The variant that is most difficult to diagnose is absence seizure, as the patient may not realize that they are having these episodes. These types of seizures are often identified by an astute teacher in the classroom, who may notice brief periods of "daydreaming" and a change in grades.

Status epilepticus is a convulsive generalized seizure or series of seizures that last more than 5 minutes or recurring seizures without a return to baseline between seizures.[118] It is considered an emergency requiring intervention. Prolonged seizure activity can result in hypoxia, hypoglycemia, hyperthermia, acidosis, electrolyte imbalance, and increased intracranial pressure.[118]

Assessment Findings and Interventions

Seizure activity in children older than age 6 presents similarly to adult seizure activity.[119] In younger children, their immature nervous system function leads to an increased propensity for seizures with subtle symptoms.

RED FLAG

Without knowledge of the unique seizure presentations in younger children, seizures and status epilepticus may go undetected. Tonic–clonic movements may be focal or generalized. These muscle contractions are usually rhythmic and repetitive, but can be slower than what is typically seen in adults. The following signs are sudden but subtle[92,119]:

- Asynchronous movements of extremities
- Behavior change, usually becoming quiet
- Bicycling of legs (neonatal seizure presentation)
- Extension of arms, head, and trunk
- Flexion of arms, head, and trunk
- Forced deviation of the eyes
- Increased muscle tone/tenseness (focal or generalized)
- Lip smacking (more common in neonatal seizure presentation)
- Loss of head control
- Loss of muscle tone (focal or generalized)
- Pallor, cyanosis
- Twitching of eyelids or extremities
- Unilateral twitching/spasms

For the child who presents with seizure activity, support the airway, breathing, and circulation. When there is no history or suspicion of trauma, place the child on their side to prevent aspiration. During the seizure, do not restrain the child or attempt to put anything in their mouth. Protect the head. Provide a safe environment and institute seizure precautions such as padding the side rails of the crib or bed, removing any clutter that could be harmful, initiating fall precautions, and having oxygen and suction readily available. Assess for hypoglycemia as a cause of the seizure or as a result of prolonged seizure activity and correct as needed.

The history will help determine whether the seizure was provoked and which diagnostics may be needed to determine the cause. Assessment questions include the length of the seizure; symptoms associated with the seizure, such as a fever or vomiting; current medications or changes in medications or dosing; triggers prior to the seizure; description of body movements, if they involved the whole body or one particular area; and any change in color. If the seizure subsided prior to arriving at the ED, ask about the child's behavior and mental status since the seizure. Ask the parent what their impression was of the event.[121]

Figure 14-4 is an example of one algorithm for managing pediatric status epilepticus. For children with epilepsy, ask caregivers what medications they are taking currently, what medications have been given for the seizure, and what medications have been used in the past to manage the child's seizures successfully. No algorithm will account for individual responses to medications; past experiences may be much more useful for guiding management.

Diabetic Ketoacidosis

In Canada and the United States, 30% of children are in diabetic ketoacidosis (DKA) when they are first diagnosed with type 1 diabetes.[32] Causes of DKA in children who are known to have diabetes include failure to administer or incorrect administration of insulin, limited access to healthcare, gastroenteritis, and unrecognized issues with insulin delivery in patients using an insulin pump.[2,32] When children in DKA are dehydrated and acidotic enough to experience cerebral injury, the mortality rate ranges from 21% to 24%.[33]

Assessment Findings and Interventions

Anorexia, nausea, vomiting, and abdominal pain may lead clinicians to suspect appendicitis or gastroenteritis. The definition of pediatric DKA is as follows[32]:

- Hyperglycemia: Blood glucose > 200 mg/dL (11 mmol/L)
- Venous pH < 7.3 or serum bicarbonate < 15 mmol/L (15 mEq/L)
- Ketonemia (blood ß-hydroxybutyrate ≥ 3 mmol/L) or ketones in the urine

Interventions are implemented to resolve the ketoacidosis and reduce the blood glucose level while correcting dehydration and electrolyte abnormalities.[113] Anticipate administration of an insulin infusion without an insulin bolus and IV fluids as indicated by the patient's hemodynamic status and degree of dehydration. Close

Pediatric Status Epilepticus Algorithm
* in children over 1 month of age

Recognition of Status Epilepticus

An unresponsive patient with either one of the following has convulsive status epilepticus:

- Seizure >5 min and/or ongoing seizure on presentation to EMS/ED

- 2 or more seizures without full recovery of consciousness between seizures

Initial Management

- Initiate ABCs, cardiorespiratory and BP monitoring
- O₂ 10-15 L/min via non-rebreather mask
- Prioritize giving the first dose of benzodiazepine as early as possible, followed by checking blood glucose
- Monitor for respiratory depression, hypotension, arrhythmias
- Give acetaminophen 15 mg/kg/dose (MAX 650 mg) PR if febrile
- **Consider other investigations:**
  - Electrolytes, blood gas, calcium, CBC, serum glucose
  - Other: anticonvulsant drug levels, LFTs, blood & urine culture

**Phase 1
5-15
min**

Prehospital

1. Give Midazolam IM/intranasal (IN) (see dosing table).
2. Check blood glucose:
   If blood glucose <3.3 mmol/L (<60 mg/dL):
   Treat with D25W 2 mL/kg/dose IV (MAX 100 mL/dose) OR
   D10W 5 mL/kg/dose IV (MAX 250 mL/dose).
3. If still seizing after 5 minutes, give Midazolam second dose.
   MAX cumulative dose 10 mg in prehospital setting.

Emergency Department (ED)

1. Give benzodiazepine if two doses not already given prior to ED arrival (see dosing table).
2. Check blood glucose if not already done. Treat hypoglycemia as above. Reassess blood glucose in 5 minutes.
3. Give second benzodiazepine dose for ongoing seizures 5 minutes after first dose. When IV/IO access available, switch to IV/IO route.

CAUTION: Do not give more than 2 doses of benzodiazepines.

First Line Agents

No IV/IO	
Midazolam IM or IN	≤13 kg: 0.2 mg/kg/dose 13-40 kg: 5 mg/dose >40 kg: 10 mg/dose MAX 10 mg/dose

IV/IO	
Lorazepam IV/IO	0.1 mg/kg/dose MAX 4 mg/dose
Midazolam IV/IO	0.1 mg/kg/dose MAX 10 mg/dose

Reassess ABCs, monitor for respiratory depression. If still seizing give one of these second-line agents:

**Phase 2
15-20
min**

Drug	Dose	Age	Comments/Cautions
Levetiracetam	60 mg/kg/dose IV/IO (MAX 3000 mg/dose) Infuse over 5 minutes	Any age	↓side effects/drug interactions, low risk of psychosis
Fosphenytoin	20 mg phenytoin equivalent (PE)/kg/dose IV/IO/IM (MAX 1000 mg PE/dose) Infuse over 10 minutes	Any age	↓BP, ↓HR, arrhythmia; avoid in toxicologic seizures; choose alternate drug if on phenytoin at home or consider partial loading dose of 10 mg PE/kg/dose
Valproic Acid	40 mg/kg/dose IV/IO (MAX 3000 mg/dose) Infuse over 10 minutes	≥2 years	In Canada, only available via Health Canada Special Access Program; caution in patients with liver dysfunction, mitochondrial disease, urea disorder, thrombocytopenia or unexpected developmental delay
Phenytoin	20 mg/kg/dose IV/IO (MAX 1000 mg/dose) **Infuse over 20 minutes**	Any age	↓BP, ↓HR, arrhythmia; avoid in toxicologic seizures; choose alternate drug if on phenytoin at home or consider partial loading dose of 10 mg kg/dose; use only if Fosphenytoin not available
Phenobarbital	20 mg/kg/dose IV/IO (MAX 1000 mg/dose) **Infuse over 20 minutes**	<6 mos	Respiratory depression, especially in combination with benzodiazepines

Reassess ABCs, monitor for respiratory depression. If still seizing:

Administer alternative second line agent (e.g., if fosphenytoin given, use levetiracetam)

Pediatric Referral Centre Discussion:

- Need for intubation vs. bag-mask ventilation; hypercapnia is common and resolves with seizure cessation and non-invasive respiratory support
- Additional work up including full septic work up, use of antibiotics/antivirals, brain imaging
- Persistent altered LOC possibly related to non-convulsive status epilepticus or severe underlying brain disorder
- Third line agent: infusion of midazolam, pentobarbital, propofol OR ketamine

 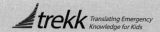

Figure 14-4 *Pediatric status epilepticus algorithm.*

Pediatric DKA Presentation

Patients with DKA may present with irritability, erratic behavior, confusion, lethargy, and coma. Obtaining a bedside glucose level for any child with altered mental status can quickly identify a hypoglycemic or hyperglycemic etiology. Other signs and symptoms of DKA include the following:

- Abdominal pain
- Anorexia
- Deep, fast breathing (Kussmaul respirations)
- Dehydration
- Fruity breath
- Incontinence, bedwetting in previously toilet-trained child
- Nausea
- Polydipsia (excessive thirst)
- Polyuria
- Vomiting
- Weight loss

In adolescents, altered mental status with fruity breath may be mistaken as alcohol intoxication. Young children who cannot express thirst or obtain their own fluids my not have notable polyuria. Additionally, diaper rash with *Candida* raises suspicion for diabetes.[32]

glucose monitoring and reevaluation of the ketoacidosis is needed to guide insulin, fluid, and dextrose administration. Initial potassium levels may be elevated but will decrease with insulin administration and will likely require supplementation. Monitor for signs and symptoms of cerebral injury such as altered mental status, urinary incontinence, new headache, or persistent vomiting. These signs of cerebral edema may be treated with mannitol or hypertonic saline.[33]

Emerging Trend

There has been a longstanding concern that initial rapid fluid boluses would increase the risk of cerebral edema in children with DKA. A recent Pediatric Emergency Care Applied Research Network (PECARN) study looked at four different approaches to fluid resuscitation in children with DKA. Rates of correction of acidosis and normalization of electrolytes were analyzed based on fluid infusion rates and sodium chloride concentrations. The recommendation is to administer fluids more quickly to normalize the anion gap sooner. There was no correlation between faster infusions and mental status changes.[82]

Electrolyte Imbalances

Electrolyte disorders require an understanding of fluid and electrolyte balance and the regulatory mechanisms that maintain homeostasis. Body fluids shift to maintain an osmolar balance. The neuron impulse transmissions responsible for functions such as cardiac conduction and muscle contraction require a normal influx of sodium, potassium, and calcium ions. Other electrolytes such as magnesium and phosphate also impact interdependent biologic functions.[99]

Assessment Findings and Interventions

Various electrolyte imbalances can present with altered mental status, weakness, fatigue, or irritability. Other common presentations are nausea, vomiting, ECG changes, and skeletal muscle weakness or twitching. The brain is particularly sensitive to sodium levels. Shifts of intracellular fluid to and from the intravascular space can cause cerebral edema and injury. Potassium and calcium disturbances can present with a dysrhythmia-induced syncopal episode or altered mental status from cardiogenic shock.[52] **Table 14-3** lists electrolyte abnormalities along with their potential causes and associated signs and symptoms.[16,35,52,64,101]

Electrolyte imbalances are gradually corrected to avoid rapid fluctuation and fluid shifts. Many electrolytes are interdependent, necessitating close monitoring and potential supplementation. Interventions may include hypotonic, hypertonic, or isotonic IV fluid infusions; limiting oral fluid intake; administering diuretics; dialysis; and further diagnostics to determine the cause of the imbalance. With the exception of calcium given for life-threatening dysrhythmias, electrolytes are infused slowly when IV administration is necessary.[35,52]

Treatment for hyperkalemia focuses on stabilizing cardiac function and shifting potassium intracellularly. The urgency of administration depends on the level of hyperkalemia, the significance of the ECG changes, and the potential for continuing potassium increases (e.g., crush injury, tumor lysis syndrome). Interventions may include the following[68,98]:

- Calcium gluconate or calcium chloride immediately stabilizes cardiac conduction by antagonizing potassium. It is the priority intervention for significant ECG changes such as a widening QRS and dysrhythmias,
- Infusion of a dextrose solution prevents hypoglycemia caused by administration of insulin.
- Insulin shifts potassium intracellularly.

TABLE 14-3   Electrolyte Imbalances

Electrolyte Imbalance	Causes	Signs and Symptoms
Hyponatremia	Adrenal insufficiency Cystic fibrosis Diarrhea Heat-related illness Long-distance running Overly diluted infant formula Syndrome of inappropriate antidiuretic hormone Vomiting Water intoxication	Ataxia Headache Lethargy Muscle cramps Nausea, vomiting Psychosis Seizure Weakness
Hypernatremia	Diabetes insipidus Diarrhea Enemas Fever Phototherapy Sodium bicarbonate administration Undiluted infant formula Vomiting	Confusion Intracranial hemorrhage Irritability Seizure Weakness
Hypokalemia	Diarrhea Diuretics DKA management Laxatives Metabolic alkalosis Vomiting	ECG changes Cardiac dysrhythmias Flattened T wave Prolonged PR interval Prolonged QT interval U waves Widened QRS Nausea, vomiting Skeletal muscle weakness
Hyperkalemia	Adrenal corticoid insufficiency Blood draw hemolysis Blood transfusion Burns Drug interactions or effects DKA Heat-related illness Hypoparathyroidism Renal failure Rhabdomyolysis Tumor lysis syndrome	ECG changes Cardiac dysrhythmias Peaked T wave Prolonged PR interval Shortened QT interval U waves Widened QRS

(continues)

TABLE 14-3   Electrolyte Imbalances (*continued*)

Electrolyte Imbalance	Causes	Signs and Symptoms
Hypocalcemia	Abnormal magnesium metabolism Fluoride poisoning Hypoparathyroidism Pancreatitis Vitamin D deficiency	Anxiety Irritability Muscle tetany Muscle twitching Facial grimacing Hyperactive deep tendon reflexes Paresthesia (mouth, hands, feet) Seizure
Hypercalcemia	Adrenal insufficiency Cancer Hyperparathyroidism Hyperthyroidism Paget's disease Pheochromocytoma Vitamin A and D toxicity	Abdominal pain Anorexia Confusion Constipation Fatigue Headache Hypotonicity Nausea, vomiting Nocturia, polyuria Seizure

Abbreviations: DKA, diabetic ketoacidosis; ECG, electrocardiogram.

Data from Chan, M., & Enarson, P. (2020). Fluid and electrolyte therapy in infants and children. In J. E. Tintinalli, O. J. Ma, D. M. Yealy, G. D. Meckler, J. Stapczynski, D. M. Cline, & S. H. Thomas (Eds.), *Tintinalli's emergency medicine: A comprehensive study guide* (9th ed., pp. 851–856). McGraw Hill; Greenbaum, L. (2020). Fluid and electrolyte disorders. In R. Kliegman & J. St. Geme (Eds.), *Nelson textbook of pediatrics* (21st ed., pp. 389–403). Elsevier; Kaplan, R. L., & Burns, R. (2021). Renal and electrolyte emergencies. In K. Shaw & R. Bachur (Eds.), *Fleisher & Ludwig's textbook of pediatric emergency medicine* (8th ed., pp. 965–989). Wolters Kluwer; Mahajan, P., & Felt, J. (2017). Fluids, electrolytes, and acid-base composition. In T. K. McInerny, H. M. Adam, D. E. Campbell, T. G. DeWitt, J. M. Foy, & D. M. Kamat (Eds.), *American Academy of Pediatrics textbook of pediatric care* (2nd ed., pp. 420–433); Swan, T. (2018). Electrolyte disturbances. In C. M. Zeretzke-Bien, T. B. Swan, & B. R. Allen (Eds.), *Quick hits for pediatric emergency medicine* (pp. 117–131). Springer International Publishing. https://doi.org/10.1007/978-3-319-93830-1_17

- Albuterol/salbutamol via inhalation shifts potassium intracellularly; it does not require IV access.
- Sodium bicarbonate may assist to shift potassium, particularly when the patient is severely acidotic.
  - Controversial and without proven benefit
  - Should not be the only therapy used
- Diuretics improve urinary excretion of potassium. Ensure adequate hydration and renal function prior to their administration.
- Sodium polystyrene sulfonate (Kayexelate) binds with potassium within the gastrointestinal tract and is eliminated in stool.
- Dialysis removes excess potassium; it is especially useful in children with renal dysfunction.

Headache

Despite advances in healthcare, headaches are one of the most frequently reported problems among school-aged children and adolescents worldwide.[71] The Global Burden of Disease study ranks headaches as the second leading cause of years lived with a disability[78] and the third leading cause of pediatric ED visits.[79] One study reported a higher incidence among girls and provided suggestions for effective coping mechanisms for stress and increased access for mental health.[50] The burden of headaches leads to frequently missed hours of school, poorer learning outcomes, and, if significant enough, the need to repeat a grade or drop out of school completely.[54]

Chvostek's and Trousseau's Signs with Hypocalcemia

- Chvostek's sign: Facial spasm induced by lightly tapping just in front of the patient's ear.
- Trousseau's sign: Carpal spasm induced after inflating a blood pressure cuff above the patient's systolic blood pressure for 3 minutes.[101]

Administration of Insulin and Dextrose for Hyperkalemia

It is always possible to suddenly lose IV access. Administer dextrose before insulin to avoid hypoglycemia with no means of IV correction in the case of IV infiltration or dislodgement.

Assessment Findings and Interventions

Headaches are classified as either primary or secondary headaches. Although life-threatening secondary headaches are most worrisome, primary headaches are more common. **Figure 14-5** depicts a broad approach to the assessment and management of pediatric headaches.

With primary headache, the headache itself is the cause of the child's pain. Such headaches have multifactorial etiologies, including psychosocial causes, and can change over time. A retrospective study of primary headaches revealed that the two most common triggers were stress (75.5%) and sleep disturbances (69.9%).[123] The most common types of primary headaches in pediatric patients are tension-type headaches and migraines.

Secondary headaches are due to an underlying condition or disease process. They are further classified as benign or life-threatening. Thunderclap headache is an acute-onset headache that reaches maximum intensity in 1 minute and is mainly associated with life-threatening causes, which require emergent interventions. Red flags such as fever, trauma, occipital headaches, and abnormalities in a neurologic examination may point to underlying diseases such as meningitis; intracerebral, subarachnoid, subdural, and epidural hemorrhages; increasing intracranial pressure; brain tumor; or stroke as being the cause of the headache. Children who present with symptoms concerning for a secondary headache often will undergo blood tests and a CT scan as part of the diagnostic process. Based on the CT findings, a lumbar puncture may be required as well.[79]

Assessment requires a thorough history related to headache frequency; symptoms surrounding the headache; pain intensity; signs of aura; abdominal involvement, including dull, diffuse abdominal pain; nausea; and vomiting to determine the type of headache. Components of a thorough history include the following:

- Headache description: Onset, duration, location, quality
- Pain: Severity using an appropriate pain scale
- Triggers and exacerbating factors: Stress and sleep patterns
- Alleviating factors

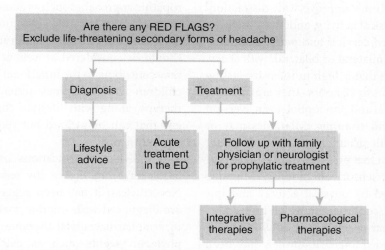

Figure 14-5 *Pediatric headache: Assessment and management.*

- Dose of medications taken to relieve the headache
- Mental health screening
- Medical history and family history

RED FLAG ⚠

Be alert for red flags while assessing the child with a headache.[79,87] The following indicators are associated with a life-threatening secondary headache:

- Abnormal eye movements
- Age < 5 years
- Altered level of consciousness
- Ataxia
- Changes or increase in severity of headache
- Comorbidities (e.g., sickle cell disease, malignancy, pregnancy, ventriculoperitoneal shunt)
- Fever
- Focal neurologic deficits
- Increased head circumference
- Occipital headache (relative red flag)
- Pain: "Worst ever" or that wakes a child from sleep
- Seizure
- Sudden onset of headache
- Trauma
- Visual field deficits

Tension-type headaches and migraines can be differentiated by presentation of symptoms. Tension headaches are mostly bilateral, dull oppressive pain that is of medium intensity, lasting anywhere from 30 minutes to 7 days. Symptoms sometimes improve with distraction, are not worsened by physical activity, and are sometimes accompanied by increased cervical and pericranial muscle tone. Migraines are unilateral or bilateral, with sharp, pulsating oppressive pain that is high in intensity, lasting anywhere from 60 minutes to 72 hours. They are often associated with photophobia and phonophobia, an aversion to smells, and nausea and vomiting. Migraines may or may not be associated with an aura. An aura is a transient focal neurologic symptom that precedes the headache; examples include visual or sensory alterations.[79] Migraine symptoms are aggravated by physical activity and improved by finding a dark, cool room in which to sleep.[71]

While in the ED, pharmaceutical options for headache treatment can be explored. Ibuprofen has been shown to provide superior headache relief as compared to acetaminophen.[79] Antiemetics and IV fluids are useful for nausea, vomiting, and dehydration. If analgesics were taken prior to presenting to the ED with little or no effect, review the dosage. Other medication options include dihydroergotamine and triptans. Dopamine receptor antagonists administered with IV ketorolac have been shown to be effective for pain and nausea relief, but clinicians must be alert for extrapyramidal reactions and excessive sedation with respiratory depression.[79]

The use of opioids is explicitly discouraged for primary headache disorders. Opioids may potentiate the migraine. More broadly, there is concern about the rising rate of opioid (mis)use and the morbidity and mortality among adolescents from opioid overdose.[79]

Treatment of headache is multifaceted and may require trialing different strategies. A combination of integrative therapies may be required. Primary headaches are often the culmination of genetics, lifestyle, stress, and environmental factors. Avoiding triggers (e.g., caffeine, monosodium glutamine, alcohol, and chocolate) and promoting adequate hydration, nutrition, and sleep are recommended.[79] Other lifestyle and nutrition strategies include the following[24]:

- Encouraging children to do the best that they can do but not pushing them to do more or achieve higher goals, to mitigate the risk of increasing migraine episodes.[71]
- Having a regular, structured day with adequate nutrition, sleep, water, and physical activity.
- Engaging in regular sports or exercise as least twice a week with a group of peers in a noncompetitive setting.

Some evidence indicates that dietary supplements such as magnesium, riboflavin, and coenzyme Q10 may lead to improvement in neuronal-based symptoms. Naturopathic approaches such as acupuncture, aroma therapy, hypnosis, and learning relaxation techniques have also been successful for some children. Psychological services should be considered as well, as depression and anxiety may contribute to the functional impairment from which children with migraines suffer.[24] Cognitive-behavioral therapy, along with lifestyle changes, is another strategy that can be utilized but requires a significant time commitment.[54]

Prophylactic medications used in the adult population have not shown any reliable results in children. Nevertheless, it has been suggested that children who are diagnosed with migraines and who do not respond to nonpharmaceutical therapies can be trialed on prophylactic agents such as calcium channel blockers, beta blockers, amitriptyline (a TCA), or topiramate (an anticonvulsant).[71,75]

Stroke

Stroke is defined as an acute neurologic deficit with imaging evidence of ischemic injury in a vascular bed. It is not a term that one often hears when referring to pediatric patients, though the incidence of pediatric stroke is on the rise. Strokes in children are not related to plaque deposits, but rather are due to underlying conditions. Such strokes can occur when a cerebral blood vessel becomes occluded, leading to ischemia distal to the occlusion, or ruptures, leading to a hemorrhage. The increased reporting of such events may be due to the fact that we have better diagnostics for detecting these incidents or the fact that we are better able to manage illnesses such as sickle cell disease and leukemia, increasing survivability and, in turn, reporting of adverse events such as a stroke.[83]

Neonatal stroke is much more common than childhood stroke, and they are very different in terms of their etiologies. Neonates present with acute encephalopathy, altered mental status, and focal seizures.[117] Typically, neonatal strokes occur in term babies with uneventful deliveries. Imaging studies suggest that these events occur prior to birth and are most often classified as a venous thrombosis. Most such strokes are due to sluggish perfusion or a hypercoagulable state. The treatment is to maintain adequate hydration and administer anticonvulsants if the stroke is associated with seizures. Prognosis is not good, with long-term sequelae being noted. Better diagnostics and management protocols are needed for patients with this condition.[83]

Assessment Findings and Interventions

Children with stroke often present with headache and vomiting followed by a seizure. Other signs and symptoms of pediatric stroke include the following[29]:

- Focal signs and symptoms
- Hemiparesis
- Speech disturbance
- Visual disturbance
- Dysphagia (difficulties with swallowing)
- Ataxia
- Nonlocalizing signs and symptoms
- Headache
- Altered mental status
- Vomiting
- Seizure

Ischemic strokes are often due to diseases that affect the vasculature or are related to coagulopathies, but may not always be identifiable. Many of the stroke treatments commonly used for adults are adapted for children despite the fact there is little evidence for their safety and effectiveness in children. Thrombolysis with fibrinolytics, antiplatelet agents, other anticoagulants, and clot retrieval may be used within the same time parameters as for adults.[83]

Hemorrhagic stroke presentations are often associated with a sudden onset of headache, vomiting, and rapid deterioration of neurologic function. Most hemorrhagic strokes are due to arteriovenous malformation, but other causes include brain tumors, coagulopathies, thrombocytopenia, and subarachnoid hemorrhages. Most often, subarachnoid hemorrhages are associated with trauma. Like adults, children can incur cerebral injury and neurologic deficits with stroke. Approximately 50% of children will develop long-term deficits from their stroke.[93]

Use the Pediatric Nursing Process to identify the need for any immediate life-saving interventions and to obtain a baseline assessment for future comparisons. Complete a history including any symptoms of weakness, headache, nausea and vomiting, changes in vision, or seizure-like activity. The National Institute of Health Stroke Scale has been adapted for use in children older than 2 years of age.[59] Ask if the onset of symptoms was gradual (which suggests the cause is an infection, metabolic abnormality, or space-occupying lesion) versus sudden (which suggests the patient has a structural lesion—that is, a stroke).[28] When immediately available and tolerated by the patient, magnetic resonance imaging (MRI) is preferred over CT with angiography.[29] Facilitate consultation with a pediatric neurologist as soon as possible to determine the most effective, regionally available intervention.

Hydrocephalus

Hydrocephalus may be either a congenital or an acquired condition. The etiology of hydrocephalus is varied, with this condition being caused by overproduction of cerebrospinal fluid (CSF), impaired circulation, inhibited absorption, or obstructed flow.[5] Presentation of hydrocephalus differs greatly depending on the age group.

Understanding the concept and symptomology of hydrocephalus requires understanding the Monro-Kellie hypothesis. The Monro-Kellie hypothesis suggests that the skull is a fixed volume that houses three components: brain, blood, and CSF. In the case of hydrocephalus, changes in the CSF volume directly affect the brain and blood volumes. Symptomology of hydrocephalus is related to ability or inability to accommodate to these changing volumes. Infants, with the exception of those who have craniosynostosis, are unique in that their skull volume is not fixed, as they have open suture lines.[80]

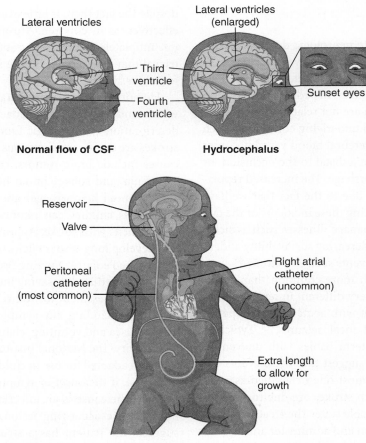

Figure 14-6 *Clinical appearance of hydrocephalus with sunset eyes and ventriculoperitoneal shunt.*

Assessment Findings and Interventions

An infant with hydrocephalus may present with symptoms that include difficulty feeding, irritability, increased or decreased temperature, higher-pitched cry, dilated scalp veins, increasing head circumference, widening cranial sutures, bulging fontanelle, and sunset eyes (**Figure 14-6**). Children and adolescents may present with nausea and vomiting, complaints of a headache, difficulties with vision, slowing of developmental progress, inability to concentrate or a decline in cognitive function, changes in personality, poor appetite, urinary incontinence, or gait abnormalities. A late sign of hydrocephalus for all age groups is seizures.[51]

Children with hydrocephalus are most often treated with a ventriculoperitoneal (VP) shunt (Figure 14-6). The shunt diverts excess CSF to another body cavity. This implanted device is usually required for life and remains in place unless there is a shunt malfunction or revisions are required.

Parents are taught to watch for signs and symptoms that may indicate a malfunctioning or infected VP shunt—for example, redness or tenderness at the site of the shunt valve, fever, abdominal pain, or return of preoperative symptoms.[94] Assessment of the VP shunt may be needed if parents present to the ED with concerns. Depending on the patient's symptoms, the integrity and position of the shunt may need to be evaluated. Radiographical assessment can be achieved with either a shunt series, head CT, or brain MRI, with the last being the gold standard.[5] If the radiological findings show a fracture or disconnection, surgical repair will be required. If an infection is suspected, CSF is obtained from a shunt tap for culture. In the case of an infection, externalization of the shunt may be required in conjunction with antibiotics and replacement of the shunt once all signs of infection are clear.[40] Over- or under-drainage can also be a complication, though with new technology and ongoing research, surgical repair to change the valve may no longer be required. Ongoing studies are investigating the use of adjustable gravitational valves[38] and the use of programmable pressure valves for patients requiring VP shunts.

Summary

Many disease processes affect the CNS, resulting in changes in level of consciousness. An altered mental status and associated conditions pose risks in terms of the patient's airway, breathing, circulation, and disability. Use the Pediatric Nursing Process to prioritize assessments and interventions, including a blood glucose measurement during the disability assessment for any change in alertness. A thorough history will help determine the potential cause for mental status changes and the need for additional diagnostics. Consult pediatric experts early when the etiology is unclear and/or the patient's diagnostic or intervention needs exceed those available at the treating facility.

References

1. Alberta Health Services. (2021, June 15). *Risk of cannabis toxicity from accidental ingestion of candy look-alike products* [Patient safety memo]. https://elmtreeclinic.ca/handouts/Safety%20at%20Home/PS%20Memo%20-%20Look%20Alike%20Candy%20Products%20April%202021%20FINAL.pdf

2. American Diabetes Association. (2021). Diabetes care in the hospital: Standards of medical care in diabetes–2021. *Diabetes Care, 44*(suppl 1), S211–S220. https://doi.org/10.2337/dc21-S015

3. American Heart Association. (2020). Managing respiratory distress and failure. In *Pediatric advanced life support provider manual* (pp. 113–128).

4. American Heart Association. (2020). Managing shock. In *Pediatric advanced life support provider manual* (pp. 201–202).

5. Ammar, A. (Ed.). (2018). *Hydrocephalus: What do we know? And what do we still not know?* Springer International Publishing.

6. Ballard, E. D., Cwik, M., Van Eck, K., Goldstein, M., Alfes, C., Wilson, M. E., Virden, J. M., Horowitz, L. M., & Wilcox, H. C. (2017). Identification of at-risk youth by suicide screening in a pediatric emergency department. *Prevention Science, 18*(2), 174–182. https://doi.org/10.1007/s11121-016-0717-5

7. Barrueto, F. (2020). Beta blocker poisoning. *UpToDate.* Retrieved March 19, 2022, from https://www.uptodate.com/contents/beta-blocker-poisoning

8. Barrueto, F. (2021). Calcium channel blocker poisoning. *UpToDate.* Retrieved March 19, 2022, from https://www.uptodate.com/contents/calcium-channel-blocker-poisoning

9. Bartlett, J. W., & Walker, P. L. (2019). Management of calcium channel blocker toxicity in the pediatric patient. *Journal of Pediatric Pharmacology and Therapeutics, 24*(5), 378–389. https://doi.org/10.5863/1551-6776-24.5.378

10. Bayram, M. T., Yıldız, G., Soylu, A., & Kavukçu, S. (2019). An adolescent patient presenting with hyponatremic seizure: Questions. *Pediatric Nephrology, 34*(8), Article 1369. https://doi.org/10.1007/s00467-019-04212-y

11. Boyer, E. W. (2021). Serotonin syndrome (serotonin toxicity). *UpToDate.* Retrieved March 10, 2022, from https://www.uptodate.com/contents/serotonin-syndrome-serotonin-toxicity

12. Brocato, C., & Paley, R. (2021). Toxidromes: Common poisonings syndromes to know. *Journal of Emergency Medical Services, 46*(2). https://www.jems.com/patient-care/common-poisoning-syndromes-to-know/

13. Bryant, S. (2019). Understanding the risk of seizure in tramadol overdose: Still a long way to go. *Clinical Toxicology, 57*(12), 1161–1162. https://doi.org/10.1080/15563650.2019.1591433

14. Canadian Association of Poison Control Centres. (2021, July). *Canadian antidote guide in acute care toxicology.* https://www.ciusss-capitalenationale.gouv.qc.ca/en/antidotes

15. Carpenter, R. W., Treloar Padovano, H., Emery, N. N., & Miranda R., Jr. (2019). Rate of alcohol consumption in the daily life of adolescents and emerging adults. *Psychopharmacology, 236*(11), 3111–3124. https://doi.org/10.1007/s00213-019-05262-8

16. Chan, M., & Enarson, P. (2020). Fluid and electrolyte therapy in infants and children. In J. E. Tintinalli, O. J. Ma, D. M. Yealy, G. D. Meckler, J. Stapczynski, J., D. M. Cline, & S. H. Thomas (Eds.), *Tintinalli's emergency medicine: A comprehensive study guide* (9th ed., pp. 851–856). McGraw-Hill.

17. Clardy, P. F., Manaker, S., & Perry, H. (2021). Carbon monoxide poisoning. *UpToDate.* Retrieved March 21, 2022, from https://www.uptodate.com/contents/carbon-monoxide-poisoning

18. Dani, C., & Corsini, I. (2020). Guidelines for management of neonatal hypoglycemia: Are they actually applicable? *JAMA Pediatrics, 174*(7), 638–639. https://doi:10.1001/jamapediatrics.2020.0632

19. Day, R., Bradberry, S. M., Thomas, S. H. L., & Vale, J. A. (2019). Liquid laundry detergent capsules (pods): A review of their composition and mechanisms of toxicity, and of the circumstances, routes, features, and management of exposure. *Clinical Toxicology, 57*(11), 1053–1063. https://doi.org/10.1080/15563650.2019.1618466

20. De Leon-Crutchlow, D. D., & Lord, K. (2021). Approach to hypoglycemia in infants and children. *UpToDate.* Retrieved March 12, 2022, from https://www.uptodate.com/contents/approach-to-hypoglycemia-in-infants-and-children

21. Department of Emergency Medicine. (2019, June). *Acute iron poisoning* [Fact sheet]. Clinical Pharmacology & Toxicology Pearl of the Week. University of Calgary. https://cumming.ucalgary.ca/sites/default/files/teams/127/pearl-ofthe-week/Iron%20overdose%20PotW%20June%202019.pdf

22. Dharmapuri, S., Miller, K., & Klein, J. D. (2020). Marijuana and the pediatric population. *Pediatrics, 146*(2), Article e20192629. https://doi.org/10.1542/peds.2019-2629

23. Dorney, K., & Agus, M. S. D. (2021). Endocrine emergencies. In K. Shaw & R. Bachur (Eds.), *Fleisher & Ludwig's textbook of*

pediatric emergency medicine (8th ed., pp. 653–679). Wolters Kluwer.

24. Esparham, A., Herbert, A., Pierzchalski, E., Tran, C., Dilts, J., Boorigie, M., Wingert, T., Connelly, M., & Bickel, J. (2018). Pediatric headache clinic model: Implementation of integrative therapies in practice. *Children*, 5(6), Article 74. https://doi.org/10.3390/children5060074

25. Evans, G. (2017, October 1). Exposures to opioid patients endanger healthcare workers. *Hospital Employee Health, 36*(10). https://www.reliasmedia.com/articles/141390-exposures-to-opioid-patients-endanger-healthcare-workers

26. Farrell, N. M., Hamilton, S., Gendron, B. J., Corio, J. L., & Lookabill, S. K. (2021). Presence of "one pill can kill" medications in medication organizers: Implications for child safety. *Journal of Pharmacy Practice*. https://doi.org/10.1177/08971900211017491

27. Fernandez, E., & Doty, C. I. (2021). Pediatric ethanol toxicity treatment & management. *Medscape*. Retrieved November 9, 2021, from https://emedicine.medscape.com/article/1010220-treatment

28. Forti, R., & Avner, J. (2017). Altered mental status. In T. K. McInerny, H. M. Adam, D. E. Campbell, T. G. DeWitt, J. M. Foy, & D. M. Kamat (Eds.), *American Academy of Pediatrics textbook of pediatric care* (2nd ed., pp. 2786–2791). American Academy of Pediatrics.

29. Fox, C., & Smith, S. E. (2022). Ischemic stroke in children: Clinical presentation, evaluation, and diagnosis. *UpToDate*. Retrieved March 26, 2022, from https://www.uptodate.com/contents/ischemic-stroke-in-children-clinical-presentation-evaluation-and-diagnosis

30. Freedman, S., Thull-Freedman, J., Lightbody, T., Prisnie, K., Wright, B., Coulombe, A., Anderson, L. M., Stang, A. S., Mikrogianakis, A., VanRiper, L., Stubbs, M., Newton, A., & Pediatric Emergency Research Canada. (2020). Introducing an innovative model of acute pediatric mental health and addictions care to pediatric emergency departments: A protocol for a multicentre prospective cohort study. *BMJ Open Quality, 9*(4). https://doi.org/10.1136/bmjoq-2020-001106

31. Garcia, D. A., & Crowther, M. (2021). Management of bleeding in patients receiving direct oral anticoagulants. *UpToDate*. Retrieved March 19, 2022, from https://www.uptodate.com/contents/management-of-bleeding-in-patients-receiving-direct-oral-anticoagulants

32. Glaser, N. (2020). Diabetic ketoacidosis in children: Clinical features and diagnosis. *UpToDate*. Retrieved March 25, 2022, from https://www.uptodate.com/contents/diabetic-ketoacidosis-in-children-clinical-features-and-diagnosis

33. Glaser, N. (2021). Diabetic ketoacidosis in children: Treatment and complications. *UpToDate*. Retrieved March 25, 2022, from https://www.uptodate.com/contents/diabetic-ketoacidosis-in-children-treatment-and-complications

34. Green, S. (2020). General management of poisoned patients. In J. E. Tintinalli, O. J. Ma, D. M. Yealy, G. D. Meckler, J. Stapczynski, D. M. Cline, & S. H. Thomas (Eds.), *Tintinalli's emergency medicine: A comprehensive study guide* (9th ed., pp. 1187–1193). McGraw-Hill.

35. Greenbaum, L. (2020). Fluid and electrolyte disorders. In R. Kliegman, & J. St. Geme (Eds.), *Nelson textbook of pediatrics* (21st ed., pp. 389–403). Elsevier.

36. Guo, C., & Sutin, K. (2018). Dantrolene sodium. In L. Nelson, M. Howland, N. Lewin, S. Smith, L. Goldfrank, & R. Hoffman (Eds.), *Goldfrank's toxicologic emergencies* (11th ed., pp. 1029–1031). McGraw-Hill.

37. Gurevich, Y., Sahn, B., & Weinstein, T. (2018). Foreign body ingestion in pediatric patients. *Current Opinion in Pediatrics, 30*(5), 677–682. https://doi.org/10.1097/MOP.0000000000000670

38. Gutowski, P., Gölz, L., Rot, S., Lemcke, J., & Thomale, U. (2020). Gravitational shunt valves in hydrocephalus to challenge the sequelae of over-drainage. *Expert Review of Medical Devices, 17*(11), 1155–1168. https://doi.org/10.1080/17434440.2020.1837622

39. Hall, J. (2018, March). *Kentucky poison control center's top calls: Cleaning products, cosmetics*. Norton Children's. https://nortonchildrens.com/news/kentucky-poison-control-centers-top-calls-2017/

40. Hanak, B. W., Bonow, R. H., Harris, C. A., & Browd, S. R. (2017). Cerebrospinal fluid shunting complications in children. *Pediatric Neurosurgery, 52*(6), 381–400. https://doi.org/10.1159/000452840

41. Health Canada. (2019, March). *Guidelines for Canadian drinking water quality: Guideline technical document—lead*. Government of Canada. https://www.canada.ca/en/health-canada/services/publications/healthy-living/guidelines-canadian-drinking-water-quality-guideline-technical-document-lead/guidance-document.html#a2.1

42. Helman, A. (Host). (2015, November). Episode 73: Emergency management of pediatric seizures [Audio podcast episode]. *Emergency Medicine Cases*. https://emergencymedicinecases.com/emergency-management-of-pediatric-seizures/

43. Helman, A. (Host). (2018, January 30). Episode 106: Toxic alcohols: Minding the gaps [Audio podcast episode]. *Emergency Medicine Cases*. https://emergencymedicinecases.com/toxic-alcohols/

44. Hendrickson, R. G., & Kusin, S. (2022). Gastrointestinal decontamination of the poisoned patient. *UpToDate*. Retrieved March 19, 2022, from https://www.uptodate.com/contents/gastrointestinal-decontamination-of-the-poisoned-patient

45. Henretig, F. M., Kirk, M. A., & McKay, C. A. (2019). Hazardous chemical emergencies and poisonings. *New England Journal of Medicine, 380*(17), 1638–1655. https://doi.org/10.1056/NEJMra1504690

46. Hincapie, M., Fontane, E., & Shiber, J. R. (2020). Toxicology and OD. In J. Shiber & S. Weingart (Eds.), *Emergency department critical care* (pp. 463–476). Springer International Publishing. https://doi.org/10.1007/978-3-030-28794-8_28

47. Hoffman, R. P. (2019). Pediatric hypoglycemia. *Medscape*. Retrieved November 8, 2021, from https://emedicine.medscape.com/article/921936-overview#a5

48. Hon, K. L., Leung, A. K., Cheung, E., Lee, B., Tsang, M. M., & Torres, A. R. (2018). An overview of exposure to ethanol-containing substances and ethanol intoxication in children

based on three illustrated cases. *Drugs in Context, 7,* Article 212512. https://doi.org/10.7573/dic.212512

49. Hoyte, C., & Dart, R. C. (2019). Transition to two-bag intravenous acetylcysteine for acetaminophen overdose: A poison center's experience. *Clinical Toxicology 57*(3), 217–218. https://doi.org/10.1080/15563650.2018.1510127

50. Isensee, C., Fernandez Castelao, C., & Kröner-Herwig, B. (2016). Developmental trajectories of paediatric headache: Sex-specific analyses and predictors. *Journal of Headache and Pain, 17*(1), Article 32. https://doi.org/10.1186/s10194-016-0627-8

51. Kahle, K. T., Kulkarni, A. V., Limbrick, D. D., & Warf, B. C. (2016). Hydrocephalus in children. *Lancet 387*(10020), 788–799. https://doi.org/10.1016/S0140-6736(15)60694-8

52. Kaplan, R. L., & Burns, R. (2021). Renal and electrolyte emergencies. In K. Shaw & R. Bachur (Eds.), *Fleisher & Ludwig's textbook of pediatric emergency medicine* (8th ed., pp. 965–989). Wolters Kluwer.

53. Kaushik, S., & Bird, S. (2021). Topical chemical burns: Initial assessment and management. *UpToDate.* Retrieved March 14, 2022, from https://www.uptodate.com/contents/topical-chemical-burns-initial-assessment-and-management

54. Klausen, S. H., Rønde, G., Tornøe, B., & Bjerregaard, L. (2019). Nonpharmacological interventions addressing pain, sleep, and quality of life in children and adolescents with primary headache: A systematic review. *Journal of Pain Research, 12,* 3437–3459. https://doi.org/10.2147/JPR.S216807

55. Kloss, B. (2020, November 30). *Anticholinergic toxidrome flashcard.* Life in the Fastlane. https://litfl.com/anticholinergic-toxidrome/

56. Knopf, A. (2020). Antidepressant, including TCA, prescribing up in Canadian children and adolescents. *Child & Adolescent Psychopharmacology Update, 22*(3), 1–5. https://doi.org/10.1002/cpu.30473

57. Koyuncu, S., Bol, O., Ertan, T., Günay, N., & Akdogan, H. İ. (2020). The detection of occult CO poisoning through noninvasive measurement of carboxyhemoglobin: A cross-sectional study. *American Journal of Emergency Medicine, 38*(6), 1110–1114. https://doi.org/10.1016/j.ajem.2019.158383

58. Lagard, C., Malissin, I., Indja, W., Risède, P., Chevillard, L., & Mégarbane, B. (2018). Is naloxone the best antidote to reverse tramadol-induced neuro-respiratory toxicity in overdose? An experimental investigation in the rat. *Clinical Toxicology, 56*(8), 737–743. https://doi.org/10.1080/15563650.2017.1401080

59. Lehman, L. L., Beslow, L. A., Steinlin, M., Kossorotoff, M., & Mackay, M. T. (2019). What will improve pediatric acute stroke care? *Stroke, 50*(2), 249–256. https://doi.org/10.1161/STROKEAHA.118.022881

60. Lucas, J. (2018). Pediatric toxicology. In C. Zeretzke-Bienm, T. Swan, & B. Allen (Eds.), *Quick hits for pediatric emergency medicine* (pp. 133–145). Springer International Publishing. https://doi.org/10.1007/978-3-319-93830-1_18

61. Lucyk, S. (2020). *Guidelines on management of acetaminophen toxicity, new concentrations 2 step NAC regimen.* Poison and Drug Information Service (PADIS).

62. Madden, M. (2018). Toxicology. In M. C. Slota (Ed.), *AACN's core curriculum for pediatric high acuity, progressive, and critical care nursing* (3rd ed., pp. 734–773). Springer Publishing.

63. Magidson, J. F., Regan, S., Powell, E., Jack, H. E., Herman, G. E., Zaro, C., Kane, M. T., & Wakeman, S. E. (2021). Peer recovery coaches in general medical settings: Changes in utilization, treatment engagement, and opioid use. *Journal of Substance Abuse Treatment, 122,* 108248. https://doi.org/10.1016/j.jsat.2020.108248

64. Mahajan, P., & Felt, J. (2017). Fluids, electrolytes and acid–base composition. In T. K. McInerny, H. M. Adam, D. E. Campbell, T. G. DeWitt, J. M. Foy, & D. M. Kamat (Ed.), *American Academy of Pediatrics textbook of pediatric care* (2nd ed., pp. 420–433). American Academy of Pediatrics.

65. Marchitelli, R. (2021, January 25). *Copycat pot edibles that look like candy are poisoning kids, doctor say.* Canadian Broadcast News Corporation. https://www.cbc.ca/news/canada/british-columbia/cannabis-gummies-poisonings-kids-illegal-sites-1.5879232

66. Mayans, L. (2019). Lead poisoning in children. *American Family Physician, 100*(1), 24–30. https://www.aafp.org/afp/2019/0701/p24.html

67. McGillis, E. (2021). *Guidelines on management of sympathomimetic drugs of abuse.* Poison and Drug Information Service.

68. McNicholas, B. A., Pham, M. H., Carli, K., Chen, C. H., Colobong-Smith, N., Anderson, A. E., & Pham, H. (2018). Treatment of hyperkalemia with a low-dose insulin protocol is effective and results in reduced hypoglycemia. *Kidney International Reports, 3*(2), 328–336. https://doi.org/10.1016/j.ekir.2017.10.009

69. Nadler, A., & Fein, D. M. (2018). Acetaminophen poisoning. *Pediatrics in Review, 39*(6), 316–318. https://doi.org/10.1542/pir.2017-0093

70. Nelson, L. S., & Hoffman, R. S. (2018). Inhaled toxins. In R. M. Walls, R. S. Hockberger, & M. Gausche-Hill (Eds.), *Rosen's emergency medicine: Concepts and clinical practice* (9th ed., pp. 1926–1936). Elsevier.

71. Nieswand, V., Richter, M., & Gossrau, G. (2020). Epidemiology of headache in children and adolescents: Another type of pandemia. *Current Pain and Headache Reports, 24,* Article 62. https://doi.org/10.1007/s11916-020-00892-6

72. Normandin, P. A., Benotti, S. A., & Mullins, M. A. (2020). Hidden danger: Pediatric acetaminophen overdose unintentional and intentional emergencies. *Journal of Emergency Nursing, 46*(6), 914–922. https://doi.org/10.1016/j.jen.2020.06.015

73. Oesterle, T. S., Thusius, N. J., Rummans, T. A., & Gold, M. S. (2019). Medication-assisted treatment for opioid-use disorder. *Mayo Clinic Proceedings, 94*(10), 2072–2086. https://doi.org/10.1016/j.mayocp.2019.03.029

74. O'Malley, G., & O'Malley R. (2020, April). *Iron poisoning.* Merck Manual Professional Version. https://www.merckmanuals.com/en-ca/professional/injuries-poisoning/poisoning/iron-poisoning?query=Iron%20Poisoning

75. Oskoui, M., Pringsheim, T., Billinghurst, L., Potrebic, S., Gersz, E. M., Gloss, D., Holler-Managan, Y., Leininger, E.,

Licking, N., Mack, K., Powers, S. W., Sowell, M., Victorio, M. C., Yonker, M., Zanitsch, H., & Hershey, A. D. (2019). Practice guideline update summary: Pharmacologic treatment for pediatric migraine prevention: Report of the Guideline Development, Dissemination, and Implementation Subcommittee of the American Academy of Neurology and the American Headache Society. *Neurology, 93*(11), 500–509. https://doi.org/10.1212/WNL.0000000000008105

76. Rahmandar, M. H., Roden, R. C., & Cottrill, C. B. (2020). Identifying and treating opioid misuse in pediatric patients. In R. Shah & S. Suresh (Eds.), *Opioid therapy in infants, children, and adolescent* (pp. 155–171). Springer International Publishing. https://doi.org/10.1007/978-3-030-36287-4_11

77. Rao, R., Hoffman, R., & Erickson, T. (2018). Cocaine and other sympathomimetics. In R. M. Walls, R. S. Hockberger, & M. Gausche-Hill (Eds.), *Rosen's emergency medicine: Concepts and clinical practice* (9th ed., pp. 1895–1904). Elsevier.

78. Raucci, U., Boni, A., Evangelisti, M., Della Vecchia, N., Velardi, M., Ursitti, F., Terrin, G., Di Nardo, G., Reale, A., Villani, A., & Parisi, P. (2021). Lifestyle modifications to help prevent headache at a developmental age. *Frontiers in Neurology, 11*, Article 618375. https://doi.org/10.3389/fneur.2020.618375

79. Raucci, U., Della Vecchia, N., Ossella, C., Paolino, M. C., Villa, M. P., Reale, A., & Parisi, P. (2019). Management of childhood headache in the emergency department: Review of the literature. *Frontiers in Neurology, 10*, Article 886. https://doi.org/10.3389/fneur.2019.00886

80. Rekate, H. L. (2020). Hydrocephalus in infants: The unique biomechanics and why they matter. *Child's Nervous System, 36*(8), 1713–1728. https://doi.org/10.1007/s00381-020-04683-7

81. Renny, M. H., O'Donnell, K. A., & Calello, D. P. (2021). Toxicologic emergencies. In K. Shaw & R. Bachur (Eds.), *Fleisher & Ludwig's textbook of pediatric emergency medicine* (8th ed., pp. 1029–1083). Wolters Kluwer.

82. Rewers, A., Kuppermann, N., Stoner, M. J., Garro, A., Bennett, J. E., Quayle, K. S., Schunk, J. E., Myers, S. R., McManemy, J. K., Nigrovic, L. E., Trainor, J. L., Tzimenatos, L., Kwok, M. Y., Brown, K. M., Olsen, C. S., Casper, T. C., Ghetti, S., Glaser, N. S., & Pediatric Emergency Care Applied Research Network (PECARN) FLUID Study Group. (2021). Effects of fluid rehydration strategy on correction of acidosis and electrolyte abnormalities in children with diabetic ketoacidosis. *Diabetes Care, 44*(9), 2061–2068. https://doi.org/10.2337/dc20-3113

83. Roach, E. S., & Swafford, C. T. (2021). Cerebrovascular disorders. In E. S. Roach (Ed.), *Pediatric neurology: Clinical assessment and management* (pp. 157–168). Demos Medical.

84. Robb, E. L. & Baker, M. B. (2021, July 26). *Organophosphate toxicity*. StatPearls Publishing. https://www.ncbi.nlm.nih.gov/books/NBK470430/

85. Saccomano, S. J. (2019). Acute acetaminophen toxicity in adults. *Nurse Practitioner, 44*(11), 42–47. https://doi.org/10.1097/01.NPR.0000586020.15798.c6

86. Safe Kids Worldwide. (2021). *Poison prevention for big kids*. https://www.safekids.org/safetytips/field_age/big-kids-5%E2%80%939-years/field_risks/poison

87. Saladino, R. A. (2021). Emergency department approach to nontraumatic headache in children. *UpToDate*. Retrieved March 26, 2022, from https://www.uptodate.com/contents/emergency-department-approach-to-nontraumatic-headache-in-children

88. Salhanic, S. D., (2020). Tricyclic antidepressant poisoning. *UpToDate*. Retrieved March 27, 2022, from https://www.uptodate.com/contents/tricyclic-antidepressant-poisoning

89. Sample, J. A. (2021). Childhood lead poisoning: Exposure and prevention. *UpToDate*. Retrieved March 21, 2022, from https://www.uptodate.com/contents/childhood-lead-poisoning-exposure-and-prevention

90. Schonfeld, D., & Schnall, B. M. (2021). Ophthalmic emergencies. In K. Shaw & R. Bachur (Eds.), *Fleisher & Ludwig's textbook of pediatric emergency medicine* (8th ed., pp. 1392–1403). Wolters Kluwer.

91. Sethuraman, K., Douglas, T., Bostick, B., Comer, A., Myers, B., & Rosenthal, R. (2020). Clinical characteristics of pediatric patients with carbon monoxide poisoning. *Pediatric Emergency Care, 36*(4), 178–181. https://doi.org/10.1097/PEC.0000000000001378

92. Shellhaas, R. (2021). Clinical features, evaluation, and diagnosis of neonatal seizures. *UpToDate*. Retrieved March 25, 2022, from https://www.uptodate.com/contents/clinical-features-evaluation-and-diagnosis-of-neonatal-seizures

93. Shih, E. K., & Beslow, L. A. (2021). Hemorrhagic stroke in children. *UpToDate*. Retrieved March 26, 2022, from https://www.uptodate.com/contents/hemorrhagic-stroke-in-children

94. Shuer, L. M., & Thakkar, R. (2021). *Hydrocephalus*. American Association of Neurological Surgeons. https://www.aans.org/Patients/Neurosurgical-Conditions-and-Treatments/Hydrocephalus

95. Singh, A., Anderson, M., & Altaf, M. A. (2019). Clinical and endoscopy findings in children with accidental exposure to concentrated detergent pods. *Journal of Pediatric Gastroenterology and Nutrition, 68*(6), 824–828. https://doi.org/10.1097/MPG.0000000000002270

96. Sjogren, P. P., Skarda, D. E., & Park, A. H. (2017). Upper aerodigestive injuries from detergent ingestion in children. *Laryngoscope, 127*(2), 509–512. https://doi.org/10.1002/lary.26184

97. Smollin, C., & Hoffman, R. (2018). Cocaine. In L. Nelson, M. Howland, N. Lewin, S. Smith, L. Goldfrank, & R. Hoffman (Eds.), *Goldfrank's toxicologic emergencies* (11th ed., pp. 1124–1134). McGraw-Hill.

98. Somers, M. J. (2020). Management of hyperkalemia in children. *UpToDate*. Retrieved March 26, 2022, from https://www.uptodate.com/contents/management-of-hyperkalemia-in-children

99. Stacy, K. M. (2022). Neurologic anatomy and physiology. In L. D. Urden, K. M. Stacy, & M. E. Lough (Eds.), *Critical care nursing: Diagnosis and management* (9th ed., pp. 534–564). Elsevier.

100. Suresh, S., & Santhanam, I. (2016). Hypoglycemia. In T. K. McInerny (Ed.), *American Academy of Pediatrics textbook of*

pediatric care (2nd ed., pp. 2881–2888). American Academy of Pediatrics.

101. Swan, T. (2018). Electrolyte disturbances. In C. M. Zeretzke-Bien, T. B. Swan, & B. R. Allen (Eds.). *Quick hits for pediatric emergency medicine* (pp. 117–131). Springer International Publishing. https://doi.org/10.1007/978-3-319-93830-1_17

102. Swan, T. (2018). Pediatric altered mental status. In C. M. Zeretzke-Bien, T. B. Swan, & B. R. Allen (Eds.), *Quick hits for pediatric emergency medicine.* (pp. 89–91). Springer International Publishing. https://doi.org/10.1007/978-3-319-93830-1_18

103. Tanverdi, M. S., & Mellion, S. A. (2020). Altered mental status in children. In J. E. Tintinalli, O. J. Ma, D. M. Yealy, G. D. Meckler, J. Stapczynski, D. M. Cline, & S. H. Thomas (Eds.), *Tintinalli's emergency medicine: A comprehensive study guide* (9th ed., pp. 902–903) McGraw-Hill.

104. Theobald, J. L., & Kostic, M. (2020). Poisoning. In R. Kliegman & J. St. Geme (Eds.), *Nelson textbook of pediatrics* (21st ed., pp. 490–510). Elsevier.

105. Theobald, J. L., & Mycyk, M. B. (2018). Iron and heavy metals. In R. M. Walls, R. S. Hockberger, & M. Gausche-Hill (Eds.), *Rosen's emergency medicine: Concepts and clinical practice* (9th ed., pp. 1912–1920). Elsevier.

106. Thom, S., (2018). Hyperbaric oxygen. In L. Nelson, M. Howland, N. Lewin, S. Smith, L. Goldfrank, & R. Hoffman (Eds.), *Goldfrank's toxicologic emergencies* (11th ed., pp. 1676–1683). McGraw-Hill.

107. Tomaszewski, C. (2018). Carbon monoxide. In L. Nelson, M. Howland, N. Lewin, S. Smith, L. Goldfrank, & R. Hoffman (Eds.), *Goldfrank's toxicologic emergencies* (11th ed., pp. 1663–1676). McGraw-Hill.

108. Topjian, A. A., Raymond, T. T., Atkins, D., Chan, M., Duff, J. P., Joyner, B. L., Lasa, J. J., Lavonas, E. J., Levy, A., Mahgoub, M., Meckler, G. D., Roberts, K. E., Sutton, R. M., Schexnayder, S. M., & Pediatric Basic and Advanced Life Support Collaborators. (2020). Part 4: Pediatric basic and advanced life support: 2020 American Heart Association guidelines for cardiopulmonary resuscitation and emergency cardiovascular care. *Circulation, 142*(16 suppl 2), S469–S523. https://doi.org/10.1161/CIR.0000000000000901

109. Tran, D. (2020). Oral hypoglycemic agent toxicity treatment and management. *Medscape.* Retrieved November 9, 2021, from https://emedicine.medscape.com/article/1010629-treatment

110. Translating Emergency Knowledge for Kids. (2020). *Pediatric status epilepticus algorithm* [Infographic]. https://trekk.ca/system/assets/assets/attachments/453/original/2020-03-09_SE_algorithm_v_3.0.PDF?1583872609

111. Valentovic, M., & Rankin, G. (2019). Essentials of toxicology. In L. Wecker, D. A. Taylor, & R. J. Theobald (Eds.), *Brody's human pharmacology* (6th ed., pp. 640–644). https://doi.org/10.1016/B978-0-323-47652-2.00074-0

112. Velez, L. I., Shepher, J. G., & Goto, C. S. (2020). Approach to the child with occult toxic exposure. *UpToDate.* Retrieved March 21, 2022, from https://www.uptodate.com/contents/approach-to-the-child-with-occult-toxic-exposure

113. Veverka, M., Marsh, K., Norman, S., Brock, M. A., Peng, M., Shenk, J., & Chen, J. G. (2016). A pediatric diabetic ketoacidosis management protocol incorporating a two-bag intravenous fluid system decreases duration of intravenous insulin therapy. *Journal of Pediatric Pharmacology and Therapeutics, 21*(6), 512–517. https://doi.org/10.5863/1551-6776-21.6.512

114. Wail, S., Ahmed, S., Abdulaziz, F., Nahla, S., & Hoda, B., Shoaebi, M., & Ibrahim, K. (2017). Computed tomography of the head prior to lumbar puncture in suspected cases of meningitis in children, in Qatar. *Academic Journal of Pediatrics & Neonatology, 5*(5), Article 555732. https://juniperpublishers.com/ajpn/AJPN.MS.ID.555732.php

115. Warshawski, T., & Warf, C. (2019). It is time for an ethical, evidence-based approach to youth presenting to the ED with an opioid overdose. *Paediatrics & Child Health, 24*(6), 374–376. https://doi.org/10.1093/pch/pxz011

116. Welker, K., & Thompson, T. (2018). Pesticides. In R. M. Walls, R. S. Hockberger, & M. Gausche-Hill (Eds.), *Rosen's emergency medicine: Concepts and clinical practice* (9th ed., pp. 1947–1956). Elsevier.

117. Westmacott, R., Waxman, J., & Dlamini, N. (2019). Pediatric stroke. In K. M. Sanders (Ed.), *Physician's field guide to neuropsychology: Collaboration through case example* (pp. 147–167). Springer. https://doi.org/10.1007/978-1-4939-8722-1_9

118. Wilfong, A. (2021). Clinical features and complications of status epilepticus in children. *UpToDate.* Retrieved March 23, 2022, from https://www.uptodate.com/contents/clinical-features-and-complications-of-status-epilepticus-in-children

119. Wilfong, A. (2021). Seizures and epilepsy in children: Classification, etiology, and clinical features. *UpToDate.* Retrieved March 23, 2022, from https://www.uptodate.com/contents/seizures-and-epilepsy-in-children-classification-etiology-and-clinical-features

120. Wilson, J. D., Berk, J., Adger, H., & Feldman, L. (2018). Identifying missed clinical opportunities in delivery of overdose prevention and naloxone prescription to adolescents using opioids. *Journal of Adolescent Health, 63*(2), 245–248. https://doi.org/10.1016/j.jadohealth.2018.05.011

121. Wolters Kluwer. (2021, September). Epilepsy, pediatric. *Lippincott Advisor.* https://advisor.lww.com/lna/document.do?bid=4&did=1064737

122. Wong, K. U., & Baum, C. R. (2019). Acute cannabis toxicity. *Pediatric Emergency Care, 35*(11), 799–804. https://doi.org/10.1097/PEC.0000000000001970

123. Yamanaka, G., Morichi, S., Suzuki, S., Go, S., Takeshita, M., Kanou, K., Ishida, Y., Oana, S., & Kawashima, H. (2020). A review on the triggers of pediatric migraine with the aim of improving headache education. *Journal of Clinical Medicine, 9*(11), 3717. https://doi.org/10.3390/jcm9113717

The Child with a Behavioral Health Concern

Roberta L. Miller, DNP, RN, CPN, CPEN, TCRN

OBJECTIVES

Upon completion of this chapter, the learner will be able to:

1. Identify signs of patient agitation and implement de-escalation techniques.
2. Describe the characteristics and selected causes of pediatric behavioral health concerns.
3. Apply the Pediatric Nursing Process to a child with behavioral health concerns.

Introduction

Families seeking care for children with behavioral health emergencies are not uncommon in the emergency department (ED). Many children and adolescents do not receive ongoing treatment for behavioral health and present to the ED for various behavioral concerns. These concerns may be related to others' safety or to the patient's safety. It is essential to maintain safety for all parties involved (staff, patients, family, visitors) while promoting a calm, accepting, and supportive environment.

Escalation Cycle

Patients with behavioral health issues who are seen in the ED are presumed to have an elevated anxiety level. Anxiety can quickly develop into agitation and aggression. Agitation puts these patients at risk for harm to themselves or to others, and appropriate de-escalation techniques are imperative for improving safety in the ED.[13] Some of the most commonly encountered symptoms of anxiety or agitation include increased repetitive motor activity such as hand wringing, fidgeting with clothes and objects, pacing, increasing irritability, and repetitive statements such as "I can't stay here."[7,28] When the patient is agitated, the use of verbal de-escalation may prevent aggressive outbursts. If the verbal de-escalation techniques prove unsuccessful and the patient becomes physically aggressive, the patient may require restraint to ensure the safety of staff and patients alike.[28]

De-escalation Techniques

Agitation is commonly encountered in the ED when caring for patients with behavioral health concerns. De-escalation techniques, which are used to calm the patient, can involve environmental changes or comfort measures.[13] De-escalation techniques include strategies for building trust with patients and caregivers to mitigate violent outbursts.[28] Successful de-escalation requires empathy, patience, and genuine interest in helping the patient while reducing agitation.[28] Verbal de-escalation can be implemented quickly and help diffuse a potentially violent situation. Verbal de-escalation techniques include the following[28]:

- Respect personal space and remain at least two arm lengths away from the agitated patient.
- Establish rapport. The patient needs to know the staff will work with them to resolve the problem.
- Avoid confrontational behavior.
  - Pay close attention to body language, keeping your own hands visible and not clenched.
  - To appear nonconfrontational, stand at an angle rather than standing directly in front of the patient. Do not turn away; that is, continue to show interest in the patient.
  - Maintain a calm facial expression.
  - Avoid folding your arms across your chest.
- Use clear, simple messages and instructions.
  - Use a soft voice.
  - Be concise.
  - Introduce yourself to the patient.
  - Reassure the patient that you want to help them regain control of the situation.
  - Speak in simple, short sentences, and avoid giving multiple directions.
  - Explain what will happen in the ED.
  - Repeat expectations if needed.
  - Set limits on unacceptable behaviors.
- Identify what it is that the patient feels, wants, or needs.
- Listen closely. Use active listening to affirm that you are hearing what the patient is saying.
  - Ask clarifying questions when necessary.
  - Use nonverbal behavior to convey that you are listening (e.g., nodding, eye contact).
- Offer strategies to help the patient calm down.
  - Oral medication is beneficial when the goal is to calm the patient, not sedate them.
  - Offer to meet the patient's physical needs, such as getting the patient a meal or a blanket.
  - Distraction turns the patient's attention away from the problem and helps de-escalate agitation.
- Meet the patient's basic needs, including provision of safe comfort items and food or drink if medically appropriate.
- Provide safe activities such as television, coloring with crayons, or playing cards.
- Allow simple choices when available (e.g., type of drink, intravenous access site).

See Chapter 17, "The Child, Family, and Healthcare Provider in Crisis," for more information about de-escalation for families.

RED FLAG

Nurses cannot always safely de-escalate a patient. Staff safety is always the priority, and it may be best to remove yourself from the situation. When entering a patient space, identify a route of escape and avoid being blocked from the exit. Use resources such as other staff, security personnel, and law enforcement personnel. Planning and implementing hospital and community policies and processes to support staff and patient safety are vital.

Restraints

Physical or chemical restraints are used when all other attempts to calm or de-escalate the patient fail. Regulations emphasize that restraints are to be used as a last resort, and only when patients pose an imminent risk to themselves or to others.[6] Restraints are not to be used for convenience or as punishment.[26] Staff who will use restraints must have training specific to safe application, monitoring, and documentation of mechanical restraints.[6] While the patient is restrained, it is crucial to perform regular checks on their respiratory, circulatory, and mental status.[26] Release the patient as soon as they are no longer at risk of causing harm. Documentation should include indications for restraints, all interventions and assessments, and all staff members involved in the restraint procedure.[15]

If time allows, it is beneficial to debrief the patient about why the restraint happened. Explore the cause of the aggressive outburst, and ask for the patient's perspective on the situation. Debriefing enables the patient to process their feelings and the staff and patient to rebuild their relationship.[9,28]

Focused Assessment

Use a calm and caring approach to complete the assessment of a patient with a behavioral health emergency. Ensure that there is no medical reason for the patient's condition, such as an electrolyte imbalance, endocrine disorder, or brain injury or infection.[6] Abnormal vital signs should not be discounted, and medical conditions must be ruled out even though tachycardia can be associated with agitation and anxiety.[30] Obtaining information from the caregivers helps determine the acuity of the patient's condition, the duration of symptoms, and the risk to self or others.[30]

Children and adolescents can be challenging to assess due to their lack of cooperation or the lack of experience on the part of the healthcare team. While assessing the child's mental status, address the following issues[30]:

- Affect
- Orientation
- Energy level
- Sleeping and eating habits
- Somatic complaints (e.g., chest pain, shortness of breath, abdominal pain)
- Substance abuse
- Emotional or physical trauma history, including past or present abuse
- Family trouble (e.g., domestic violence, marital problems, or substance abuse)
- Risky behaviors

Assess the child or adolescent for signs of poor hygiene and self-harm. Note the pattern of thinking, especially for children or adolescents who could be experiencing hallucinations or delusions. Symptoms of disorganized thinking include slowness to respond to questions, pressured speech, flight of ideas, muteness, and loose associations.[33(Ch8)]

Appropriate Interventions

The main focus of appropriate interventions is creating a safe environment. Pediatric patients experiencing behavioral health emergencies require a calm environment, which may necessitate moving them to an area of the ED that is less busy.[32] If the patient expresses suicidal or homicidal ideation, assign a staff member to continuously observe the patient.[5] Assist the patient when changing into a gown, and remove any harmful objects from the patient's possession.[18] Follow organizational policies to search personal belongings for weapons, medications, or anything the patient could use for self-harm. Remove the patient's belongings from the room, including the patient's cell phone. Limit the number of visitors, and ensure those visitors do not bring anything into the room that poses a safety risk.[18] Specific interventions relate to the patient's condition; however, interventions must safeguard patients, staff, and visitors from harm.

Inpatient behavioral health beds are often unavailable immediately, so that children requiring behavioral health admission may be held in the ED for extended periods of time. Creative measures such as telepsychiatry and mobile crisis teams are evolving to meet the needs of these patients. The Emergency Nurses Association (ENA) has created an infographic entitled *Providing a Safe Environment for Pediatric Behavioral Health Patients in the ED* with suggestions for daily routines to guide care (**Figure 15-1**).

Selected Conditions

Children often have difficulty explaining their feelings or symptoms and may present to the ED with somatic complaints. Adolescents may be unable to articulate their feelings and regulate their emotions.[6] Compared with pediatric patients seen in other healthcare settings, pediatric patients receiving care in the ED have a higher risk of behavioral health disorders, including depression, anxiety, post-traumatic stress disorder (PTSD), and substance abuse.[6] These conditions may remain unrecognized due to the presenting complaint being vague somatic complaints, such as headaches, gastrointestinal complaints, or pain unrelated to an injury.[6]

Development and implementation of screening tools can improve recognition of behavioral health disorders.[12] EDs strive to safely manage patients with behavioral health disorders with dignity and detect previously undiagnosed mental health illnesses.[1] When caring for such patients, consider the possibility of suicidal ideation, escalating aggression, self-harm, mood disorders, autism, and other mental health disorders.[1] Ask these patients about symptoms of depression or thoughts of harming themselves, using facility-approved tools.[16]

Depression

Over the past decade, the prevalence of depression among children and adolescents doubled.[12] These increased rates of psychiatric disorders are linked to evolving changes in social interactions related to technology use, bullying, gender identity, sexual orientation, family discord, poverty, and racism.[12] Unfortunately, depression often goes undiagnosed and untreated. Untreated depression can lead to long-term adverse health and social outcomes, including self-injury, risk-taking behaviors, and poor social interactions.[19] Untreated depression in childhood and adolescents contributes to migraines, anxiety, unemployment, and other social issues in adulthood.[19]

Children and adolescents with depression often present with other mental health disorders, including anxiety, substance abuse, attention-deficit/hyperactivity disorder (ADHD), eating disorders, PTSD, and conduct disorders.[27] Compared to their peers without depression, children and adolescents with depression visit the ED and require hospital admission more often.[34] The reasons for seeking care may range from vague somatic symptoms to suicidal ideation.[34] Signs and symptoms of depression vary among different age groups but frequently include significant dysfunctions in regular activities and social interactions. Young children may present with irritability or anxiety or mood swings.[31(Ch12)]

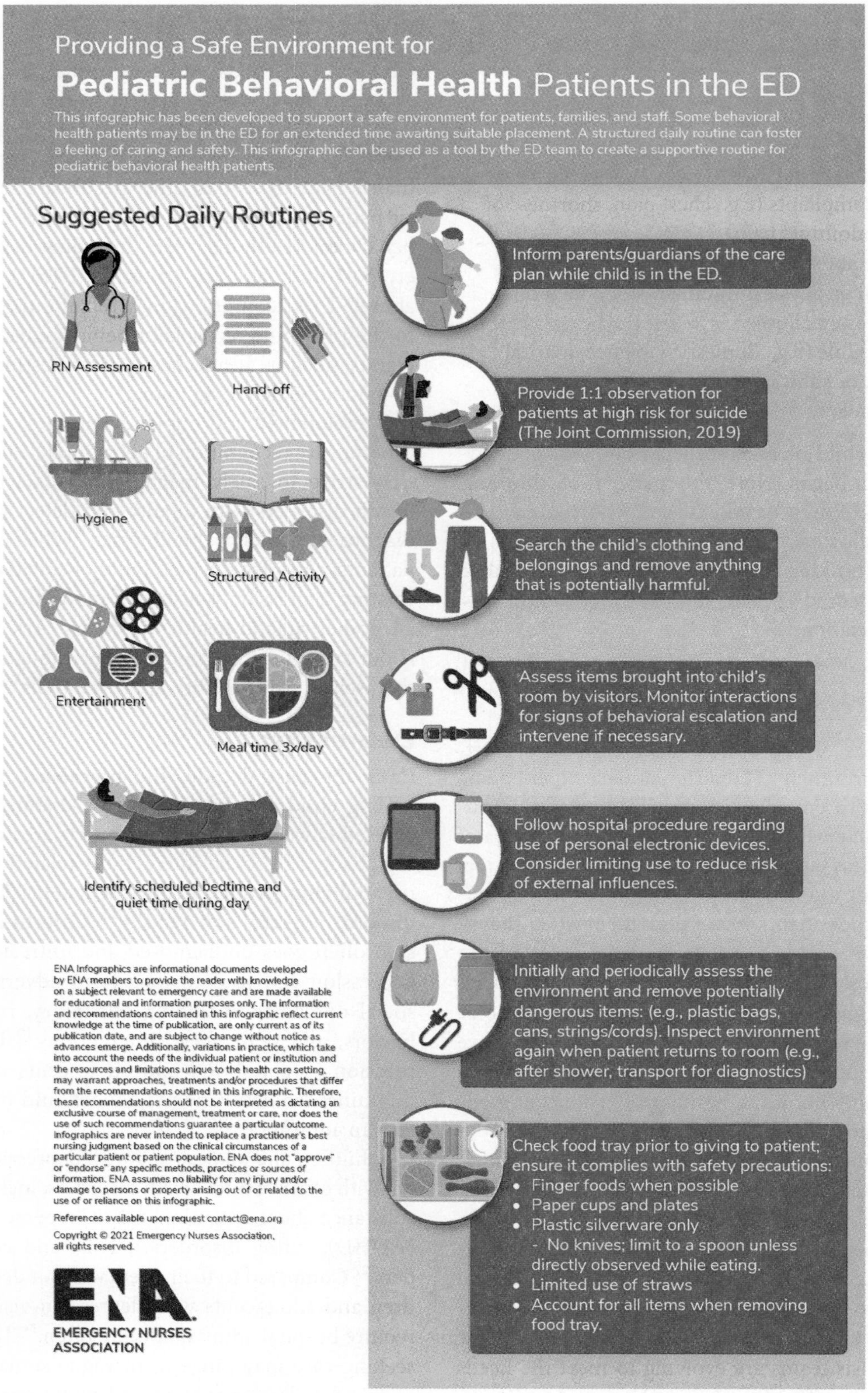

Figure 15-1 *Providing a Safe Environment for Pediatric Behavioral Health Patients in the ED infographic.*

Reprinted with permission from the Emergency Nurses Association.

Appropriate Interventions

Consider the following interventions for pediatric patients with known or suspected depression[26,31(Ch12)]:

- Ask direct questions about suicidal ideation.
- Perform a complete physical examination and further diagnostic studies if there is no known preexisting medical condition.
- Obtain a complete blood count to rule out anemia, and measure thyroid levels to rule out hypothyroidism.
- After eliminating physical causes, request a consultation with a mental health professional when possible.
- Consider suicide precautions and provide a safe environment.

Suicidal Ideation

Suicide rates among both children and adolescents have increased over the past decade. Today, approximately half of the referrals to the ED for behavioral health evaluations are related to suicidal ideation.[32] Suicide is a leading cause of death in children and adolescents worldwide.[30] Suicidal ideation can be associated with other behavioral health conditions, such as depression, anxiety, ADHD, substance abuse, and mood disorders.[16]

Asking children and adolescents whether they have suicidal thoughts can help them feel understood and provides opportunities for introducing resources.[32] Multiple screening tools exist to facilitate the assessment of suicide risk in pediatric patients, and a facility-approved assessment tool should be used to identify patients with increased suicide risk.[32]

It is essential to differentiate between suicidal ideation and suicide attempt when screening for risk and planning treatment. A suicide attempt includes action intended to harm oneself, whereas suicide ideation is thinking about or planning to harm oneself.[15] For patients who have made suicide attempts, medical stabilization is the priority and one-to-one observation can maintain patient safety.[15]

When suicidal ideation is identified, ask the patient what they have thought about or planned to do to kill themselves to further evaluate risk and plan appropriate interventions.[15] Females are more likely to attempt suicide, but males are more likely to die by suicide—a difference that reflects the lethality of methods used by females versus males.[6] The most common means of suicide involve medication overdose, firearms, hanging, and ingestion of poisonous substances.[30]

Screening for Suicidal Ideation

Asking questions to screen for suicide risk is imperative to identifying children and adolescents at risk for suicide. The first step is to ask about suicidal risk factors, thoughts, and intent.[15] When screening for suicide risk, interview patients and caregivers both together and separately to gain insights into the patient's state of mind and details of the ideation or attempt.[6] Multiple screening tools exist that can improve the assessment of suicide risk (**Table 15-1**).[31(Ch80),32(pp11–12)] Ask the screening questions in a direct, simple, and nonthreatening manner to facilitate an accurate assessment of the suicide risk.[30]

Risk factors for suicide include the following[6,15,16,30,33]:

- History of chronic or terminal illness or psychiatric diagnosis
- Previous suicide attempts
- Non-heterosexual orientation
- Male gender
- Transgender
- A family member, classmate, or friend who died by suicide
- History of being abused or bullied
- Feelings of helplessness
- Homelessness
- Depression or other mood disorders
- Impulsive behavior
- Runaway
- Social isolation
- Access to a firearms
- Barriers to or unwillingness to seek mental health care

If suicidal ideation is identified, implement safety measures as directed by your institution. Recommendations for patient safety include having the patient remove their clothing and dress in hospital clothing. Perform a safety search per organizational policy, and remove all dangerous items from the room. Direct and constant observation is a priority, so as to increase patient safety.

Self-Harm

Self-harm is an intentional injury to one's body, such as cutting or burning, without suicidal intent.[5] Pediatric patients who engage in self-harm may have recent stressors in their lives and indicate that these behaviors help to relieve their stress.[5] The incidence of self-harm among children with behavioral health disorders continues to increase as behavioral health ED visits increase.[27] Although self-harm is often not intended to be lethal, it can cause serious health complications if not addressed.[31(Ch14)] The most common injuries are to the wrists, arms, legs, stomachs, and hands.[31(Ch14)] The most common forms of self-harm are cutting, scratching, or burning the skin and hitting or biting the body.

TABLE 15-1	Suicidal Ideation Screening Tools	
Screening Tool	**Availability**	**Additional Details**
Ask Suicide Screening Questions (ASQ)	Free: Full toolkit is available online	› Four questions about risk factors and three questions about suicidal ideation › Tested tool for assessing suicide factors › Recommended for pediatric patients in the ED
Suicide Assessment Five-Step Evaluation and Triage	Free: Full toolkit is available online	› Three sets of questions about risk, protective factors, and suicide inquiry › Five-step screen that walks the screener through a comprehensive suicide assessment and triage process
Columbia Suicide Severity Rating Scale (C-SSPS)	Free: Available online	› Two to six questions › Assesses the severity of suicidal ideation › Validated for use with adolescents in the ED setting › Significant predictor of suicide attempt at return visit for adolescents
Suicide Ideation Questionnaire (SIQ) and SIQ-Junior	Available for purchase	› SIQ: 30 items for children in grades 10–12 › SIQ-Junior: 15 items for grades 7–9 › Has utility for adolescents to address suicide risk factors, especially in association with depression and/or alcohol abuse

Data from Shatkin, J. P. (2015). *Child & adolescent mental health: A practical all-in-one guide.* Norton & Company; and United States Department of Health and Human Services, Health Resources and Services Administration, & Maternal and Child Health Bureau. (2019). *Critical crossroads: Pediatric mental health care in the emergency department: A care pathway resource toolkit.*

Appropriate Interventions

Children who present with injuries from self-harm need screening for suicidal risk. Complete a physical assessment to identify and provide appropriate interventions for any injuries. Ensure a safe environment where all harmful objects are removed. Discuss other stress management alternatives.

Risk of Harm to Others

The overall goal of treatment for patients at risk for harm to others in the ED is to manage the behavior in the least restrictive manner and to maintain safety.[16] Aggressive behaviors can be related to medical conditions; therefore, medical conditions must be considered and addressed in case of a violent or aggressive patient.[32] Staff should implement de-escalation techniques to help patients regain control of their behavior and to prevent injuries.[16] Methods for successful de-escalation include decreasing sensory stimulation, removing triggers, and ensuring safer rooms.[6] Remove or secure all objects that might be used as weapons

to make rooms safer, and never let the child get between the healthcare professional and the door.[6] Triggers may include an argumentative caregiver or a confrontational staff member.[6] When available, child life specialists are an excellent resource for calming an agitated child.

Anxiety Disorders

Anxiety disorders are the most common mental health disorder in adolescents.[8] Risk factors for anxiety disorders include having a parent with an anxiety disorder and environmental factors, including parental responses to behavior, traumatic events, and difficulty controlling emotions.[8] When children and adolescents cannot obtain outpatient mental health support, their parents may seek care for them in the ED.

Anxiety disorders can occur concurrently with ADHD, substance abuse, suicidal ideation, and depression.[33] Many pediatric patients will seek care for anxiety disorders or experience anxiety related to physical complaints.[31(Ch10)] They will often complain of headaches, stomach pain, nausea, diarrhea, chest pain, fatigue or exhaustion, irritability, or sleep disturbances.[31(Ch10)] Adolescents may struggle to explain their emotions and complain of similar symptoms. In addition, adolescents may present with increased oppositional or disruptive behaviors. Anxiety may escalate to agitation if it is not managed appropriately.[33]

Appropriate Interventions

Some providers choose to treat anxiety with pharmacologic interventions. Long-term treatment involves regularly scheduled therapy sessions with a mental health professional to help the patient and caregivers learn to manage anxiety.[31(Ch10)] Pediatric patients who present with anxiety require a full assessment, and medical conditions must be ruled out.[31(Ch10)] Offer empathetic responses, validate feelings, offer choices, and provide a distraction to help the patient gain a sense of control and manage anxiety.[33]

Agitated Delirium

Agitated delirium can be associated with multiple medical or behavioral disorders. Early identification of its cause and treatment can reduce the adverse effects of prolonged delirium.[32] Conditions related to agitated delirium include exacerbation of psychiatric disorders, drug or alcohol intoxication, and altered mental status caused by shock or metabolic imbalance.[23] Behavioral health disorders associated with delirium include bipolar disorder, depression, anxiety, PTSD, and schizophrenia.[31]

Symptoms of delirium include disorientation, hallucinations, incoherent speech, and extreme agitation.[23] Identifying hallucinations in children can be a challenge and will vary based on the patient's developmental level. For example, a younger child experiencing hallucinations may express symptoms relating to common childhood fears (e.g., seeing a monster in the room). In contrast, adolescents are more likely to experience complex hallucinations such as hearing voices commanding that they harm themselves or someone else or a voice consistently belittling their self-esteem.[10]

Appropriate Interventions

It is a priority to rule out medical reasons for agitated delirium to prevent long-term sequelae. Consider the following diagnostic studies[10,23]:

- Bedside glucose to identify hypoglycemia or hyperglycemia
- Complete blood count (CBC) and blood culture to help identify infection
- Complete metabolic panel to identify electrolyte imbalances and organ dysfunction

- Ammonia level to identify metabolic disorders, any disorder affecting the liver, and Reye's syndrome
- A drug screen, urinalysis, and urine culture can help identify drug or toxin ingestion and infection

Patient and staff safety remains a priority for the patient experiencing agitated delirium. Remove any objects that may cause injury from the room, maintain a calm environment, and limit stimuli.[10] Provide support to any patient who is actively hallucinating, as this can be a frightening experience. Other interventions may include the administration of antipsychotic medications. The patient with agitated delirium will likely require admission.

Bipolar Disorder

Bipolar disorder is a mood disorder characterized by cycles of mania and depression.[31(Ch13)] A chronic condition, it requires long-term treatment.[33] Bipolar disorder is often challenging to diagnose in the pediatric population. Children with bipolar disorder frequently present with other conduct disorders or ADHD.[33] To differentiate between occasional spontaneous childhood behaviors and symptoms of bipolar disorder, obtain a history of the behaviors, including their frequency, intensity, number, and duration.[33]

Symptoms associated with mania in children include the following[33]:

- Euphoric mood
- Irritable mood
- Grandiosity
- Decreased need for sleep
- Pressured speech
- Racing thoughts
- Distractibility
- Increased psychomotor agitation
- Involvement in risky behaviors
- Psychosis
- Suicidality

Appropriate Interventions

Assess the patient for high-risk behaviors, including impulsivity and suicidal ideation. Also assess for agitation and irritability while providing a safe environment.[31(Ch13)] Involve the caregivers in the treatment plan when possible. Pharmacologic treatment is the most common intervention to prevent relapses; therefore, compliance with the treatment plan is essential to improving long-term outcomes.[33]

Schizophrenia

Schizophrenia causes disruptions in thought processes, perception, and daily functioning.[33] Approximately 1%

of the population is affected by schizophrenia, and symptoms most commonly emerge in late adolescence to early adulthood.[33] The development of symptoms before the age of 13 is referred to as *very early-onset schizophrenia*.[33] Characteristics of this disorder include auditory and visual hallucinations with illogical and disorganized thinking, delusions, and lack of engagement with others and the environment.[31(Ch15)] Pediatric patients with schizophrenia may present to the ED for various reasons, including delusions, hallucinations, or adverse medication reactions.[31(Ch15)] The caregivers of these patients may report hygiene problems and difficulty completing daily living activities, and note that the patient verbalizes seeing or hearing things that are not there.

Assessment of the patient with schizophrenia is a complex process due to the difficulty of obtaining information and building trust.[33]

Appropriate Interventions

The potential for suicide or violence toward others is a significant concern for children and adolescents with schizophrenia.[33] Intervene at the first sign of increased anxiety or agitation by setting limits, reinforcing instructions, and meeting basic needs.[33] Do not validate hallucinations. Encourage the patient to recognize that the hallucinations are not real so as to decrease the patient's anxiety and agitation.[33]

Schizophrenia is treated with antipsychotic medications that can have serious side effects. The most commonly used first-generation antipsychotic medications include chlorpromazine and haloperidol.[33] Second-generation antipsychotic medications include clozapine, risperidone, olanzapine, quetiapine, and ziprasidone. Second-generation antipsychotics present less risk of adverse side effects, but may still have serious unwanted effects.[31(Ch15)] Specifically, antipsychotic medications may have the following side effects[33]:

- Weight gain
- Type 2 diabetes
- Sedation
- Dry mouth
- Dizziness
- Nausea

In severe cases, patients can develop serious side effects known as extrapyramidal symptoms (EPS). These symptoms include the following[31(Ch15)]:

- Dystonia: Muscle contractions that cause distorted posture, excessive blinking, or eyes rolling back into head

- Dyskinesia: Repetitive movements of the face, lips, torso, or legs
- Akathisia: Internal restlessness, inability to sit still
- Pseudoparkinsonism: Tremors, stiffness, rigidity, and unsteady posture

EPS become irreversible if left untreated; therefore, symptoms must be treated immediately upon their recognition.[31(Ch15)] These symptoms are often successfully treated with diphenhydramine or benztropine. Obtain medication blood levels when possible to ensure the concentration of the medication is at a therapeutic level.[31(Ch15)]

Autism

Autism is a spectrum of disorders characterized by impaired social interaction and communication skills.[33] Autism spectrum disorders (ASD) include a range of conditions (**Table 15-2**), and the specific diagnosis depends on severity, verbal abilities, genetic disorders, and intellectual disability.[33]

Recognizing symptoms of autism and beginning early treatment improves the quality of life for children with autism and their families.[33] Not meeting developmental milestones is one of the first symptoms of autism. Red flags for ASD in young children include the following[2]:

- Not responding to their name by 12 months of age
- Not reaching for objects by 14 months of age
- Not engaging in make-believe games by the age of 18 months
- Getting upset by minor changes
- Repetitive movements
- Intense reactions to smells, tastes, or textures

Appropriate Interventions

Although there is no cure for ASD, patients can experience decreased severity or improvement of symptoms with early diagnosis and treatment. Treatment includes exercises for improving coping skills, skill development, special training for caregivers, occupational therapy, and social skills training.[2] Incorporate caregivers in the plan of care and provide information about ways of decreasing patient anxiety and agitation.[33] Children with ASD have difficulty expressing thoughts and describing symptoms. Agitation may indicate fear or pain.[2]

In the ED, the loud and often chaotic environment found there can increase anxiety levels in these patients. Use these strategies when caring for children with ASD in the emergency setting[20,26,33]:

- Place the patient in a room that is protected from sound and away from main hallways.

TABLE 15-2 Autism Spectrum		
Level 1: "Requiring Support"	**Level 2: "Requiring Substantial Support"**	**Level 3: "Requiring Very Substantial Support"**
› The least severe; functioning improves with support. › Deficits in social communication cause noticeable impairment, and inflexibility of behaviors causes significant interference with functioning in one or more areas. › Difficulty initiating social interactions; responds inappropriately to social interactions. May have decreased interest in social interactions. › Problems with organization, switching between activities.	› Obvious deficits in verbal and nonverbal social communication skills, social impairments with limited initiation of social interactions. › Inflexible behaviors, difficulty coping with change, restrictive or repetitive movements. › Distress and/or difficulty changing focus or action.	› Most severe. › Severe deficits in verbal and nonverbal communication and functioning; very limited initiation of social interactions. › Inflexible behavior, extreme difficulty coping with change, restrictive or repetitive behaviors interfere with functioning. › Marked distress or difficulty changing focus or activities.

Data from American Psychiatric Association. (2021). *Autism*. https://www.psychiatry.org/patients-families/autism/what-is-autism-spectrum-disorder; and Shatkin, J. P. (2015). Autism spectrum disorders. In *Child & adolescent mental health: A practical all-in-one guide* (pp. 114–144). Norton & Company.

- Recognize the risk for self-harm and provide safety.
- Ask caregivers for details on the best techniques to gain cooperation for examination and treatment.
- Assess for common sources of pain.
- Maintain consistent treatment team members.
- Avoid touching the child until after a complete health history has been obtained.
- Explain procedures using visual cues.
- Move slowly through the exam and avoid sudden changes.

Attention-Deficit/Hyperactivity Disorder

ADHD is a neurodevelopmental disorder characterized by hyperactivity, high levels of inattention, and impulsivity.[26] Young children may present to the ED due to a crisis, aggressive behaviors, and issues associated with impulse control, such as injuries or substance abuse.[21] Notably, children with ADHD have a higher attempted and completed suicide rate than children without this disorder.[30] Children with ADHD find it difficult to function in social settings and experience conflict with caregivers and peers because they often exhibit disruptive behavior, social immaturity, and learning difficulties.[2] Problems with interpersonal relationships and poor impulse control increase the risk of self-harm for children with ADHD.

ADHD is associated with several mental health disorders and harmful behaviors. The following list includes comorbidities or harmful behaviors associated with ADHD[17,33]:

- Risk for traumatic injury
- Anxiety disorder
- Bipolar disorder
- Depression
- Increased risk of addiction
- Risk of being a victim of physical or sexual abuse
- High risk for eating disorders

Appropriate Interventions

EDs must provide safe and culturally sensitive care to children with ADHD or symptoms of ADHD. Provide a calm, nonjudgmental environment and remove any harmful objects. Apply cultural considerations when assessing and obtaining a history, including culturally appropriate practices for addressing behavioral concerns.[22]

Frequently, medication is used to manage symptoms of ADHD. Central nervous system (CNS) stimulants can effectively activate the dopamine receptors in the basal ganglia and thalamus to depress motor activity.[33] Monitor children who are being treated with CNS stimulants for palpitations, tachycardia, hypertension, and overstimulation.[33] Long-term side effects can include insomnia, weight loss, dependence, and severe liver damage.[33]

Eating Disorders

Eating disorders, such as anorexia nervosa and bulimia nervosa, are chronic conditions that may cause severe physical ailments.[24] The typical onset of eating disorders is during adolescence. Although these disorders occur in both males and females, they affect substantially more females than males.[25] Children with eating disorders often experience significant associated medical comorbidities and mental health problems.[25]

The two most common eating disorders are anorexia nervosa and bulimia nervosa. Characteristics of anorexia nervosa include a disproportionate fear of obesity, distorted body image, preoccupation with food, and refusal to eat.[33] Assessment findings include the following[33]:

- Excessive weight loss
- Hypothermia and hypotension
- Dependent edema
- Decreased renal function
- Bradycardia and other cardiac dysrhythmias
- Amenorrhea
- Anemia and osteoporosis
- Hormonal abnormalities

Bulimia nervosa is a compulsion to rapidly consume large amounts of food followed by purging the body of the excess calories.[33] Food consumed during binges is usually high-calorie and sweet. Binging and purging episodes generally occur in private without others being aware of them.[33] Purging may include self-induced vomiting; use of laxatives, enemas, or diuretics; and excessive exercise or fasting.[33] Children and adolescents with bulimia nervosa are typically average weight and have weight fluctuations surrounding the episodes of binging and purging.[33] Assessment findings include the following[33]:

- Calloused hands and erosion of enamel on teeth from forcing vomiting episodes
- Esophageal and gastric erosion
- Dehydration
- Cavities
- Bradycardia and other cardiac dysrhythmias
- Hypotension
- Electrolyte disturbances (e.g., hypocalcemia, hypochloremia, hypokalemia)

Physical complications of the eating disorder may be the primary reason for seeking care in the ED.

Appropriate Interventions

In the ED, treatment for eating disorders focuses on managing the physical complications. Assess the patient for physical findings or self-harm risks.[33] For complaints of dizziness or lightheadedness, consider baseline laboratory testing and an electrocardiogram to rule out electrolyte imbalances and rhythm disturbances.[33] Address any physical findings.

Pediatric patients with eating disorders often hide the disorder by reporting an intake higher than their actual intake or denying excessive exercising or purging.[33] Obtaining a thorough history from the patient and caregivers is essential to identifying these behaviors.[33] Anxiety levels may be higher in children with eating disorders in the ED setting. They may be reluctant to change into a gown, be weighed, or receive help due to insecurities with their body image.[33] When possible, offer choices to enable these patients to regain a sense of control.[31(Ch17)] Emergency interventions for eating disorders include rehydrating the patient, correcting electrolyte and metabolic imbalances, and monitoring for cardiac dysrhythmias and hypotension.[31(Ch17)]

Post-Traumatic Stress Disorder

PTSD is a specific form of anxiety disorder occurring in children and adolescents who experienced or witnessed a traumatic event. It can occur in conjunction with traumatic life events, such as actual or potential threat of death, disasters, serious accidental injury, abuse, or physical or sexual violence.[2] PTSD is related to one significant event and differs from the psychological symptoms experienced by children and adolescents affected by ongoing abuse.[33] Symptoms of PTSD include impaired executive functioning, reexperiencing the trauma, elevated anxiety levels, nightmares, and difficulty remembering events.[33] Symptoms of depression are common and can be severe.[33]

For all children and adolescents, the criteria for diagnosis of PTSD include the following[33]:

- Exposure to the traumatic event, either witnessed or directly involved
- One or more of the following intrusion symptoms:
  - Recurrent and interfering memories of the event
  - Recurring dreams of the event
  - Flashbacks
  - Emotional distress after being reminded of the event
  - Avoidance of activities, places, people, or conversations that remind the patient of the event
  - Inability to remember important aspects of the event
  - Distorted perception of the cause of the event, leading to self-blame and guilt
  - Lack of interest in previously enjoyed activities or decreased play

- One or more of the following increased arousal symptoms:
  - Increased irritability, anger, or temper tantrums
  - Inability to relax and increased startle response
  - Difficulty concentrating and inability to sleep

Symptoms must be present for more than 1 month and significantly impact the patient's relationships, schoolwork, and home life to merit the PTSD diagnosis.[33]

The child's or adolescent's response to a traumatic event will depend on several factors, including age, developmental age, presence or absence of a support system, prior experiences with traumatic events, and whether any loss occurred because of the event.[33] A child with PTSD will often present to the ED with signs of regression, including bedwetting, encopresis (fecal incontinence), sleep disturbances, and appetite changes.[2] Children and adolescents with this disorder may exhibit a variety of mental and emotional disturbances. The associated behaviors include separation anxiety, attachment to strangers, increased aggression, and risky behaviors.[33] Concurrent mental health disorders include anxiety disorders, mood disorders, eating disorders, substance abuse disorders, and self-injurious behaviors.[33]

Appropriate Interventions

Children and adolescents with PTSD have difficulty building relationships and asking for help. The nurse needs to establish trust and maintain an attitude of acceptance.[33] See Chapter 17, "The Child, Family, and Healthcare Team in Crisis," for more information on trauma-informed care.

Interventions include the following[33]:

- Provide a safe environment and remain sensitive when discussing the traumatic event.
- Ask permission before touching the patient.
- Offer as much choice as possible during assessments.
- Avoid changing staff, when possible, to maintain trust.
- Provide an age-appropriate overview of the assessments to be performed.

CLINICAL PEARL

Disclosure of Physical or Sexual Maltreatment

If the patient discloses physical or sexual maltreatment, the presence of a trained forensic interviewer or pediatric sexual assault nurse examiner will be invaluable.

Substance Abuse/Misuse

Although their rates are still low compared to those for adults, substance abuse is more common in adolescents than in young children. Approximately 20% of adolescents ages 12 to 17 report using alcohol or illicit drugs at least once.[29] Substance abuse/misuse negatively impacts social and cognitive development due to increased high school dropout rates, depression, risky behaviors, and elevated suicide rates.[29] Adolescents may begin by experimenting with an occasional illicit substance, which leads to regular use, which then leads to harmful use.[33]

Appropriate Interventions

Children and adolescents with substance abuse problems may present to the ED while acutely intoxicated. They also tend to engage in dangerous activities while intoxicated. Immediately address any physical concerns, including injuries, CNS depression, psychosis, withdrawal, or fluid and electrolyte imbalances.[33] Screen for alcohol and substance abuse if pediatric patients express mental health or behavioral health problems, as patients with these conditions are more likely to experiment with illicit substances.[31(Ch16)] Consider screening all adolescents for substance use.

Administer naloxone intravenously, intranasally, or intramuscularly to reverse the harmful effects of opioids, such as respiratory depression.[14] In any cases of suspected opioid ingestion involving respiratory depression, consider the administration of this medication.

Bullying/Cyberbullying

Bullying and cyberbullying have negative impacts on pediatric mental, physical, and emotional health. Bullying consists of repeated exposure to negative interactions with others who aim to either assert power or intimidate their target.[4(Ch1)] Cyberbullying is characterized by use of electronic devices or social media to intimidate, spread rumors, or tease.[4(Ch1)] The anonymity provided by fake accounts and profiles prevents the victim from knowing who is doing the bullying.[4(Ch2)]

Victims of bullying may present to the ED with vague somatic symptoms or symptoms of other behavioral health disorders. Potential symptoms include anxiety, depression, low self-esteem, stomach pain, decreased appetite, sleep disturbances, bedwetting, fatigue, headache, and poor school performance or high absentee rates.[4(Ch3)] Cyberbullying can involve multiple people focused on one victim and lead to severe depression, self-harm, and suicide.[4(Ch3)]

Prevention

Prevention of bullying and cyberbullying is difficult but can be accomplished. Steps geared toward prevention include recognizing signs of aggression in the bully and ensuring the victim feels confident enough to report the bullying.[4(Ch10)] Most schools have established anti-bullying programs along with anti-aggression curricula and a safe method for children or families to report bullying or cyberbullying.[4(Ch11)] It is vital for children and adolescents to feel comfortable reporting episodes of bullying to caregivers and school officials. If a patient reports being a victim, immediately notify the caregivers to take the necessary steps to protect the patient. It may benefit children and adolescents who are already being cyberbullied to block offenders on social networking sites and change phone numbers, email addresses, and online profiles.[4(Ch12)]

Considerations for Transfer

It is essential to assess for and treat any underlying medical conditions in children and adolescents seeking care for behavioral health emergencies. Medical conditions, such as electrolyte imbalances or neurologic disorders, may require hospital admission. Pediatric psychiatric admissions are indicated for immediate safety concerns, medication regulation, stabilization of behavior, and inpatient therapy. Collaboration with local behavioral health resources is vital.

Discharge Teaching

General therapeutic approaches can benefit the child or adolescent by improving coping mechanisms, social interactions, and daily living skills. Types of therapy include behavioral therapy, family therapy, and psychopharmacology.[33] Eye movement desensitization and reprocessing (EMDR) therapy and trauma-focused cognitive-behavioral therapy are evidence-based interventions that incorporate the trauma-informed care approach.[11] Ensure the patient and family have appropriate behavioral health follow-up care. Emphasize the importance of maintaining a consistent medication regimen and keeping regular therapy appointments.[33]

Ensure that the pediatric patient is not having active suicidal ideation at the time of discharge. If a patient expresses suicidal ideation while in the ED, obtain a behavioral health evaluation before discharge and establish a safety plan to use at home.[32] Provide written instructions for safety measures to apply in the home, including proper storage of medications, sharp objects, and firearms.[15] Emphasize the need for caregivers to notify authorities of any potential threat the child might pose to self or others.

Safety, Injury Prevention, and Health Promotion

Promoting home safety is an essential component of protecting children and adolescents with behavioral health emergencies from harm. Encourage the caregivers to remove or secure harmful items at home. Firearms are especially lethal if used in a suicide attempt. If these weapons are kept in the home, instruct caregivers that they need to be locked in a safe place with no access by children and adolescents.

Medication overdose is a common mechanism for suicide attempts. Children and adolescents with diagnosed mental illnesses often have access to potentially lethal medications. Instruct caregivers to secure all home medications in a cabinet or box with a lock to prevent overdoses, including over-the-counter medications.[15]

Many outreach programs emphasize support for patients with behavioral health disorders, aiding them in developing coping skills and improving interpersonal communication.[33] These programs identify at-risk youth through schools and healthcare settings for early interventions. Successful programs help children and adolescents identify strengths and positive coping skills, teaching them how to communicate, problem-solve, and regulate emotions.[31(Ch2)]

Summary

Children with behavioral health emergencies present differently than adults with such conditions. In many cases, their symptoms may be vague and somatic in nature. The first step is to complete an assessment, obtain a thorough history, and rule out medical causes of the behavior. After physical causes are ruled out, it is appropriate to consider a behavioral health problem. Provide a calm environment and develop rapport. Involve family members as much as possible in therapy and treatments. Behavioral health disorders require long-term care and family education and support. Screening for abuse, violence in the home, and human trafficking is crucial. The priority is always to keep the patient safe.

References

1. American College of Emergency Physicians. (2019). Pediatric mental health emergencies in the emergency department. *Annals of Emergency Medicine*, 73(3), e33–e36. https://doi.org/10.1016/j.annemergmed.2018.11.005

2. American Psychiatric Association. (2022). Neurodevelopmental disorders. *Diagnostic and statistical manual of mental disorders* (5th ed. Text Revision).

3. American Psychiatric Association. (2021). *Autism.* https://www.psychiatry.org/patients-families/autism/what-is-autism-spectrum-disorder

4. Bartlett, C. P. (2019). *Predicting cyberbullying: Research, theory, and intervention.* Academic Press.

5. Carbone, J. T., Jackson, D. B., Holzer, K. J., & Vaughn, M. G. (2021). Childhood adversity, suicidality, and non-suicidal self-injury among children and adolescents admitted to emergency departments. *Annals of Epidemiology, 60,* 21–27. https://doi.org/10.1016/j.annepidem.2021.04.015

6. Chun, T. H., Mace, S. E., & Katz, E. R. (2016). Evaluation and management of children and adolescents with acute mental health or behavioral problems. Part 1: Common clinical challenges of patients with mental health and/or behavioral emergencies. *Pediatrics, 138*(3), Article e20161570. https://doi.org/10.1542/peds.2016-1570

7. Coleman, K. D., Chow, Y., Jacobson, A., Hainsworth, K. R., & Drendel, A. L. (2021). An evaluation of short anxiety measures for use in the emergency department. *American Journal of Emergency Medicine, 50,* 679–682. https://doi.org/10.1016/j.ajem.2021.09.028

8. Creswell, C., Waite, P., & Hudson, J. (2020). Practitioner review: Anxiety disorders in children and young people: Assessment and treatment. *Journal of Child Psychology and Psychiatry, 61*(6), 628–643. https://doi.org/10.1111/jcpp.13186

9. Davids, J., Murphy, M., Moore, N., Wand, T., & Brown, M. (2021). Exploring staff experiences: A case for redesigning the response to aggression and violence in the emergency department. *International Emergency Nursing, 57,* Article 101017. https://doi.org/10.1016/j.ienj.2021.101017

10. Gerson, R., Malas, N., Feuer, V., Silver, G. H., Prasad, R., & Mroczkowski, M. M. (2019). Best practices for evaluation and treatment of agitated children and adolescents (BETA) in the emergency department: Consensus statement of the American Association for Emergency Psychiatry. *Western Journal of Emergency Medicine, 20*(2), 409–418. https://doi.org/10.5811/westjem.2019.1.41344

11. Goddard, A., Janicek, E., & Etcher, L. (2022). Trauma-informed care for the pediatric nurse. *Journal of Pediatric Nursing, 62,* 1–9. https://doi.org/10.1016/j.pedn.2021.11.003

12. Gonzalez, K., Patel, F., Cutchins, L. A., Kodish, I., & Uspal, N. G. (2020). Advocacy to address emergent pediatric mental health care. *Clinical Pediatric Emergency Medicine, 21*(2), Article 100778. https://doi.org/10.1016/j.cpem.2020.100778

13. Gottlieb, M., Long, B., & Koyfman, A. (2018). Approach to the agitated emergency department patient. *Journal of Emergency Medicine, 54*(4), 447–457. https://doi.org/10.1016/j.jemermed.2017.12.049

14. Gupta, R., Shah, N. D., & Ross, J. S. (2016). The rising price of naloxone: Risks to efforts to stem overdose deaths. *New England Journal of Medicine, 375*(23), 2213–2215. https://doi.org/10.1056/NEJMp1609578

15. Kennebeck, S., & Bonin, L. (2020). Suicidal ideation and behavior in children and adolescents: Evaluation and management. *UpToDate.* Retrieved January 24, 2022, from https://www.uptodate.com/contents/suicidal-ideation-and-behavior-in-children-and-adolescents-evaluation-and-management

16. Knopf, A. (2016). AAP issues guidance to EDs on acute pediatric mental health conditions. *Brown University Child & Adolescent Behavior Letter, 32*(10), 1–7. https://doi.org/10.1002/cbl.30156

17. Korczak, D. J., Finkelstein, Y., Barwick, M., Chaim, G., Cleverley, K., Henderson, J., Monga, S., Moretti, M. E., Willan, A., & Szatmari, P. (2020). A suicide prevention strategy for youth presenting to the emergency department with suicide related behaviour: Protocol for a randomized controlled trial. *BMC Psychiatry, 20*(1), Article 20. https://doi.org/10.1186/s12888-019-2422-y

18. Lawrence, R. E., Fuchs, B., Krumheuer, A., Perez-Coste, M., Loh, R., Simpson, S. A., & Stanley, B. (In press). Self-harm during visits to the emergency department: A qualitative content analysis. *Journal of the Academy of Consultation-Liaison Psychiatry.* https://doi.org/10.1016/j.jaclp.2021.10.003

19. Lu, W. (2019). Adolescent depression: National trends, risk factors, and healthcare disparities. *American Journal of Health Behavior, 43*(1), 181–194. https://doi.org/10.5993/AJHB.43.1.15

20. Lunsky, Y., Tint, A., Weiss, J., Palucka, A., & Bradley, E. (2018). A review of emergency department visits made by youth and adults with autism spectrum disorder from the parent perspective. *Advances in Autism, 4*(1), 10–18. https://doi.org/10.1108/AIA-08-2017-0019

21. Lynch, S., Bautista, M., Freer, C., Kalynych, C., Cuffe, S., & Hendry, P. (2016). Toward effective utilization of the pediatric emergency department: The case of ADHD. *Social Work in Public Health, 31*(1), 9–18. https://doi.org/10.1080/19371918.2015.1087909

22. Mattox, G. A., & Vinson, S. Y. (2018). Culturally competent approaches to ADHD: Issues in African-American populations. *Psychiatric Times, 35*(9), 19–20. https://www.psychiatrictimes.com/view/culturally-competent-approaches-adhd-issues-african-american-populations

23. Miner, J. R., Klein, L. R., Cole, J. B., Driver, B. E., Moore, J. C., & Ho, J. D. (2018). The characteristics and prevalence of agitation in an urban county emergency department. *Annals of Emergency Medicine, 72*(4), 361–370. https://doi.org/10.1016/j.annemergmed.2018.06.001

24. Munkholm, A., Olsen, E. M., Rask, C. U., Clemmensen, L., Rimvall, M. K., Jeppesen, P., Micali, N., & Skovgaard, A. M. (2016). Early predictors of eating problems in preadolescence: A prospective birth cohort study. *Journal of Adolescent Health, 58*(5), 533–542. https://doi.org/10.1016/j.jadohealth.2016.01.006

25. Pinhas, L., Nicholls, D., Crosby, R. D., Morris, A., Lynn, R. M., & Madden, S. (2017). Classification of childhood onset eating disorders: A latent class analysis. *International*

Journal of Eating Disorders, 50(6), 657–664. https://doi.org/10.1002/eat.22666

26. Pon, N., Asan, B., Anandan, S., & Toledo, A. (2015). Special considerations in pediatric psychiatric populations. *Emergency Medicine Clinics of North America, 33*, 811–824. https://doi.org/10.1016/j.emc.2015.07.008

27. Randall, M. M., Parlette, K., Reibling, E., Chen, B., Chen, M., Randall, F., & Brown, L. (2020). Young children with psychiatric complaints in the pediatric emergency department. *American Journal of Emergency Medicine, 46*, 344–348. https://doi.org/10.1016/j.ajem.2020.10.006

28. Roppolo, L. P., Morris, D. W., Khan, F., Downs, R., Metzger, J., Carder, T., Wong, A. H., & Wilson, M. P. (2020). Improving the management of acutely agitated patients in the emergency department through implementation of Project BETA (Best Practices in the Evaluation and Treatment of Agitation). *Journal of the American College of Emergency Physicians Open, 1*(5), 898–907. https://doi.org/10.1002/emp2.12138

29. Sakai-Bizmark, R., Webber, E. J., Estevez, D., Murillo, M., Marr, E. H., Bedel, L. E. M., Mena, L. A., Felix, J. C. D., & Smith, L. M. (2021). Health care utilization due to substance abuse among homeless and nonhomeless children and young adults in New York. *Psychiatric Services, 72*(4), 421–428. https://doi.org/10.1176/appi.ps.202000010

30. Santillanes, G., & Gerson, R. S. (2017). Special considerations in the pediatric psychiatric population. *Psychiatric Clinics of North America, 40*(3), 463–473. https://doi.org/10.1016/j.psc.2017.05.009

31. Shatkin, J. P. (2015). *Child and adolescent mental health: A practical all-in-one guide.* W. W. Norton & Company.

32. U.S. Department of Health and Human Services, Health Resources and Services Administration, Maternal and Child Health Bureau. (2019). *Critical crossroads: Pediatric mental health care in the emergency department: A care pathway resource toolkit.* https://www.hrsa.gov/sites/default/files/hrsa/critical-crossroads/critical-crossroads-tool.pdf

33. Videbeck, S. L. (2017). *Psychiatric–mental health nursing* (7th ed.). Wolters Kluwer.

34. Vish, N. L., & Stolfi, A. (2020). Relationship of children's emotional and behavioral disorders with health care utilization and missed school. *Academic Pediatrics, 20*(5), 687–695. https://doi.org/10.1016/j.acap.2020.02.017

The Child with a Suspicious Presentation

Shannon Miller, SANE-P, TNS, CPNP-PC, DNP

OBJECTIVES

Upon completion of this chapter, the learner will be able to:

1. Integrate the evaluation of child maltreatment into daily nursing practice.
2. Identify the risk factors, key indicators, common physical injuries, and long-term consequences of child maltreatment.
3. Recognize the importance of screening, evaluation, and appropriate nursing interventions for victims of child maltreatment.
4. Appreciate the value of documentation, evidence collection, and reporting suspected child maltreatment to appropriate local authorities.

Introduction

Child maltreatment is a significant cause of pediatric morbidity and mortality and is associated with major physical and mental health problems that can extend into adulthood. The Child Abuse Prevention and Treatment Act defines child abuse as follows: "any recent act or failure to act on the part of a parent or caretaker, which results in death, serious physical or emotional harm, sexual abuse or exploitation, or an act or failure to act which presents an imminent risk of serious harm."[14]

Most jurisdictions recognize four major types of maltreatment: neglect, physical abuse, psychological abuse, and sexual abuse.[29,31,37] Each specific type may be observed independently, but very frequently allegations of child maltreatment involve more than one type.[31,37,49]

Forms of Child Maltreatment

Unfortunately, there are many forms of maltreatment that fall within the four main types. Some are more subtle than others, but all are damaging. Awareness of the various forms enables nurses to identify the potential for harm and intervene.

Neglect

Among the types of child maltreatment, neglect is the most common and accounts for more than half of all confirmed cases.[37,49] Neglect is the failure to provide for a child's basic physical, emotional, or educational needs or to protect a child from harm or potential harm.[15] Within this child maltreatment type, there are several defined subtypes and categories within the subtypes (**Table 16-1**).[16]

TABLE 16-1 Types of Neglect

Types of Neglect	Subcategories of Neglect
Physical neglect	*Abandonment:* The desertion of a child without arranging for their reasonable care or supervision
	Expulsion: The blatant refusal of custody without adequately arranging for their care by others or the refusal to accept custody of a returned runaway
	Shuttling: When a child is repeatedly left in the care of others for days or weeks at a time
	Nutritional neglect: When a child is undernourished or is repeatedly hungry for extended periods of time, sometimes evidenced by poor growth
	Clothing neglect: When a child lacks appropriate clothing, such as not having appropriately warm clothes or shoes in the winter
	Other physical neglect: Includes inadequate hygiene and forms of reckless disregard for the child's safety and welfare (e.g., driving while intoxicated with the child, leaving a young child in a car unattended)
Medical neglect	*Denial of healthcare:* The failure to provide or to allow needed care as recommended by a competent healthcare professional
	Delay in healthcare: The failure to seek medical care for a serious health problem that any reasonable person would recognize as needing attention
Inadequate supervision	*Lack of appropriate supervision:* Some jurisdictions specify the amount of time children at different ages can be left unsupervised
	Exposure to hazards: Safety hazards, smoking, guns or weapons, unsanitary household conditions, or lack of car safety restraints
	Inappropriate caregivers: Leaving the child in the care of someone who either is unable or not trustworthy to provide care for a child
	Other inadequate supervision: Leaving a child with an appropriate caregiver, but without proper planning or consent; leaving the child with a caregiver who is not adequately supervising the child; and permitting or not keeping the child from engaging in risky, illegal, or harmful behaviors
Environmental neglect	A lack of environmental or neighborhood safety, opportunities, or resources
Emotional neglect	*Inadequate nurturing or affection:* Persistent, marked inattention to the child's needs for affection, emotional support, or attention
	Inadequate nurturing or affection: Persistent, marked inattention to the child's needs for affection, emotional support, or attention
	Chronic or extreme intimate-partner abuse: Exposure to chronic or extreme intimate-partner abuse or other domestic violence
	Permitted drug or alcohol abuse: Encouragement or permission by the caregiver of drug or alcohol use by the child
	Other permitted maladaptive behavior: Encouragement of or permission for other maladaptive behavior (e.g., chronic delinquency, assault)

Types of Neglect	Subcategories of Neglect
Educational neglect	*Permitted, chronic truancy:* Permitting habitual absenteeism from school averaging at least 5 days a month
	Failure to enroll or other truancy: Failing to homeschool, to register, or to enroll a child of mandatory school age, causing the child to miss at least 1 month of school without valid reasons
	Inattention to special education needs: Refusing to allow or failing to obtain recommended remedial education services
Newborns addicted or exposed to drugs	Women who use drugs or alcohol during pregnancy can put their unborn children at risk for mental and physical disabilities

Data from Child Welfare Information Gateway. (2018, July). *Acts of omission: An overview of child neglect.* https://www.childwelfare.gov/pubPDFs/acts.pdf

Physical Abuse

The signs and injuries involved in physical abuse make detection much more objective than other forms of abuse, but the challenge is differentiating between unintentional and intentional injuries. Determining whether a fracture or bruise is the result of normal childhood activity or the result of an abuser is seldom easy unless a thorough physical assessment is performed that incorporates the past medical history as well as the history of the injury as told by the caregivers and the child. While the "story" may initially seem extremely plausible and well articulated, the explanation of how a child was injured may evolve. It is important to monitor for signs of discrepancies throughout the visit.[50,51]

Psychological Abuse

Psychological abuse, which includes emotional abuse, is intentional behavior on the part of the caregiver that conveys to a child that they are worthless, flawed, unloved, unwanted, endangered, or valued only in meeting another's needs. Psychological and emotional abuse are perpetrated through verbal abuse, cruelty, and threats.[47] Because of the variability in pediatric psychosocial development and abusers' ability to alter their interactions in public, psychological maltreatment is difficult to pinpoint. This is particularly true with the episodic and unpredictable nature of care provided in emergency departments (EDs): In large facilities, it may be possible for a child and their abuser to present several times without ever encountering any of the same care providers.

Sexual Abuse

Child sexual abuse includes physical sexual contact as well as sexual exploitation, exhibitionism, voyeurism, trafficking, and being shown pornography with or without physical contact.[5,47] Seeking treatment for sexual abuse can be a traumatizing experience. Adolescents often disclose their mistreatment to a friend or peer, rather than a parent or a mandated reporter. This often delays follow-up post disclosure, presenting complications because often the parents are not aware of the abuse.[21] Many children are fearful of "breaking the rules" and do not want to upset or disappoint the abuser, which is why so many of these cases go unreported into adulthood. The combination of the child's dependence on caregivers and the child's developmental age and cognitive ability creates an opportunity for offenders to manipulate and silence children.

Advocate for the patient and family through appropriate examination techniques, providing emotional support, and referring to crisis and community services.[10] Patients who have experienced sexual abuse require consistent, objective, and immediate medical care, with forensic evidence collected by emergency nurses and medical providers trained in jurisdictional guidelines and protocols. Whenever possible, forensic nurses, physicians, social workers, child life specialists, and advanced practice providers with specialized training in pediatric sexual assault are consulted for children for whom there is concern for or disclosure of sexual abuse.[4,11,32]

Human Trafficking

Human trafficking involves the use of force, fraud, or coercion to obtain some type of labor or commercial sexual act. Traffickers use manipulation, violence, substance dependency, threats, fear of law enforcement, false promises of well-paying jobs, basic human needs (food, shelter, clothing), and romantic relationships to lure children. Trafficking is a global problem for millions of people of varying ages, races, genders, and nationalities.[7] When a suspicion for human trafficking arises, make every effort to talk to the person alone and offer resources. If they are not ready to disclose, ensure the person is aware that a hospital is a safe place to which they can return. In the United States, resources include the National Human Trafficking hotline (1-888-373-7888) and texting "BeFree" (233733). Small downloadable information cards are available in multiple languages (https://www.dhs.gov/blue-campaign/materials/indicator-card).

> **RED FLAG** ⚠
>
> Several red flags can help identify human trafficking[6]:
>
> - Are there signs of physical or psychological abuse?
> - Are there unreasonable security measures?
> - Does the child defer to another person?
> - Does the child have unique tattoos?
> - Does the child seem fearful, timid, or submissive?
> - Has there been a sudden or dramatic behavior change?
> - Is the child confused or disoriented?
> - Is the child engaging in sexual acts?
> - Is the child regularly attending school?
>
> Data from Blue Campaign. (n.d.). Indicators of human trafficking. U.S. Department of Homeland Security. https://www.dhs.gov/blue-campaign/indicators-human-trafficking

Medical Child Abuse

Medical child abuse occurs when a child receives unnecessary, harmful, or potentially harmful medical care at the instigation of a caretaker. Since 1977, when it was first described among the medical community, this condition has been referred to by various names, including Munchausen syndrome by proxy, factitious disorder imposed on another, factitious disorder by proxy, doctor shopping, caregiver-fabricated illness, and pediatric condition falsification. Medical child abuse entails a combination of physical and psychological abuse. Severe cases are noted in the literature, but the true prevalence of medical child abuse is unknown.[27,45]

Caregivers who are committing medical child abuse tend to "doctor shop," choosing physicians who recommend repeated testing and invasive procedures and removing their children from the care of physicians who refuse to escalate treatment. Any presentation is possible, but commonly reported symptoms include bleeding, seizures, lethargy, apnea, diarrhea, vomiting, fever, and rash. These symptoms may occur only in the presence of the caregiver. The abuse may begin with fabricated symptoms and progress to the caregiver inducing the symptoms. Chronic laxative administration, adding salt to infant formula, and substance injection are just three of many documented symptom-induction methods.[27,45]

The caregiver's motivation to inflict this form of abuse may be a need for attention or to covertly manipulate or deceive authority figures. The power of this attention cannot be underestimated or overlooked as a small consolation given the amount of time medical child maltreatment may involve. This can be an extremely dangerous form of child maltreatment with severe physical and psychological consequences and is most life-threatening when caregivers induce symptoms.[27]

Epidemiology of Child Maltreatment

The vast majority of children who are subjected to maltreatment are under-identified.[31,37,49] More than 70% of U.S. fatalities from child maltreatment occur in children younger than 3 years[17] and parents—acting alone or with another parent—were responsible for 79.7% of child maltreatment or neglect fatalities.[49] Globally, 20% of women and 7.7% of men report being sexually abused as a child, and 300 million children between the ages of 2 and 4 regularly experience physical punishment and/or psychological abuse from caregivers.[52]

Long-Term Consequences of Maltreatment

Children thrive in environments where they feel safe. A landmark study conducted at Kaiser Permanente in the 1990s[22] found a significant relationship between the number of adverse childhood experiences (ACEs) a person experienced and a variety of negative outcomes in adulthood, including poor physical and mental health, substance use, and risky behaviors. The more ACEs experienced, the greater the risk for these outcomes becomes. An emerging body of evidence shows that ACEs, including all forms of maltreatment, influence biological adaptations associated with how the brain, neuroendocrine stress response, and immune system function. Children who endure repeated abuse and neglect may experience cognitive challenges, social difficulties, compromised mental health, and chronic illness as an adult.[28]

Risk Factors for Maltreatment

Numerous risk factors for child maltreatment have been identified, and awareness of child maltreatment is a fundamental part of the emergency assessment of children.

TABLE 16-2	Factors and Characteristics That Place a Child at Risk for Maltreatment	
Child	**Parent**	**Environment (Community and Society)**
Chronic illness	Low self-esteem	Conflict and negative communication styles
Developmental disabilities	Depression or other mental illness	Family or intimate-partner violence
Emotional/behavioral difficulties	Negative perception of normal child behavior	Food insecurity
Younger than 4 years of age		High violence and crime rates
Physical disabilities	Parent abused as a child	Incarcerated family members
Preterm birth	Poor knowledge of child development or unrealistic expectations for child	Lack of youth community activities
Unplanned pregnancy		Limited educational and economic opportunities
Unwanted child	Poor impulse control	Poverty
	Single parent	Non-biologically related male living in the home
	Substance/alcohol abuse	
	Young parental age	Social isolation

Data from Centers for Disease Control and Prevention. (2021). *Child abuse and neglect: Risk and protective factors.* https://www.cdc.gov/violenceprevention/childabuseandneglect/riskprotectivefactors.html; Giardino, A. P., Giardino, E. R., & Moles, R. L. (2017). Physical child abuse. *Medscape.* Retrieved December 14, 2021, from https://emedicine.medscape.com/article/915664-overview

Children with disabilities are victims of abuse at a greater frequency than children in the general population, and their vulnerabilities allow abuse to continue into adulthood.[3,36] More than 77% of U.S. children subjected to maltreatment are maltreated by one or both parents.[49] **Table 16-2** lists numerous factors and characteristics that place a child at increased risk for child maltreatment.[12,23]

In addition to individual factors and characteristics that put a child at increased risk for maltreatment, there are many "red flags" to alert the emergency nurse to the possibility of abuse. **Table 16-3** lists common indications of child maltreatment.[9,20,43] The use of specific and directed screening protocols may help in the identification of these patients.

Selected Maltreatment Topics

While most injuries in children are not the result of abuse or neglect, simply asking a verbal child, "What happened?" creates the opportunity for the child to interact with the nurse, gathering more information than if specific targeted questions are asked. Children are also more apt to describe the story behind an injury when the injury is not the result of abuse. Comparing the caregiver and patient explanations with the injuries identified by the physician or advanced practice provider will also help to identify discrepancies.

Bruises

Bruises are the most common injuries resulting from physical abuse. A heightened level of suspicion for abuse is warranted if bruises are noted where they are not likely the result of normal child activity, such as bruises on the torso (including genitals), ears, or neck in a child younger than 4 years or any bruising in a child younger than 4 months. Using the mnemonic "TEN-4 FACES P" can be helpful for identifying suspicious bruising, where "TEN" refers to bruising to the torso, ear, or neck, "4" refers to age younger than 4 years or 4 months, and "FACES P" refers to bruising of the frenulum, angle of the jaw/auricular area (ear), cheek, eyelid, subconjunctivae, and assessing for patterned injuries.[44]

Fractures

Other injuries commonly seen in ambulatory children include fractures, which are the second most common presentation of child maltreatment, following soft-tissue bruising.[25] Fractures raise concerns about physical abuse in nonambulatory children with no clear history of how the injury occurred. **Table 16-4** lists fractures that heighten the suspicion of child maltreatment.[9,46]

Further radiographic studies are indicated if there is any degree of uncertainty as to the cause of a fracture. A skeletal survey is used to evaluate suspicious injuries in any child, particularly in those who are younger than 2 years, unable to communicate, with an altered level of

TABLE 16-3 Red Flags for Child Maltreatment

History of Present Illness	Physical Examination Findings	Radiologic Findings
Behavior changes	Any bruise in a nonexploratory location (especially torso, ears, and neck) in children younger than 4 years	Any fracture in a nonambulating infant
Changing history		Dislocations
Chronic medical conditions		Metaphyseal fractures (corner fractures)
Delay in seeking care	Any bruise in any nonambulating child	
Domestic violence in home		Rib fractures (especially posterior) in infants
Low birth weight or intrauterine growth restriction	Bruises, marks, or scars in patterns that suggest hitting with an object	Subdural hematoma and/or subarachnoid hemorrhage on neuroimaging in young children, particularly in the absence of skull fracture (children younger than 1 year)
Fear of going home	Difficulty ambulating	
Inconsistent history	Failure to thrive, poor growth patterns	
No history		
Premature infant (< 37 weeks' gestation)	Large heads in infants (consider measuring head circumference in children younger than 1 year)	
Prior emergency department visit	New and healing lacerations, abrasions, bruises, burns	Undiagnosed healing fracture
Recurrent urinary tract infections	Red, swollen genitalia	
Submersion injuries	Sexually transmitted infections	
Substance abuse	Torn frenulum	
Suicide attempt	Welts	
Unwitnessed injury		

Data from Boos, S. C. (2022). Physical child abuse: Recognition. *UpToDate*. Retrieved March 7, 2022, from https://www.uptodate.com/contents/physical-child-abuse-recognition; Escobar, M. J., Pflugeisen, B. M., Duralde, Y., Morris, C. J., Haferbecker, D., Amoroso, P. J., & Pohlson, E. C. (2016). Development of a systematic protocol to identify victims of non-accidental trauma. *Pediatric Surgery International*, 32(4), 377–386. https://doi.org/10.1007/s00383-016-3863-8; Perkins, A. (2018). The red flags of child abuse. *Nursing Made Incredibly Easy*, 16(2), 34–41. https://doi.org/10.1097/01.NME.0000529946.76463.6b

TABLE 16-4 Skeletal Injury in Intentional Trauma

Skeletal Injury	Correlate Mechanism of Injury with Physical Finding
Long bones	Epiphyseal/metaphyseal "bucket handle" or "corner" fracture at the end of long bones. This fracture often occurs secondary to pulling, twisting, or shaking, but can also be caused by natural shearing forces.
	Spiral fractures may be suspicious for abuse but can be seen with rotational forces (e.g., "toddler's fracture" of tibia).
Ribs, sternum, scapula, or spinous process	Posterior nondisplaced rib fractures due to severe squeezing of the rib cage. These fractures may not be visible on plain film until callus formation occurs.
Skull	Fractures more than 3 mm wide, complex fractures, bilateral fractures, and non-parietal fractures, particularly in children younger than 18 months of age, suggest forces greater than that of minor household trauma.

Data from Boos, S. C. (2022). Physical child abuse: Recognition. *UpToDate*. Retrieved March 7, 2022, from https://www.uptodate.com/contents/physical-child-abuse-recognition; Scherl, S. A. (2020). Orthopedic aspects of child abuse. *UpToDate*. Retrieved March 7, 2022, from https://www.uptodate.com/contents/orthopedic-aspects-of-child-abuse

consciousness, or younger than 5 years with a distracting injury.[8,47] **Figures 16-1** through **16-4** depict radiographic evidence of child abuse.[48] Comparing the stated mechanism of injury with the imaging results provides the necessary perspective to identify fractures resulting from abuse rather than from normal childhood activity.

Abusive Head Trauma

Abusive head trauma (AHT), formerly known as shaken baby syndrome, is the leading cause of death from child maltreatment.[18,51] Its presentation may be subtle, with no outward signs of physical trauma, and may mimic other medical or neurologic conditions. Vomiting, irritability, decreased oral intake, respiratory distress without respiratory illness, seizures, behavioral changes, and delayed development are common. A child with a significant alteration in mental status and no overt findings is a red flag for conducting further diagnostics, including an urgent ophthalmology assessment and skeletal survey. Classic findings in AHT include the absence of a history to support the injury, subdural hemorrhage, retinal hemorrhage, abnormal bruising, complex skull fractures, rib fractures, and long bone fractures.[18,51]

Burns

Whether their injuries occur from touching hot objects, hot liquids, or fire, many children sustain unintentional burns. However, it has been estimated that as many as 20% of pediatric burns are associated with abuse.[34] Several characteristics of the history and burn injury are associated with a significantly higher perceived likelihood of abuse, including children with reported inflicted injury, absent or inadequate explanation, hot water as agent, immersion scald, a bilateral/symmetric burn pattern, 10% or more of the total body surface area affected, full-thickness burns, and coexistent injuries.[39] Inflicted burns are generally deeper than unintentional burns and more severe because of a delay in seeking care. Unintentional

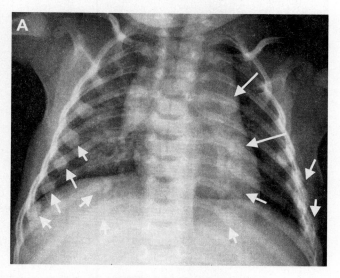

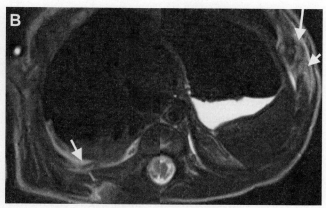

Figure 16-2 *A 2-month-old male patient presented with a witnessed history of shaking and punching injury.* **A.** *Twenty-nine healing rib fractures were identified on the chest radiograph. Some of the rib fractures are indicated with arrows.* **B.** *Magnetic resonance imaging of the spine juxtaposing two different levels of the chest demonstrated the healing rib fractures with callus formation bilaterally (arrows).*

Reproduced from Tun, K., Choudhary, A. K., Methratta, S., & Boal, D. K. (2013). Featured article: Radiological features of nonaccidental injury. *Journal of Radiology Nursing*, 323–329. https://doi.org/10.1016/j.jradnu.2012.08.005

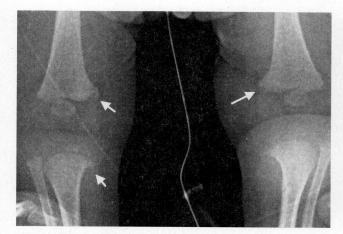

Figure 16-1 *A 5-month-old female patient presented with unexplained cardiopulmonary arrest at home and was found to have diffuse hypoxic–ischemic encephalopathy of the brain with multiple healing rib fractures. Radiograph of the bilateral femurs demonstrates metaphyseal fractures of the bilateral distal femurs and right proximal tibia (arrows).*

Reproduced from Tun, K., Choudhary, A. K., Methratta, S., & Boal, D. K. (2013). Featured article: Radiological features of nonaccidental injury. *Journal of Radiology Nursing*, 323–329. https://doi.org/10.1016/j.jradnu.2012.08.005

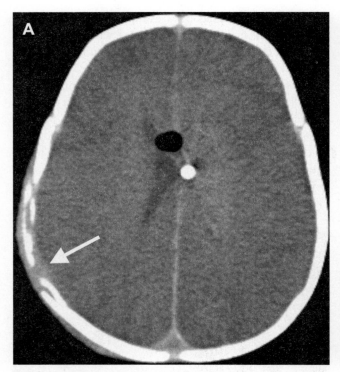
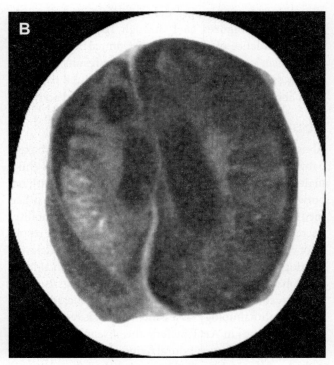

Figure 16-3 A. *Head computed tomography scan on a 2-month-old male patient presenting with seizures demonstrates complex skull fracture (arrow) with diffuse changes of hypoxic–ischemic encephalopathy (HIE) with loss of gray white matter differentiation of the brain.* **B.** *A follow-up head computed tomography scan at 2 years demonstrates diffuse encephalomalacia and volume loss of the brain reflecting the diffuse HIE at presentation.*

Reproduced from Tun, K., Choudhary, A. K., Methratta, S., & Boal, D. K. (2013). Featured article: Radiological features of nonaccidental injury. *Journal of Radiology Nursing,* 323–329. https://doi.org/10.1016/j.jradnu.2012.08.005

scald burns with a spill, splash, or pull-down mechanism have a typical burn pattern. These injuries have irregular margins and non-uniform depth, with downward flow evident by deeper burns in the superior regions, becoming shallower as the fluid cools. Inflicted immersion burns characteristically have sharp lines of demarcation and often involve the genitals and the lower extremities in symmetric distributions. The area burned in submersion burns may occur in a location covered by a sock or a glove, with a characteristic line at the wrist or ankle. Immersions that are deliberate incur burns of uniform depth with distinct borders and skin-fold sparing.[39]

Bite Marks

Bite marks may be inflicted by an adult, another child, an animal, or the patient. They may have the appearance of an oval or round area of bruising with wounds of various shapes surrounding the bruise, or there may be clearly defined teeth impressions on the surface of the skin. Bite marks may provide important evidence, especially if the injury is recent and the wound has not been thoroughly

cleaned. Clinicians and law enforcement with training and expertise in forensics are involved in the delicate and precise process of photographic and DNA evidence collection.[19]

Evaluation of Child Maltreatment

Child maltreatment screening is a systematic process at many pediatric referral centers and has been demonstrated to lead to improved patient outcomes.[29] However, not every ED has adopted this approach. A clinical report from the American Academy of Pediatrics entitled "The Evaluation of Suspected Child Physical Abuse" may be used to help guide a facility in developing such a protocol.[19]

As part of child maltreatment screening, provide a relaxed environment for obtaining the medical history from children and their caregivers. Interview the caregiver and child separately.[41] The use of open-ended questions with the child is extremely important. "Yes" or "no" questions

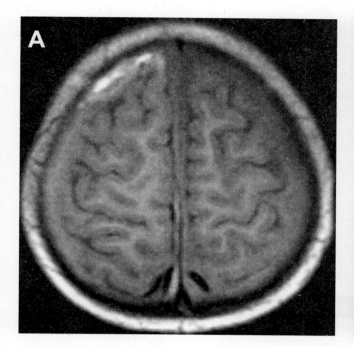

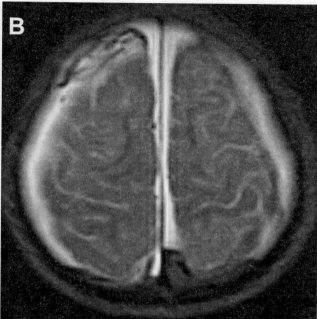

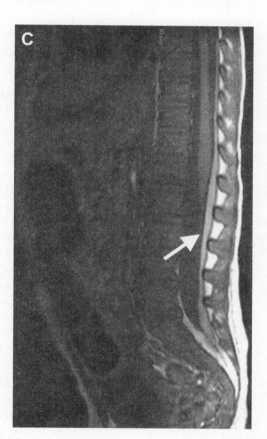

Figure 16-4 A–B. *A 20-month-old female patient who presented with altered mental status and seizures demonstrates bilateral subdural hemorrhage. This patient also had multiple rib fractures and metaphyseal fractures.* **C.** *Magnetic resonance imaging of the spine demonstrates T1 spinal subdural hemorrhage (arrow).*

are easy to ask and answer, but are much less useful in terms of the information they yield. In one study, children who were interviewed using open-ended questions provided significantly more details during the interview as compared with children who were interviewed with direct questions.[2]

Comprehensive and accurate documentation of the history and physical examination is essential, including exact quotes from the history and photographs of injuries using appropriate forensic methods.[41] The extent of diagnostic testing depends on several factors, including the severity of the injury, type of injury, and age and developmental level of the child.[19] Whenever possible, involve clinicians with advanced training in child abuse evaluation and forensic evidence collection.

Conditions Mistaken for Child Maltreatment

Being aware of and sensitive to cultural healing practices and maintaining a nonjudgmental attitude will aid in obtaining an accurate history and examination and in differentiating manifestations of cultural healing practices from signs of physical abuse. These situations also provide an opportunity to educate the family in a nonjudgmental manner in methods that may be more effective. Some traditional healing practices are briefly outlined in **Table 16-5**.[30]

In addition to cultural healing practices, numerous medical conditions may be mistaken for child maltreatment. Some examples are listed in **Table 16-6**.[1,23,38,42]

TABLE 16-5	Cultural Healing Practices Often Mistaken for Child Maltreatment		
Practice	**Origin**	**Signs**	**Description**
Caogio, coining	Vietnam, Laos, Cambodia	Linear erythematous patches, petechiae, or purpura, particularly on the posterior thorax, shoulders, chest, temples, and forehead	Dermabrasion therapy, which involves intense rubbing of the skin.
Guasha, spooning	China	Skin eruptions may be generated that resemble a pine tree pattern, with long vertical marks along the spine and paralleling the ribcage	Water is applied to the back, neck, shoulders, chest, or forehead, after which the area is pinched or massaged until it reddens. It is then scratched with a spoon or spoon-like instrument, made of porcelain, jade, bone, horn, or similar material, until bruises appear.
Hijama, cupping	Middle East, Asia, Latin America, Russia, Eastern Europe	Multiple, grouped circular ecchymoses or petechiae, particularly on the back, neck, shoulders, and extremities	An open-mouthed vessel is heated and then applied to the skin. Suction is produced by the cooling and contracting of the heated air; it is thought to "draw out" the ailment as the heated air and the rim of the cup burn the skin.
Moxibustion	Asia	A pattern of "discrete circular, target-like burns" that may be confused with cigarette burns from child maltreatment	Considered a form of acupuncture. The burning of rolled pieces of moxa herb (mugwort or *Artemisia vulgaris*) directly over the skin above acupuncture points and allowing the herb to burn near the skin's surface. The moxa herb is burned onto the skin with a piece of yarn or incense near the area of pain.

Data from Killion, C. M. (2017). Cultural healing practices that mimic child abuse. *Annals of Forensic Research and Analysis, 4*(2), 1042. https://www.jscimedcentral.com/Forensic/forensic-4-1042.pdf

TABLE 16-6   Medical Conditions Often Mistaken for Child Maltreatment

Condition	Signs	Description
Capillary hemangiomas, vascular malformations	Tangled blood vessels exhibit rapid growth during the first few months of life.	Well demarcated and present in the neonatal period, lesions may present as bruising or ulceration.
Dermal melanocytosis (formerly known as Mongolian spots)	Benign, irregularly shaped, blue-gray or green, nontender macules present in the neonate.	Located primarily over the sacrum and buttocks; also shoulders, arms, wrists, and ankles.
Epidermolysis bullosa (EB)	Blistering lesions that share characteristics of second- and third-degree burns, found in an otherwise healthy child.	Ranging from mild to severe, all forms of EB are marked by skin fragility and formation of bullous lesions secondary to minimal or absent mechanical friction.
Incontinentia pigmenti (IP)	Blistering lesions may be mistaken for burns, and a distinct whorl or streak-like pattern of hyperpigmentation over the trunk and extremities may be mistaken for bruising.	In addition to cutaneous manifestations, IP can be associated with neurologic findings including seizure and cerebral edema, which may raise suspicion for abusive head trauma.
Phytophotodermatitis	A condition caused by the combination of exposure to phototoxic substances and ultraviolet radiation, with a spectrum of clinical appearances from minor dermatitis to full-thickness burn-like wounds.	The severity of some of these lesions can mimic an abusive burn, particularly with an absence of a relevant history. Inducing substances in children include lime and lemon juice, fig leaf sap, and hogweed.
Urticaria pigmentosa (UP)	The development of localized urticaria and erythema following scratching or stroking of the skin lesions.	The lesions of UP are characterized by reddish-brown macules or minimally raised papules found primarily on the limbs and thorax.
Factor deficiencies, platelet disorders, fibrinogen defects	Variable severity of bleeding, ranging from epistaxis to hemarthroses, but cutaneous bruising is common and spontaneous intracranial hemorrhage is rare in all forms.	Heritable hematologic disorders are frequently causes of cutaneous bruising; such bruising can occur on any region of the body, including areas suspicious for abuse.
Ehlers-Danlos syndrome	Poor weight gain, bone fractures or skin lesions that look like bruises or burns, fragile skin that bruises or tears easily, poor and slow healing of wounds, and widened atrophic scars with the formation of cigarette paper–like scars.	A collagen disorder that is characterized by hyperextensibility and fragility of the skin, with easy bruising and hypermobility of the joints.

(continues)

TABLE 16-6	Medical Conditions Often Mistaken for Child Maltreatment (*continued*)	
Condition	**Signs**	**Description**
Osteogenesis imperfecta (OI)	Physical findings suggestive of OI include short stature, blue-gray sclera hue, blue-gray/yellow-brown/translucent teeth, ligamentous laxity, and other signs of connective tissue abnormality.	Children with OI are more susceptible to fractures; they are most likely to sustain midshaft fractures, where the bones are most fragile.
Henoch-Schönlein purpura (HSP)	Symmetrical bruises on the buttocks and extensor surfaces of the arms and legs.	HSP is a fairly common pediatric disease that typically presents in a child with a history of a recent upper respiratory infection.

Data from Alwan, R. M., & Atigapromoj, N. S. (2021). Child maltreatment and neglect. *Emergency Medicine Clinics of North America, 39*(3), 589–603. https://doi.org/10.1016/j.emc.2021.04.009; Giardino, A. P., Giardino, E. R., & Moles, R. L. (2017). Physical child abuse. *Medscape.* Retrieved December 14, 2021, from https://emedicine.medscape.com/article/915664-overview; Patel, B., & Butterfield, R. (2015). Common skin and bleeding disorders that can potentially masquerade as child abuse. *American Journal of Medical Genetics: Part C, Seminars in Medical Genetics, 169*(4), 328–336. https://doi.org/10.1002/ajmg.c.31462; Pereira, E. M. (2015). Clinical perspectives on osteogenesis imperfecta versus non-accidental injury. *American Journal of Medical Genetics: Part C, Seminars in Medical Genetics, 169*(4), 302–306. https://doi.org/10.1002/ajmg.c.31463

Sentinel Injuries

Infants are at greatest risk for fatal abuse but often present to the medical team multiple times before abuse is identified. Sentinel injuries are visible but subtle findings that are poorly explained and increase the suspicion for child maltreatment. Such injuries include bruising, subconjunctival hemorrhage, and frenulum tears. Conducting a thorough physical exam and being aware of injuries highly associated with abuse provide an opportunity to prevent further harm. Sentinel injuries should prompt a further evaluation for abuse, including consideration of a skeletal survey or other imaging.[24]

Nursing Interventions

Nursing interventions for the child with a suspicious presentation involve evidence collection/preservation, documentation, and mandatory reporting to regional authorities.

Evidence

Evidence is any data presented to a court or jury to prove or disprove a claim. It may include physical evidence, words spoken during an interaction, and observations of the child and family in the ED. Physical evidence is tangible and can be measured, visualized, or analyzed. While evidence is important, patient care takes precedence over forensic evidence collection.[11,40]

The safeguarding of evidentiary materials is a component of emergency nursing practice. If it is necessary to cut clothing from the patient, avoid cutting through blood, stains, spatter, or holes. Clothes placed on the floor may be contaminated. Each piece of clothing needs to be placed in a separate clean paper bag to avoid moisture condensation and degradation of evidence.[40]

The Emergency Nurses Association (ENA) has published a position statement entitled *Forensic Evidence Collection in the Emergency Care Setting*. It states:

Collaborating with community partners such as criminal justice system providers, law enforcement, and advocacy agencies will help to create evidence collection and preservation guidelines consistent with jurisdictional needs and patient rights. Physical evidence, including but not limited to, clothing, bullets, physical injuries, etc., should be handled and documented with details to prevent disruption of the chain of custody or contamination of evidence. Subjective evidence—i.e., anything the patient or witness discloses about the injury—requires documentation in fine detail using verbatim words as often as possible. Education and protocols that detail evidence collection procedures, patient rights, healthcare responsibilities, and the legal process are critical for emergency nurses to feel comfortable caring for this patient population. Annual refreshers can aid in increasing skills and comfort levels in facilities where staff do not often use these skills. In cases where forensic evidence collection is warranted, both the legal system and the patient rely upon emergency nursing documentation and evidence preservation in the external court proceedings.[11(p2)]

The ENA position statement also prioritizes nursing assessments and interventions over evidence collection as indicated by the patient's clinical condition.

Documentation

Patients and caregivers alike can mislead the emergency nurse, provide inaccurate history, and omit critical information.[35] Despite these challenges, the nurse should document as much information as possible without interjecting personal, subjective opinions. If there is no answer to an assessment query, document the question and lack of response. If the story changes, document exactly what the patient and/or caregiver tells you each time. Use descriptive details for voice volume, response to touch, eye contact, body positioning, and other physical behaviors and observations to give the reader the most accurate picture of the patient interaction. This may also help the nurse recall events years later if a case goes to court. Document the exact words of the patient and caregivers in quotes, even if slang, violent terms, or vulgar terms are used.[40]

CLINICAL PEARL

How to Document Objectively and Descriptively

Consider the differences in the following statements:

- "The patient refused to answer."
- "The patient did not answer when asked, 'What happened today?' The patient was looking down and did not make eye contact with the parent or this RN. The patient's arms were crossed, and one knee was bouncing up and down with both feet on the floor."

Now compare these statements:

- "The parent yelled at the nurse."
- "While making direct eye contact and standing within 6 inches [15 cm] of Joseph Black, RN, the patient's mother, Jane Doe, stated loudly, 'Get out of here. I better not see you anywhere near my child.'"

Mandated Reporting

In accordance with regional law, many professionals in regular contact with children—such as nurses, physicians, advanced practice providers, and teachers—are mandated reporters for any reasonable suspicion of child abuse or neglect. Every state in the United States and a growing number of countries have mandatory reporting laws for physicians and nurses.[33] Regional child protective services agencies and procedures vary, but this legal requirement protects vulnerable children. Failure to report suspicious presentations places children at risk for continued abuse, immediate physical harm, long-term physical and psychological difficulties, and death.[41,51]

In cases in which a child does not have obvious signs of abuse, emergency nurses may be less inclined to report. The fear of over-reporting and adding to an already overburdened system may be a deterrent. **Box 16-1** cites other reasons that have been given for failing to report suspected abuse. Confidence in the ability to recognize

---

BOX 16-1   Failure to Report Child Abuse

A study of nurses from Taiwan, Australia, and the United States found that one in five had failed to report suspected child abuse in the past. Reasons for not reporting child abuse include the following[13]:

- Concern for insufficient evidence or incorrect clinical judgment
- Insecurities about personal and legal consequences
- Fear of making the patient situation worse
- Colleague disagreement with their assessment
- Lack of knowledge, and poor recognition of abuse and the impact of abuse

In the United States, the courts have been clear that a reasonable suspicion for abuse mandates a report. In other words, reporting does not require a high degree of certainty.[33]

Data from Chan, A. C. Y., Cheng, W. L., Lin, Y. N., Ma, K. W., Mark, C. Y., Yan, L. C., Yim, K. W., Yim, P. Y., & Ho, G. W. K. (2020). Knowledge and perceptions of child protection and mandatory reporting: A survey of nurses in Hong Kong. *Comprehensive Child and Adolescent Nursing, 43*(1), 48–64. https://doi.org/10.1080/24694193 .2018.1561763; Narang, S. K. (2021). Child abuse: Social and medicolegal issues. *UpToDate.* Retrieved March 8, 2022, from https://www.uptodate.com/contents/child -abuse-social-and-medicolegal-issues#H4

child maltreatment may assist healthcare providers to take necessary action and report their suspicions. It is crucial to note that a reasonable suspicion is all that is needed—the threshold for reporting does not require a high degree of certainty.[33]

Safety, Injury Prevention, and Health Promotion

The ED is a common entry point into the healthcare system and, as such, is an ideal setting for implementing primary and secondary prevention efforts for children at risk of maltreatment before a devastating outcome occurs.[29] The emergency nurse might note caregivers demonstrating concerning interactions with their children that do not constitute child maltreatment but indicate a need for caregiver education and support. The emergency nurse can provide resources nonjudgmentally to caregivers who may not otherwise be aware of healthier ways to raise their children.

Summary

Emergency nurses are in a crucial position to identify children at risk for maltreatment and perform a more comprehensive evaluation to determine whether they are in a safe situation. It is well documented that healthcare providers who have had education related to child maltreatment are more likely to recognize and report their findings.[29] Healthcare providers at every point in the care process must effectively identify and intervene on behalf of children, all of whom deserve a life free from abuse.[26]

References

1. Alwan, R. M., & Atigapromoj, N. S. (2021). Child maltreatment and neglect. *Emergency Medicine Clinics of North America, 39*(3), 589–603. https://doi.org/10.1016/j.emc.2021.04.009

2. Anderson, G. D., Anderson, J. N., & Gilgun, J. F. (2014). The influence of narrative practice techniques on child behaviors in forensic interviews. *Journal of Child Sexual Abuse, 23*(6), 615–634. https://doi.org/10.1016/s0140-6736(13)62183-2

3. Australian Bureau of Statistics. (2019). *Characteristics and outcomes of childhood abuse.* https://www.abs.gov.au/articles/characteristics-and-outcomes-childhood-abuse#how-many-australian-adults-have-experienced-childhood-abuse-

4. Bechtel, K., & Bennett, B. L. (2020). Management and sequelae of sexual abuse in children and adolescents. *UpToDate.* Retrieved March 6, 2022, from https://www.uptodate.com/contents/management-and-sequelae-of-sexual-abuse-in-children-and-adolescents

5. Bechtel, K., & Bennett, B. L. (2021). Evaluation of sexual abuse in children and adolescents. *UpToDate.* Retrieved March 5, 2022, from https://www.uptodate.com/contents/evaluation-of-sexual-abuse-in-children-and-adolescents

6. Blue Campaign. (n.d.). *Indicators of human trafficking.* U.S. Department of Homeland Security. https://www.dhs.gov/blue-campaign/indicators-human-trafficking

7. Blue Campaign. (n.d.). *What is human trafficking?* U.S. Department of Homeland Security. https://www.dhs.gov/blue-campaign/what-human-trafficking#

8. Boos, S. C. (2021). Physical child abuse: Diagnostic evaluation and management. *UpToDate.* Retrieved March 7, 2022, from https://www.uptodate.com/contents/physical-child-abuse-diagnostic-evaluation-and-management

9. Boos, S. C. (2022). Physical child abuse: Recognition. *UpToDate.* Retrieved March 7, 2022, from https://www.uptodate.com/contents/physical-child-abuse-recognition

10. Bush, K. (2016). *Care of prepubescent pediatric sexual abuse patients in the emergency care setting* [Joint position statement]. Emergency Nurses Association & International Association of Forensic Nurses. https://enau.ena.org/Users/LearningActivityAssetSingleViewer.aspx?LearningActivityAssetID=a5%2byNkQjxs5Cnf8%2bc3SCIA%3d%3d

11. Bush, K. (2018). *Forensic evidence collection in the emergency care setting* [Position statement]. Emergency Nurses Association. https://enau.ena.org/Users/LearningActivityAssetSingleViewer.aspx?LearningActivityAssetID=3AtkzqLQuToJkZc%2fOBDZrQ%3d%3d

12. Centers for Disease Control and Prevention. (2021). *Violence prevention: Risk and protective factors.* https://www.cdc.gov/violenceprevention/childabuseandneglect/riskprotectivefactors.html

13. Chan, A. C. Y., Cheng, W. L., Lin, Y. N., Ma, K. W., Mark, C. Y., Yan, L. C., Yim, K. W., Yim, P. Y., & Ho, G. W. K. (2020). Knowledge and perceptions of child protection and mandatory reporting: A survey of nurses in Hong Kong. *Comprehensive Child and Adolescent Nursing, 43*(1), 48–64. https://doi.org/10.1080/24694193.2018.1561763

14. Child Abuse Prevention and Treatment Act (CAPTA), 42 U.S.C.A. § 5106g. (2022). Chapter 67: Child Abuse Prevention and Treatment Adoption Reform. https://uscode.house.gov/view.xhtml?path=/prelim@title42/chapter67&edition=prelim

15. Child Welfare Information Gateway. (n.d.). *Identification of neglect.* https://www.childwelfare.gov/topics/can/identifying/neglect/

16. Child Welfare Information Gateway. (2018, July). *Acts of omission: An overview of child neglect.* https://www.childwelfare.gov/pubPDFs/acts.pdf

17. Child Welfare Information Gateway. (2021, March). *Child abuse and neglect fatalities 2019: Statistics and interventions.* U.S. Department of Health and Human Services, Children's Bureau. https://www.childwelfare.gov/pubpdfs/fatality.pdf

18. Christian, C. (2021). Child abuse: Evaluation and diagnosis of abusive head trauma in infants and children. *UpToDate.* Retrieved March 7, 2022, from https://www.uptodate.com/contents/child-abuse-evaluation-and-diagnosis-of-abusive-head-trauma-in-infants-and-children

19. Christian, C. W. (2015). The evaluation of suspected child physical abuse. *Pediatrics, 135*(5), e1337–e1354. https://doi.org/10.1542/peds.2015-0356

20. Escobar, M. J., Pflugeisen, B. M., Duralde, Y., Morris, C. J., Haferbecker, D., Amoroso, P. J., & Pohlson, E. C. (2016). Development of a systematic protocol to identify victims of non-accidental trauma. *Pediatric Surgery International, 32*(4), 377–386. https://doi.org/10.1007/s00383-016-3863-8

21. Fehler-Cabral, G., & Campbell, R. (2013). Adolescent sexual assault disclosure: The impact of peers, families, and schools. *American Journal of Community Psychology, 52*(1–2), 73–83. https://doi.org/10.1007/s10464-013-9577-3

22. Felitti, V., Anda, R., Nordenberg, D., Edwards, V., Koss, M., & Marks, J. (1998). Relationship of childhood abuse and household dysfunction to many of the leading causes of death in adults. *American Journal of Preventative Medicine, 14*(4), 245–258.

23. Giardino, A. P., & Giardino, E. R., & Moles, R. L. (2017). Physical child abuse. *Medscape.* Retrieved December 14, 2021, from https://emedicine.medscape.com/article/915664-overview

24. Henry, K., & Wood, J. (2021). What is in a name? Sentinel injuries in abused infants. *Pediatric Radiology, 51*(6), 861–865. https://doi.org/10.1007/s00247-020-04915-7

25. Hernandez, B. S. (n.d.). *Child abuse (non-accidental trauma).* Clerkship Directors in Emergency Medicine. https://www.saem.org/about-saem/academies-interest-groups-affiliates2/cdem/for-students/online-education/peds-em-curriculum/gu-ob/child-abuse-(non-accidental-trauma)

26. Hoft, M., & Haddad, L. (2017). Screening children for abuse and neglect: A review of the literature. *Journal of Forensic Nursing, 13*(1), 26–34. https://doi.org/10.1097/JFN.0000000000000136

27. Hornor, G. (2021). Medical child abuse: Essentials for pediatric health care providers. *Journal of Pediatric Health Care, 35*(6), 644–650. https://doi.org/10.1016/j.pedhc.2021.01.006

28. Jones, C. M., Merrick, M. T., & Houry, D. E. (2020). Identifying and preventing adverse childhood experiences: Implications for clinical practice. *Journal of the American Medical Association, 323*(1), 25–26. https://doi.org/10.1001/jama.2019.18499

29. Jordan, K. S., & Steelman, S. H. (2015). Child maltreatment: Interventions to improve recognition and reporting. *Journal of Forensic Nursing, 11*(2), 107–113. https://doi.org/10.1097/jfn.0000000000000068

30. Killion, C. M. (2017). Cultural healing practices that mimic child abuse. *Annals of Forensic Research and Analysis, 4*(2), Article 1042. https://www.jscimedcentral.com/Forensic/forensic-4-1042.pdf

31. Mathews, B., Pacella, R., Dunne, M., Scott, J., Finkelhor, D., Meinck, F., Higgins, D. J., Erskine, H., Thomas, H. J., Haslam, D., Tran, N., Le, H., Honey, N., Kellard, K., & Lawrence, D. (2021). The Australian Child Maltreatment Study: Protocol for a national survey of the prevalence of child abuse and neglect, associated mental disorders and physical health problems and burden of disease. *BMJ Open, 11*, Article e047074. https://doi.org/10.1136/bmjopen-2020-047074

32. Molnar, J., O'Connell, M. S., Mollen, C., & Scribano, P. (2021). Sexual assault: Child and adolescent. In K. N. Shay & R. G. Bachur (Eds.), *Fleisher & Ludwig's textbook of pediatric emergency medicine* (8th ed., pp. 1448–1459). Wolters Kluwer.

33. Narang, S. K. (2021). Child abuse: Social and medicolegal issues. *UpToDate.* Retrieved March 8, 2022, from https://www.uptodate.com/contents/child-abuse-social-and-medicolegal-issues#H4

34. Nigro, L. C., Felfman, M. J., Foster, R. L., & Pozez, Al. L. (2018). A model to improve detection of nonaccidental pediatric burns. *American Medical Association Journal of Ethics, 20*(6), 552–559. https://doi.org/10.1001/journalofethics.2018.20.6.org1-1806

35. Normandin, P. A. (2016). Hidden child abuse identification in the emergency department. *Journal of Emergency Nursing, 42*(2), 181–182. https://doi.org/10.1016/j.jen.2016.02.006

36. Nowak, C. B. (2015). Recognition and prevention of child abuse in the child with disability. *American Journal of Medical Genetics: Part C, Seminars in Medical Genetics, 169*(4), 293–301. https://doi.org/10.1002/ajmg.c.31458

37. Office for National Statistics. (2020). *Child abuse in England and Wales: March 2020* [Statistical bulletin]. https://www.ons.gov.uk/peoplepopulationandcommunity/crimeandjustice/bulletins/childabuseinenglandandwales/march2020

38. Patel, B., & Butterfield, R. (2015). Common skin and bleeding disorders that can potentially masquerade as child abuse. *American Journal of Medical Genetics: Part C, Seminars in Medical Genetics, 169*, 328–336. https://doi.org/10.1002/ajmg.c.31462

39. Pawlik, M. C., Kemp, A., Maguire, S., Nuttall, D., Feldman, K., & Lindberg, D. (2016). Children with burns referred for child abuse evaluation: Burn characteristics and co-existent injuries. *Child Abuse & Neglect, 55*, 52–61. https://doi.org/10.1016/j.chiabu.2016.03.006

40. Pedrotty, C. M. (2020). Forensic nursing in the emergency department. In V. Sweet & A. Foley (Eds.), *Sheehy's emergency nursing: Principles and practice* (7th ed., pp. 594–606). Elsevier.

41. Pekarsky, A. R. (2016). Overview of child maltreatment. *Merck Manual Professional Edition.* Retrieved December 14, 2021, from http://www.merckmanuals.com/professional/pediatrics/child-maltreatment/overview-of-child-maltreatment

42. Pereira, E. M. (2015). Clinical perspectives on osteogenesis imperfecta versus non-accidental injury. *American Journal of Medical Genetics: Part C, Seminars in Medical Genetics, 169*(4), 302–306. https://doi.org/10.1002/ajmg.c.31463

43. Perkins, A. (2018). The red flags of child abuse. *Nursing Made Incredibly Easy, 16*(2), 34–41. https://doi.org/10.1097/01.NME.0000529946.76463.6b

44. Pierce, M. C., Kaczor, S., O'Flynn, J., & Lorenz, D. J. (2021). Validation of a clinical decision rule to predict abuse in young children based on bruising characteristics. *Journal of the American Medical Association Network Open, 4*(4), e215832. https://doi.org/10.1001/jamanetworkopen.2021.5832

45. Roesler, T. A., & Jenny, C. (2020). Medical child abuse (Munchausen syndrome by proxy). *UpToDate.* Retrieved March 6, 2022, from https://www.uptodate.com/contents/medical-child-abuse-munchausen-syndrome-by-proxy

46. Scherl, S. A. (2020). Orthopedic aspects of child abuse. *UpToDate.* Retrieved March 7, 2022, from https://www.uptodate.com/contents/orthopedic-aspects-of-child-abuse

47. Slingsby, B. (2022). Child abuse and neglect. In F. F. Ferri (Ed.), *Ferri's clinical advisor 2022* (pp. 362.e2–362.e7). Elsevier.

48. Tun, K., Choudhary, A. K., Methratta, S., & Boal, D. K. (2013). Featured article: Radiological features of nonaccidental injury. *Journal of Radiology Nursing*, 323–329. https://doi.org/10.1016/j.jradnu.2012.08.005

49. U.S. Department of Health and Human Services, Administration for Children and Families, Administration on Children, Youth and Families, Children's Bureau. (2021). *Child maltreatment 2019.* https://www.acf.hhs.gov/sites/default/files/documents/cb/cm2019.pdf

50. Wilkins, G. G., Ball, J., Mann, N. C., Nadkarni, M., & Meredith, J. W. (2016). Increased screening for child physical abuse in emergency departments in a regional trauma system: Response to a sentinel event. *Journal of Trauma Nursing, 23*(2), 77–82. https://doi.org/10.1097/jtn.0000000000000190

51. Wood, J. N., Connelly, J., Callahan, J. M., & Christian, C. W. (2021). Child abuse/assault. In K. N. Shay & R. G. Bachur (Eds.), *Fleisher & Ludwig's textbook of pediatric emergency medicine* (8th ed., pp. 620–633). Wolters Kluwer.

52. World Health Organization. (2020, June 8). *Child maltreatment* [Fact sheet]. https://www.who.int/news-room/fact-sheets/detail/child-maltreatment

The Child, Family, and Healthcare Team in Crisis

Roberta L. Miller, DNP, RN, CPN, CPEN, TCRN

OBJECTIVES

Upon completion of this chapter, the learner will be able to:

1. Identify factors that affect the human response to crisis and trauma.
2. Assess pediatric patients, families, and healthcare team members for behavioral or physical indications of crisis and distress.
3. Describe therapeutic interventions for patients, families, and healthcare team members experiencing crisis and trauma.

Introduction

The emergency department (ED) is a high-stress area with a fast pace and often critically ill patients. Pediatric injuries and illnesses treated in the ED are challenging for patients, families, and healthcare teams alike. Critical illness and injury are particularly stressful and require recognizing distress and intervening appropriately.[25] Although the ED is prepared to function during a crisis, traumatic events involving pediatric patients can increase distress for all involved. The unexpected nature of the event, previous experiences, and risk of loss of life significantly affect reactions to the event.[25] Exposure to the suffering or death of a child is distressing to healthcare professionals, who may experience burnout or post-traumatic distress syndrome (PTSD).[33] It is essential to use developmentally appropriate approaches when treating pediatric patients in a crisis, to allow family involvement, and to provide updates.[25] Recognizing and

responding to signs of healthcare team distress is equally, if not more, essential.

Adverse Childhood Experiences

Adverse childhood experiences (ACEs) are stressful and traumatic events occurring in childhood that have a significant long-term impact on health and well-being. ACEs include various aspects of family dysfunction, such as sexual abuse, physical or emotional abuse, neglect, or witnessing violence.[31,38] They are associated with life-long psychological and stress-related health problems, including heart disease, stroke, chronic lung disease, or diabetes later in life.[38] Exposure to ACEs can lead to immune system, brain function, and genetic changes. Experiencing ACEs within the first 5 years of life can lead to exaggerated stress responses and changes in brain development.[31] These changes in brain development can then negatively affect educational attainment, physical and mental health, and life opportunities.[30] Such changes are even associated with a greater propensity to commit crimes. Children who have experienced adverse events, such as abuse or violence, may not feel safe even in a safe environment and will require reassurance and patience.[28] They may exhibit high levels of anxiety and heightened emotional responses to life events.[28]

While caring for patients who have experienced an ACE, it is important to provide the patient with as much control as possible, acknowledge grief and loss, and provide reassurance to help build a trusting relationship. These therapeutic interventions can lessen the negative outcomes associated with ACEs.[28] Nurses can also effect change by increasing awareness of the lasting impact of ACEs on health, with a focus on health promotion through ACE prevention.

Medical Illness or Injury

The circumstances that bring a child to an ED and the frightening and painful experiences involved with medical care can become an ACE. Visits to the ED are frequently unexpected, which causes increased stress levels for patients and families. The pediatric patient and family are likely to have increased anxiety during a traumatic event. Subsequently, children and adolescents may experience increased anxiety in the ED due to the loud and confusing environment. Fear of medical procedures and the unknown can make physical assessment difficult.[24] Previous experiences with healthcare can increase anxiety in the child and adolescent. For example, previous negative experiences, such as uncontrolled pain or a traumatic event involving a loved one, can increase anxiety and compromise coping mechanisms.[24] Avoid unnecessary invasive procedures to help decrease anxiety, such as repeated blood draws in addition to initiation of intravenous access.

The presence of pain in the pediatric patient increases anxiety for the patient as well as for caregivers, due to the child's visible distress.[3] Pediatric patients will benefit from having a caregiver at the bedside. Family presence at the bedside decreases the pain and anxiety felt by pediatric patients during treatment.[34] Anxiety is known to increase pain in the pediatric patient, so early and adequate pain control is vital to enabling the nurse to carry out a complete physical examination and implement needed interventions without causing undue trauma.[3] After identifying and managing life-threatening conditions, the primary assessment prioritizes pain assessment and management. Using developmentally appropriate means to diminish pain and anxiety can minimize the possibility of the ED experience becoming an ACE. See Chapter 3,

"Pediatric Differences," for more information on pediatric pain. Pain management and other therapeutic approaches fall under the umbrella of trauma-informed care.

Trauma-Informed Care

Children in crisis react differently than adults in similar situations. Children have difficulty expressing emotions and describing feelings. They are often more traumatized by a crisis due to their inadequate coping skills and an inability to describe fears or concerns.[37] Adults may show signs of depression and preoccupation with the event. In contrast, children may experience nightmares, startle easily, have difficulty sleeping, and have angry outbursts.[37] Children may also manifest physical complaints, such as pain, in response to their psychological distress.[37] For example, children and adolescents may complain of headaches, abdominal pain, constipation, and other vague somatic symptoms.

Experiencing or witnessing a traumatic event impacts perceptions of life and may have a negative impact on the future well-being of the pediatric patient and family. Whether the trauma is related to a single traumatic event, a disaster, or ongoing abuse, it influences the child's emotions and behaviors.[7] Implementing trauma-informed care in the ED improves outcomes and cognitive development of children experiencing complex trauma.[2] Trauma-informed care is an approach to understanding the psychological, neurologic, and social effects that trauma has on patients.[7]

Retraumatization occurs when someone relives a trauma either consciously or subconsciously. Situations, interactions, or activities can cause intense reactions, such as anger, fear, or defensive behaviors, from the person experiencing this phenomenon.[2] Maintain a supportive approach to patients who have experienced a traumatic event.

Trauma-informed care also recognizes compassion fatigue or secondary trauma as a serious concern. Secondary trauma results from perceived or actual loss or caring for someone who has lived through a traumatic event.[32]

Trauma-Informed Care Approach

Several trauma-informed care strategies exist for fostering a caring and inclusive environment and avoiding acute distress or retraumatization of pediatric patients. During the critical event, providing emotional support, maintaining a calm environment, and using family-centered care will improve long-term psychological outcomes.[2] The trauma-informed care approach integrates knowledge about trauma into all aspects of care and avoids retraumatization.[7]

Trauma-informed care allows staff to create a safe environment for patients. It changes the focus of care from "What is wrong with you?" to "What happened to you?"[42] Patients with complex health and social needs often have been exposed to traumatic events in their lives. Children or adolescents may become fearful or agitated in stressful situations or in situations that remind them of previous traumatic events.[42] Healthcare professionals who understand how life experiences impact behavior can implement more effective and therapeutic interventions in such cases.

Looking at behaviors from a different perspective often improves patient care. When a child or adolescent exhibits attention-seeking behaviors, such as throwing tantrums or fabricating illnesses, it may be because they do not receive attention at home.[26] The child or adolescent needs communication about what to expect, updates if they will be left alone, and regular check-ins during the visit.[26] When patients exhibit disruptive behaviors, the team should work to understand the behavior instead of trying to control the behavior using the trauma-informed care approach.[42] Key components of such care include the following[41]:

- Ensure safety, both physically and emotionally, by establishing trust and boundaries.
- Allow the individual to make choices.
- Use the least restrictive options for care.
- Ensure basic needs are met, such as hydration, nutrition, and toileting.

The acuity of the illness or injury and the high-stress environment increase the challenges of emergency care for patients, families, and healthcare teams. Implementing family-centered care enables caregivers to be involved in the child's care, which is comforting to the patient and helps the family rebuild their sense of control.[30] Incorporate the following points into the care of pediatric patients in crisis[13,30]:

- Patients and caregivers in crisis may have low attentiveness and altered memory. Provide frequent updates or have a staff member stay with the family for support.
- Allow a family member to remain at the bedside when it does not interfere with care.
- An unconscious and critically injured pediatric patient may benefit from a caregiver at the bedside.
- A calm caregiver's presence greatly helps a pediatric patient who is fearful or in pain.
- Allow choices when appropriate.
- Keep the environment as calm as possible to avoid increased anxiety.
  - Place the patient in a private room when possible.

- Consider creating a pediatric area featuring colorful walls, furniture, and pictures.
  - Use games, toys, and other age-appropriate distractors when possible.
- Consistently reassess pain and provide comfort measures.

Involve a child life specialist, if available, to help calm and prepare pediatric patients before and during procedures. Child life specialists provide support using developmentally appropriate techniques that aim to decrease children's anxiety and improve their cooperation.[35] The intervention techniques they use can help pediatric patients cope with traumatic experiences, but are not available at all facilities.[35] If a child life specialist is not available in your facility, nurses can assist by incorporating calming techniques into the care plan. Commonly used methods include the following[20]:

- Distraction: Singing songs, blowing bubbles, looking at pictures, searching pictures for specific items, videos, asking questions about favorite activities.
- Deep breathing: Younger children can blow bubbles, inhaling in for a count of two and exhaling for a count of four.
- Guided imagery: "You told me your favorite place is the beach. What do the waves sound like? What do the birds do when the water leaves the sand? What does the sand feel like on your toes? Is it warm? Rough? Soft?"

De-escalation

Caregivers may display a variety of reactions to the event. Some family members may experience intense feelings and anxiety related to the actual or thought of the loss of a child. Their response to the crisis will depend on the severity of the child's illness or injury, whether they witnessed the traumatic event, their own mental health and coping skills, and the chaos level in the emergency environment.[15] In addition, external factors can impact how the person reacts to the situation. Factors unrelated to the event that can affect the family's response include stress at work, major illness or injury of a loved one, divorce, moving, and stress in the home.

During a critical event, caregivers of pediatric patients are placed in an unfamiliar, stressful environment and may feel pressured to make decisions about the child's care.[15] Under such conditions, an event that may seem minor to the healthcare team might be perceived as a crisis based on an individual's history, experiences, and coping mechanisms. Some individuals have aggressive stress responses. Every effort should be made to prevent escalation of a situation to aggressive behavior by involving the family in care and providing frequent updates.[15]

Appropriate Interventions

The emergency nurse must remain aware of escalating behaviors. Signs of escalation include refusal to answer questions, impatience, and blaming others.[19] De-escalation techniques include maintaining a nonjudgmental attitude, allowing personal space to decrease anxiety, using nonthreatening nonverbal communication, and remaining calm.[6] Signs of escalation include changes in posture, threatening statements, pointing fingers, and shouting.[19] When a person is angry or becomes confrontational, do not argue with them. Instead, listen, acknowledge, and address feelings.[6] Some people have difficulty processing and communicating what is happening, so use supportive words and body language. Set limits by letting them know which behaviors are unacceptable.[6] Nurses can also attempt to take a more objective view and acknowledge whether their behaviors are contributing to the escalation, removing themselves from the situation if appropriate. If de-escalation techniques are unsuccessful and behaviors put patients, staff, or others in danger, notify security personnel or take other appropriate action as determined by the facility. See Chapter 15, "The Child with a Behavioral Health Concern," for more information about de-escalation with pediatric patients who have behavioral health emergencies.

Homelessness

The number of children aged 5 to 18 years who are homeless in the United States is estimated at more than 100,000.[18] Lack of stable housing and safety negatively impacts children's health.[18] Children who are homeless have higher morbidity and mortality rates and are at higher risk for developmental, emotional, and behavioral problems.[18] The transient nature of homelessness is a barrier to obtaining preventive care and maintenance care for chronic conditions.[16] Adolescents who are homeless are at increased risk for drug misuse and abuse, sexually transmitted infections, pregnancy, and involvement in sex trafficking.[18] Recent eviction and homelessness contribute to high anxiety levels, depression, and heat- or cold-related injuries.[16] Children and adolescents experiencing homelessness may present to the ED for severe illness, malnutrition, or as victims of violence.[18]

Appropriate Interventions

Homelessness in children and adolescents is associated with adverse health outcomes. Nurses must build trust with patients and families experiencing homelessness

and provide care without judgment.[22] They may be reluctant to disclose their living situation for fear of such judgment from providers.[18] Many patients who are homeless return to the ED multiple times for the same complaint due to the inability to fill prescriptions, complete follow-up visits, or obtain food and supplies when needed.[22]

Assessment of these patients should include open-ended questions, a multidisciplinary approach, and a non-blaming attitude.[16] Families who are homeless are more likely to experience heightened anxiety and stress levels, and they require emotional support and referrals and resources for obtaining food, shelter, and health care.[36] Many communities have shelters, low-income housing, and other resources available.[36] Involving social workers or case managers in these patients' care can help children and adolescents experiencing homelessness find valuable resources for improving their physical and mental health.[36]

Death of a Pediatric Patient

The death of a child in the ED is one of the most challenging events possible for both the family and the healthcare team. The death of a pediatric patient is typically sudden and unexpected. The Emergency Nurses Association (ENA) supports family presence during the resuscitation efforts and recommends providing a support person who can provide updates on the patient's treatment and condition.[13] When explaining to caregivers that their child is dying or has died, speak in simple, straightforward sentences and avoid euphemisms. It is typically the physician's responsibility to inform the caregivers of the child's death. However, as a nurse, it is crucial to be prepared to speak to the family in such a case.

Regardless of who informs the family, healthcare personnel should provide a dedicated support person to accompany the caregivers and family members.[23] Caregivers may experience guilt or concerns over ways the death could have been prevented, even when they had no control over the event.[23] The healthcare team should remain supportive and nonjudgmental. Provide information, being conscious of the family's potentially limited ability to process and comprehend that information. Ask the family what they understand so clarification can be provided as needed. Know that there is nothing the nurse can do or say to "fix" the situation, but that nursing presence and support, even without words, facilitates the family's grieving process.

Bereavement Strategies

Although nurses must be aware of and comply with local laws or regulations regarding autopsy and forensic evidence requirements, allow the family to be present at the bedside of the deceased child if at all possible. Consider caregiver cultural differences in the grieving process and provide ample time for immediate grieving practices.[29] Some families may wish to participate in memory-making activities such as collecting locks of hair and making hand molds, but be aware that some caregivers may choose not to participate in these activities. Allow siblings and other family members to join in memory-making activities if they are willing.

Caregivers may request help in relaying news of the death to other family members, especially siblings of the deceased child. The loss of a sibling has a significant impact, producing a variety of emotions, such as anger, fear, or guilt.[29] Offer the caregiver and other family members the option to schedule follow-up appointments with bereavement teams, family physicians, or pediatricians before leaving the hospital. Involve social services if appropriate to help arrange follow-up or support services. Many families find comfort in small gestures, including cards or a phone call after the child's death.[29]

Legal Responsibilities

Be aware of the local laws related to patient death. Required notifications may include the medical examiner, coroner, children's services, and law enforcement.[29] Required reporting is done before memory-making activities and allowing the family to hold the deceased patient.[29] Memory-making activities are initiated only if the authorities grant permission. If law enforcement is involved, follow all requests to obtain and maintain evidence using proper chain-of-custody procedures. Notify the local organ procurement organization, if appropriate.

The Pause

The Pause is a period of silence observed by the team at the time of a patient's death. This practice, which was created by healthcare professionals, involves taking 30 seconds to a minute after a patient's death to honor the life and the team who worked to save them.[8] In essence, it highlights the human aspect of healthcare. The Pause helps provide closure for families and the healthcare team. The patient's life is honored, and the Pause gives everyone time to recognize the loss of life. It provides an opportunity for the team to process the event, decompress afterward, and be more present for the next patient. The practice helps to foster staff well-being.

Health Promotion for Healthcare Providers

Traumatic events, including injuries from natural disasters, traumatic injuries, and critical illnesses, are common in the ED; however, a critical event involving a child can significantly impact the healthcare team. Unsuccessful pediatric resuscitation can take an emotional and physical toll on ED staff.[4] It is normal to express emotions and react with compassion when witnessing the incident and the grieving family. However, repeated exposure to traumatic events without acknowledgment or treatment of the stresses created by such events can negatively impact job performance, job satisfaction, mental and physical health, and patient outcomes.[14,21]

Supporting the grieving family and witnessing their emotional reactions can be emotionally draining for the healthcare team.[20] Dealing with child maltreatment is also beyond the normal daily human work experience. The healthcare team can develop compassion fatigue, burnout, or secondary traumatic stress related to repeated exposure to critical illness, injuries, and loss.[13] If not recognized and treated, such stress disorders can lead to long-term physical and mental distress and decreased empathy.[14] **Table 17-1** summarizes the various types of stress disorders.

Recognizing signs of distress in self and others is essential for initiating treatment. Signs of a stress reaction include the following[14]:

- Headaches, stomach aches
- Short attention span
- Fatigue
- Forgetfulness
- Negative self-esteem
- Depression
- Anxiety

RED FLAG

Suicide risk has been shown to be higher for physicians globally[12] and for nurses in the United States.[9] While more research is needed for all healthcare disciplines, the need for action is obvious. The Dr. Lorna Breen Healthcare Provider Protection Act was passed in 2021 to promote behavioral health support, provide suicide and burnout prevention education, and increase awareness.[11]

If you or someone you know is in immediate danger, call your local emergency number.

Findahelpline.com enables you to search, by country, for free, confidential support via phone, text, or webchat. Many countries have national suicide hotlines.

The United States introduced 988 as a three-digit phone number that routes callers directly to the National Suicide Prevention Lifeline (1-800-273-TALK [8255]).

- Social withdrawal
- Inappropriate anger and irritability
- Increased alcohol intake
- Strain in relationships

- Difficulty separating personal and professional life
- Impaired clinical decisions
- Negativity toward work and patients
- Absenteeism

TABLE 17-1	Types of Stress Disorders		
Disorder	**Causes**	**Signs and Symptoms**	**Interventions**
Compassion fatigue	› Repeated exposure to traumatic events › Repeated exposure to ill and injured patients › Providing emotional support to grieving families › Perfectionist › Confusion over emotional boundaries › Frustration with not being able to help others	› Loss of interest in previously pleasurable activities › Reduced productivity › Lack of empathy › Oversensitivity › Avoidance of socialization › Depression › Poor concentration › Restlessness › Mood swings	› Define boundaries for expectations of self › Counseling › Support groups › Debriefing sessions › Education regarding compassion fatigue
Burnout	› Feelings of professional inadequacy › High patient acuity › Increased patient volumes › Inadequate staffing › Frequent or multiple changes in the work environment › Increased workload	› Develops gradually › Irritability › Frustration › Anger › Depression › Decreased sense of accomplishment	› Prioritize sleep › Support from leadership › Education related to the recognition of burnout signs and symptoms › Set boundaries between work and personal life › Practice self-care
Secondary traumatic stress/vicarious traumatization	› Stress-type response caused by repetitive exposure to traumatized or suffering individuals	› Physical symptoms of stress › Depression › Anger or guilt › Fear › Difficulty sleeping or nightmares › Decreased concentration › Anxiety › Impaired immunity (frequent illness)	› Relaxation techniques and self-care › Counseling › Encourage peer-to-peer support › Education related to risk factors and symptoms › Provide a safe environment in which to disclose feelings › Support from leadership for debriefing

Data from Emergency Nurses Association. (2020). *Compassion fatigue* [Topic brief]. https://enau.ena.org/Users/Learning ActivityAssetSingleViewer.aspx?LearningActivityAssetID=3khnIoBEUvDvZf%2bdH%2bkTNQ%3d%3d; Jackson, B. L. (2017). Bereavement in the pediatric emergency department: Caring for those who care for others. *Pediatric Nursing, 43*(3), 113–119; and Morrison, L. E., & Joy, J. P. (2016). Secondary traumatic stress in the emergency department. *Journal of Advanced Nursing, 72*(11), 2894–2906. https://doi.org/10.1111/jan.13030

Secondary Traumatic Stress

Secondary traumatic stress (STS) can occur when nurses repeatedly care for traumatized patients. The terms *secondary trauma* and *vicarious traumatization* are often used interchangeably. STS refers to the stress created by caring for traumatized patients, as the provider internalizes the events and experiences compassion fatigue.[14] STS results from helping or wanting to help a traumatized patient and can be heightened by poor or unknown outcomes.[27] Notably, the stressful environment that accompanies exposure to death and violence in the ED puts the healthcare team at risk for STS.[27] This risk increases with the unexpectedness of pediatric traumatic events. The fast-paced ED often requires the team to continue taking care of patients without time to stop and discuss a traumatic event, which can itself lead to increased stress.[27]

ED leaders can help healthcare personnel in this setting by fostering a supportive environment, including allowing staff to take a few minutes for informal debriefing immediately after an event.[27] Colleagues can incorporate a quick check-in, asking if others need some time to compose themselves before continuing work and planning to touch base after work. Publicly acknowledging that it is normal to struggle after vicarious traumatization encourages conversations and shared coping mechanisms. Neglecting to talk about these normal reactions to extraordinary experiences perpetuates a culture of secrecy and shame that prevents healthcare providers from seeking help.

Healthcare professionals can be alert for signs of STS in themselves and their coworkers. Staff who experience STS are more likely to engage in harmful behaviors, including illegal drug use, alcohol abuse, short-temperedness, high anxiety, and sleep disorders.[27] Support from peers can help staff to recognize distress in their teammates and themselves and to implement self-care measures.

NOTE

Asking for Help Is Not a Sign of Weakness

The critical need for healthcare provider support has been spotlighted by the COVID-19 pandemic, but it is not a new phenomenon. Innovative peer-to-peer and other support mechanisms beyond traditional employee assistance programs and critical incident stress management methods are becoming more readily available. Most important is the widespread message that healthcare providers are not expected to manage stress alone.

Appropriate Interventions for Managing Stress in Healthcare Providers

Healthcare professionals need to recognize and manage stress if they are to provide safe, quality, empathetic care to all patients.[14] Recognizing the signs of elevated stress, compassion fatigue, and STS is the first step in improving health and well-being.[14] Providing educational support and methods for stress management can mitigate the long-term physical and emotional effects of working in the high-pressure environment of the ED.[21] Strategies to manage stress include the following[4,14,21,27]:

- Engage in physical activities, such as sports and exercise.
- Practice other self-care techniques, such as meditation and other relaxation techniques.
- Take part in holistic and wellness activities, such as massage, sensory deprivation tanks, and laughter.
- Conduct an informal debriefing or diffusion immediately after the event to discuss thoughts and emotions right away.
- Obtain support from the organization for debriefings or other resources for healthcare professionals involved in the care of the patient.
- Provide additional support for those persons at higher risk of compassion fatigue and STS, such as a place where staff can step away from the chaos of the ED and debrief.
- Educate and train staff related to bereavement support, self-care, and recognizing compassion fatigue and STS signs. Provide resources for first responder or ED counselors.
- Encourage teamwork, empathy, praise, and recognition for staff successes.
- Encourage peer-to-peer relationships to provide additional perspectives, support, and valuable insights that may help prevent compassion fatigue and STS.
- When signs of compassion fatigue or STS are recognized in oneself or others, seek or encourage professional guidance from someone trained in caring for healthcare providers.

While widely used, the practice of critical incident stress debriefing is not without controversy. The American Red Cross[1] and the World Health Organization[44] conducted scientific reviews to evaluate psychological debriefings after trauma. Both concluded that evidence of efficacy was lacking and there was evidence of potential harm. Luckily, the COVID-19 pandemic has inspired innovative approaches to this problem and more research on effective stress management and nursing resiliency.

Eye movement desensitization and reprocessing (EMDR) therapy has been used to help resolve unprocessed traumatic memories and is considered a first-line treatment for military veterans with PTSD.[43] EMDR has been shown to be more effective than critical incident stress debriefing in one study of workplace violence victims, and it may be effectively delivered via telemedicine for healthcare workers caring for COVID-19 patients.[39,40] Nurses today have many options available to manage their stress, and they are encouraged to find what works for them to ensure they can continue to provide effective care to others.

> **NOTE**
>
> ### Resilience
>
> Nursing resiliency was mentioned in the literature prior to the COVID-19 pandemic but gained quite a bit of traction as staffing reached crisis levels during this healthcare challenge. Nurses can incorporate simple resilience exercises throughout their day, no matter what the setting.
>
> Examples of quick resilience-builders include the following:
>
> · Ask colleagues to share five things that went right after a resuscitation.
> · Think of three things to be grateful for every morning or evening.
> · Incorporate 30- to 60-second bursts of physical activity throughout the day (run in place, jump rope, pretend to box).
> · Tense the muscles in one part of your body. Notice how it feels when the muscles relax.
> · Concentrate on something visual. First notice the details. Then let your eyes lose focus.
> · Take a deep breath and hold it. Breathe in a bit more. Release the breath slowly.
> · Take a deep breath while raising your arms over your head. Release the breath as you drop your arms and bend forward.
> · Write down your beliefs, things you know to be true, or what gives you purpose.
> · Think of advice an older version of yourself would give you right now.

Moral Injury and Empowerment

The chaotic and challenging environment in the ED exposes the healthcare team to moral injury—that is, the team's struggle when they cannot provide the high-quality care and healing they are trained to do.[17] Moral injury results from exposure to events that violate one's beliefs. In healthcare, it is often evident in the challenge posed by the moral obligation of providing the care the patient needs and the inability to provide that care for reasons beyond the healthcare provider's control.[10] Signs of moral injury are similar to burnout; however, burnout relates to excessive workload, staffing issues, and processes, rather than emotional factors.[17] Emotional responses to moral injury include cynicism, grief, guilt, remorse, and outrage. Moral injury may manifest as depression, self-harm, aggression toward others, flashbacks, and social isolation.[17] Team members who experience moral injury need emotional support and counseling to help them improve their coping.

Addressing moral injury requires investigating the processes involved in and barriers to delivering high-quality care.[10] Empowerment—defined as the ability to provide care in a meaningful way[17]—increases job satisfaction while combating moral injury. The healthcare team is empowered to advocate for the patient. Leadership should promote an environment in which staff are involved in policy development, confidently share concerns, and have access to resources, education, and support.[5] Empowered staff demonstrate higher levels of engagement and improved clinical performance.[17]

Summary

The ED is a fast-paced, often chaotic environment. Pediatric patients add challenges to the burdens of already stressed caregivers and staff. A crisis event involving a pediatric patient intensifies the emotional response of the healthcare team and their caregivers. Family members may exhibit various maladaptive behaviors as they try to cope with the stresses of this setting. Healthcare professionals may experience increased stress levels as they strive to provide safe, quality, and compassionate care. That care should include measures to prevent further traumatization of the pediatric patient and caregivers.

The increased stress and emotional demands they face put healthcare professionals at risk for developing compassion fatigue, secondary traumatic stress, burnout, and moral injury. Peer support and engaging in self-care can help mitigate their emotional distress. Organizational support for meeting healthcare providers' educational and emotional needs can help them more effectively manage stress disorders. Building resilience to stress helps address the challenges of practicing in an emergency care environment.

References

1. American Red Cross Advisory Council on First Aid, Aquatics, Safety and Preparedness. (2010). *Critical incident stress debriefing* [Scientific review]. https://www.redcross.org/content/dam/redcross/Health-Safety-Services/scientific-advisory-council/Scientific%20Advisory%20Council%20SCIENTIFIC%20REVIEW%20-%20Critical%20Incident%20Stress%20Debriefing.pdf

2. Bartlett, J. D., Griffin, J. L., Spinazzola, J., Fraser, J. G., Norona, C. R., Bodian, R., Todd, M., Montagna, C., & Barto, B. (2018). The impact of a statewide trauma-informed care initiative in child welfare on the well-being of children and youth with complex trauma. *Children and Youth Services Review*, *84*, 110–117. https://doi.org/10.1016/j.childyouth.2017.11.015

3. Brody, A., & Sethuraman, U. (2019). Optimizing the treatment of pain and anxiety in pediatric emergencies: The role of accreditation. *Israel Journal of Health Policy Research*, *8*(1), 1–3. https://doi.org/10.1186/s13584-019-0305-9

4. Clark, P. R., Polivka, B., Zwart, M., & Sanders, R. (2019). Pediatric emergency department staff preferences for a critical incident stress debriefing. *Journal of Emergency Nursing*, *45*(4), 403–410. https://doi.org/10.1016/j.jen.2018.11.009

5. Connolly, M., Jacobs, S., & Scott, K. (2018). Clinical leadership, structural empowerment and psychological empowerment of registered nurses working in an emergency department. *Journal of Nursing Management*, *26*(7), 881–887. https://doi.org/10.1111/jonm.12619

6. Crisis Prevention Institute. (2020). *De-escalation tips*. https://institute.crisisprevention.com/Refresh-De-Escalation-Tips.html

7. Crisis Prevention Institute. (2021). *Trauma-informed care: Resources guide*. https://www.crisisprevention.com/CPI/media/Media/download/PDF_TICRG.pdf

8. Cunningham, T., Ducar, D. M., & Keim-Malpass, J. (2019). "The pause": A Delphi methodology examining an end-of-life practice. *Western Journal of Nursing Research*, *41*(10), 1481–1498. https://doi.org/10.1177/0193945919826314

9. Davidson, J. E., Proudfoot, J., Lee, K., Terterian, G., & Zisook, S. (2020). A longitudinal analysis of nurse suicide in the United States (2005–2016) with recommendations for action. *Worldviews on Evidence-Based Nursing*, *17*(1), 6–15. https://doi.org/10.1111/wvn.12419

10. Dean, W., Talbot, S., & Dean, A. (2019). Reframing clinician distress: Moral injury not burnout. *Federal Practitioner*, *36*(9), 400–402. https://www.ncbi.nlm.nih.gov/pmc/articles/PMC6752815/

11. Dr. Lorna Breen Heroes' Foundation. (2021). *The legislation*. https://drlornabreen.org/about-the-legislation/

12. Dutheil, F., Aubert, C., Pereira, B., Dambrun, M., Moustafa, F., Mermillod, M., Baker, J. S., Trousselard, M., Lesage, F. X., & Navel, V. (2019). Suicide among physicians and health-care workers: A systematic review and meta-analysis. *PLoS One*, *14*(12), Article e0226361. https://doi.org/10.1371/journal.pone.0226361

13. Emergency Nurses Association. (2017). *Family presence during invasive procedures and resuscitation* [Clinical practice guideline]. https://enau.ena.org/Users/LearningActivityAssetSingleViewer.aspx?LearningActivityAssetID=qz2OSKwM1yTamRXhrpwBYA%3d%3d

14. Emergency Nurses Association. (2020). *Compassion fatigue* [Topic brief]. https://enau.ena.org/Users/LearningActivityInformation.aspx?LearningActivityID=d5HmNmfhgfFtTgMC6Boskg%3d%3d

15. Foster, K., Mitchell, R., Young, A., Van, C., & Curtis, K. (2019). Resilience-promoting factors for parents of severely injured children during the acute hospitalization period: A qualitative inquiry. *Injury*, *50*(5), 1075–1081. https://doi.org/10.1016/j.injury.2018.12.011

16. Graffy, P., McKinnon, S., Lee, G., & Remington, P. (2019). Life outside: A narrative ethnographic inquiry into the determinants of homelessness. *Journal of Poverty*, *23*(3), 202–228. https://doi.org/10.1080/10875549.2018.1550133

17. Griffin, B. J., Purcell, N., Burkman, K., Litz, B. T., Bryan, C. J., Schmitz, M., Villierme, C., Walsh, J., & Maguen, S. (2019). Moral injury: An integrative review. *Journal of Traumatic Stress*, *32*(3), 350–362. https://doi.org/10.1002/jts.22362

18. Gultekin, L. E., Brush, B. L., Ginier, E., Cordom, A., & Dowdell, E. B. (2020). Health risks and outcomes of homelessness in school-age children and youth: A scoping review of the literature. *Journal of School Nursing*, *36*(1), 10–18. https://doi.org/10.1177/1059840519875182

19. Hallett, N., & Dickens, G. L. (2017). De-escalation of aggressive behavior in healthcare settings: Concept analysis. *International Journal of Nursing Studies*, *75*, 10–20. https://doi.org/10.1016/j.ijnurstu.2017.07.003

20. Hanrahan, K., Kleiber, C., Miller, B. J., Davis, H., & McCarthy, A. M. (2018). The Distraction in Action Tool©: Feasibility and usability in clinical settings. *Journal of Pediatric Nursing*, *41*, 16–21. https://doi.org/10.1016/j.pedn.2017.11.002

21. Jackson, B. L. (2017). Bereavement in the pediatric emergency department: Caring for those who care for others. *Pediatric Nursing*, *43*(3), 113–119.

22. Lee, S. M. (2016). Review of children living in transition: Helping homeless and foster care children and families. *Journal of Youth and Adolescence*, *45*(2), 423–426. https://doi.org/10.1007/s10964-015-0372-3

23. Lindsay, J., & Heliker, D. (2018). The unexpected death of a child and the experience of emergency service personnel. *Journal of Emergency Nursing*, *44*(1), 64–70. https://doi.org/10.1016/j.jen.2017.06.002

24. Longobardi, C., Prino, L. E., Fabris, M. A., & Settanni, M. (2019). Soap bubbles as a distraction technique in the management of pain, anxiety, and fear in children at the paediatric emergency room: A pilot study. *Child: Care, Health and Development*, *45*(2), 300–305. https://doi.org/10.1111/cch.12633

25. Manguy, A. M., Joubert, L., Oakley, E., & Gordon, R. (2018). Psychosocial care models for families of critically ill children in pediatric emergency department settings: A scoping review. *Journal of Pediatric Nursing*, *38*, 46–52. https://doi.org/10.1016/j.pedn.2017.10.014

26. Moore, C. (2020). *"What if?" Using a trauma-informed lens to reframe behavior in the classroom* [Blog post]. https://www

.epinsight.com/post/what-if-using-a-trauma-informed-lens -to-reframe-behaviour-in-the-classroom

27. Morrison, L. E., & Joy, J. P. (2016). Secondary traumatic stress in the emergency department. *Journal of Advanced Nursing, 72*(11), 2894–2906. https://doi.org/10.1111/jan.13030

28. National Child Traumatic Stress Network. (2020). *About child trauma.* https://www.nctsn.org/what-is-child-trauma/about -child-trauma

29. O'Malley, P., Barata, I., & Snow, S. (2014). Death of a child in the emergency department. *Pediatrics, 134*(1), e313–e330. https://doi.org/10.1542/peds.2014-1246

30. Phillips, B. E., Theeke, L. A., & Sarosi, K. M. (2021). Relationship between negative emotions and perceived support among parents of hospitalized, critically ill children. *International Journal of Nursing Sciences, 8*(1), 15–21. https:// doi.org/10.1016/j.ijnss.2020.10.001

31. Ports, K. A., Tang, S., Treves-Kagan, S., & Rostad, W. (2021). Breaking the cycle of adverse childhood experiences (ACEs): Economic position moderates the relationship between mother and child ACE scores among Black and Hispanic families. *Children and Youth Services Review, 127,* Article 106067. https://doi.org/10.1016/j.childyouth.2021.1060677

32. Racco, A., & Vis, J. A. (2015). Evidence based trauma treatment for children and youth. *Child & Adolescent Social Work Journal, 32*(2), 121–129. https://doi.org/10.1007/s10560-014-0347-3

33. Rodríguez-Rey, R., Palacios, A., Alonso-Tapia, J., Pérez, E., Álvarez, E., Coca, A., Mencía, S., Marcos, A., Mayordomo-Colunga, J., Fernández, F. Gómez, E., Cruz, J., Ordóñez, O., & Llorente, A. (2019). Burnout and posttraumatic stress in pediatric critical care personnel: Prediction from resilience and coping styles. *Australian Critical Care, 32*(1), 46–53. https://doi.org/10.1016/j.aucc.2018.02.003

34. Sağlık, D. S., & Çağlar, S. (2019). The effect of parental presence on pain and anxiety levels during invasive procedures in the pediatric emergency department. *Journal of Emergency Nursing, 45*(3), 278–285. https://doi-org.org/10.1016/j.jen.2018.07.003

35. Sanchez, C. N., Staab, J., Chatham, R., Ryan, S., McNair, B., & Grubenhoff, J. A. (2018). Child life reduces distress and pain and improves family satisfaction in the pediatric emergency department. *Clinical Pediatrics, 57*(13), 1567–1575. https:// doi.org/10/1166/00092818798286

36. Sheller, S. L., Hudson, K. M., Bloch, J. R., Biddle, B., Krauthamer Ewing, E. S., & Slaughter-Acey, J. C. (2018). Family care curriculum: A parenting support program for families experiencing homelessness. *Maternal & Child Health Journal, 22*(9), 1247–1254. https://doi.org/10.1007/s10995-018-2561-7

37. Simmons, K. T., & Douglas, D. Y. (2018). After the storm: Helping children cope with trauma after natural disasters. *Communique, 46*(5), 23–25.

38. Soares, S., Rocha, V., Kelly-Irving, M., Stringhini, S., & Fraga, S. (2021). Adverse childhood event and health biomarkers: A systematic review. *Frontiers in Public Health, 9,* Article 649825. https://doi.org/10.3389/fpubh.2021.649825

39. Tarquinio, C., Brennstuhl, M. J., Rydberg, J. A., Bassan, F., Peter, L., Tarquinio, C., Auxèmèry, Y., Rotonda, C., & Tarquinio, P. (2021). EMDR in telemental health counseling for healthcare workers caring for COVID-19 patients: A pilot study. *Issues in Mental Health Nursing, 42*(1), 3–14. https://doi.org/10.1080/016 12840.2020.1818014

40. Tarquinio, C., Rotonda, C., Houllé, W. A., Montel, S., Rydberg, J. A., Minary, L., Dellucci, H., Tarquinio, P., Fayard, A., & Alla, F. (2016). Early psychological preventive intervention for workplace violence: A randomized controlled explorative and comparative study between EMDR-recent event and critical incident stress debriefing. *Issues in Mental Health Nursing, 37*(11), 787–799. https://doi.org/10.1080/01612840.2016.1224282

41. The Institute on Trauma and Trauma Informed Care. (2021). *What is trauma-informed care?* Buffalo Center for Social Research. http://socialwork.buffalo.edu/social-research/institutes-centers /institute-on-trauma-and-trauma-informed-care/what-is-trauma -informed-care.html

42. Trauma-Informed Care Implementation Resource Center. (2021). *What is trauma-informed care?* Center for Health Care Strategies. https://www.traumainformedcare.chcs.org/what -is-trauma-informed-care/

43. Wininger, B. (2022). Posttraumatic stress disorder. In F. F. Ferri (Ed.), *Ferri's clinical advisor* (2022 ed., pp. 1241–1243). Elsevier.

44. World Health Organization. (2012). Psychological debriefing in people exposed to a recent traumatic event. https:// www.who.int/mental_health/mhgap/evidence/resource/other _complaints_q5.pdf?ua=1

CHAPTER

18

The Child with Special Healthcare Needs

Kimberly MacKeil-White, MSN, BN, RN, CPEN, NPD-BC

OBJECTIVES

Upon completion of this chapter, the learner will be able to:

1. Define the term *children with special healthcare needs*.
2. Describe characteristics and needs associated with selected pediatric syndromes and conditions.
3. Differentiate between person-first and identity-first language.

Introduction

Many pediatric patients are thriving while living with a multitude of rare conditions that are beyond the scope of this course. This chapter provides an overview of selected conditions. It is not expected that the nurse be well versed in every condition, but every nurse needs to recognize how to tailor their care to meet these patients' needs and when expert consultation is required.

The definition of *children with special healthcare needs* (CSHCN) was revised in 1998 for the purpose of planning and developing services for this population:

> Children with special health care needs are those who have or are at increased risk for a chronic physical, developmental, behavioral, or emotional condition and who also require health and related services of a type or amount beyond that required by children generally.[26]

Variations on this definition are often used to determine eligibility for governmental services. When CSHCN present to the emergency department (ED), the nurse can adapt care to best support the patient and family by being cognizant of these needs.

Family as Experts

CSHCN are familiar—and sometimes frequent—visitors to the ED. EDs are a resource and a source of expertise when caregivers need care more immediately than they are sometimes able to get otherwise. Because of the variety of knowledge and skills available from the ED providers, as well as a need for quicker access to specialty providers, caregivers will often present to the ED when they have exhausted their ability to manage care in the home environment.

To partner with the patient and family is to ensure a good understanding of the concerns the parents have when presenting to the ED. Communication regarding baseline behavior and the differences that prompted the current visit is essential to understanding why the caregivers are bringing the child in for evaluation. Caregivers are typically well versed in the patient's history and medical needs, making them expert historians. CSHCN can all be quite different at baseline, but the caregiver's information can ensure the exceptions are identified and included in the plan of care. Partnering with the caregivers in the plan of care will ensure collaboration and a cohesive relationship aimed at ensuring quality care for the child. This, in turn, establishes a trusting relationship that will aid future healthcare visits as well.

Glossary of Conditions with Nursing Considerations

The conditions discussed in this section are more commonly seen in children visiting the ED, but are not meant to be an exhaustive list of all possibilities. A knowledge base regarding those conditions seen more frequently gives the nurse more opportunity to provide safer and better-quality care.

RED FLAG

Fever is an emergent condition in many CSHCN. Immunocompromise can be caused by the disease itself or by medical management of the disease, such as chemotherapy for cancer, immunosuppressant drugs given post transplant, and immunologic therapies for autoimmune conditions and asthma.

Cancer

After traumatic injury, pediatric cancer is the second leading cause of death in children.[35] Occasionally, pediatric patients will receive a new cancer diagnosis in the ED (**Box 18-1**). More commonly, children with cancer will seek care for treatment-related complications or side effects. These visits are increasing as more effective cancer treatments and home therapies have evolved.[35]

Presentations During Treatment

The cancer itself may cause bleeding, anemia, and cardiorespiratory compromise. Chemotherapy, immunotherapy, radiation, and surgical resection are just a few cancer therapies with complications that may necessitate an ED visit.

BOX 18-1 New Cancer Diagnosis

Childhood cancer can be difficult to detect early. Parents may have multiple interactions with medical providers in which symptoms are overlooked or attributed to more common conditions. The following signs and symptoms are associated with a new diagnosis of cancer[35,36]:

- Abdominal pain
- Blood count abnormalities
- Bruising
- Fatigue
- Headache
- Limping
- Long bone pain
- Lump or swelling
- Pallor
- Persistent fever, nausea, or vomiting
- Vision changes
- Weight loss

Sometimes, imaging or blood work will suggest or confirm a cancer diagnosis. At other times, follow-up with a pediatric oncologist is required for definitive diagnosis. Partner with the physician or advanced practice provider to have a private discussion with the parents. Work with the parents to determine the best age-appropriate manner (with consideration of how, who, and when) to inform the child. Delayed information sharing fosters anxiety and distrust; effective communication is key to creating a trusting relationship. Be prepared for the family and child to be overwhelmed. Provide supportive information, balancing uncertainty with hope.[17,35]

Data from Stephanos, K., & Picard, L. (2018). Pediatric oncologic emergencies. *Emergency Medicine Clinics of North America, 36*(3), 527–535. https://doi.org/10.1016/j.emc.2018.04.007; Steuber, C. P. (2021). Overview of common presenting signs and symptoms of childhood cancer. *UpToDate.* Retrieved March 9, 2022, from https://www.uptodate.com/contents/overview-of-common-presenting-signs-and-symptoms-of-childhood-cancer; Dobrozsi, S., Trowbridge, A., Mack, J. W., & Rosenberg, A. R. (2019). Effective communication for newly diagnosed pediatric patient with cancer: Considerations for the patients, family members, providers, and multidisciplinary team. *American Society of Clinical Oncology Educational Book, 39*, 573–581. https://doi.org/10.1200/EDBK_238181

Chemotherapy and radiation target rapidly growing cancer cells, but also damage healthy cells such as those found in gastric mucosa and blood. Mouth sores, nausea, and vomiting may lead to dehydration. Neutropenia places children at high risk for infection. Immunotherapy, while meant to boost the immune system's ability to attack tumor cells, can cause allergic reactions and cytokine release syndrome. Fever, tachycardia, and hypotension are symptoms of cytokine release syndrome.[27] Tumor lysis syndrome results in the release of intracellular contents into the bloodstream, leading to significant electrolyte disturbances, cardiac dysrhythmias, and renal failure.[1,34,35]

Late Effects of Treatment

With access to the latest therapies, 80% of children with cancer will survive the disease.[28] Unfortunately, cancer treatment is associated with adverse health effects long after therapy is completed. Approximately 60% to 90% of children who survive cancer may develop chronic health conditions.[28] Late effects include alterations in growth and development, organ dysfunction, diminished reproductive capacity, secondary cancers, and psychosocial sequelae.[28] Such late effects can impact every body system. Take these effects into consideration when assessing the potential for significant illness in children who have been told they are in remission, cancer-free, or without any evidence of cancer.

Cerebral Palsy

Cerebral palsy is a neuromuscular disorder characterized mainly by movement limitations and spasticity, which typically results from prenatal or postnatal brain injuries. As a result of these injuries, coordination and muscle tone can be altered, with effects ranging from mild to severe, so that the child's ability to control their body movements is affected to the point they are sometimes nonambulatory. Other functions can be affected as well, such as sensation, perception, communication, and behavior.[22] Note, however, that more than 50% of patients with cerebral palsy are of at least normal intelligence; thus, these patients should be included, along with their caregivers, in all communication and plans of care.[12]

Patients with cerebral palsy often present to the ED for certain conditions that are especially common among this population. An alteration in ability to control secretions and swallow correctly due to muscle weakness and spasticity can make aspiration an issue, thereby increasing the work of breathing and increasing the risk of pneumonia. With overabundance of secretions being a norm for some patients, baseline assessment and history through the caregivers is a necessity. Seizure activity is common, as 25% to 45% of children with cerebral palsy also have epilepsy.[12] Typically, when epilepsy maintenance medication levels become altered, seizure activity may increase at home and may become uncontrollable with home medications. ED assistance may be sought to bring seizures under control if there is an increase in frequency or intensity or if status epilepticus is present.

Cystic Fibrosis

Cystic fibrosis is an autosomal recessive condition in which a defective gene alters the ability to regulate chloride and sodium channels in the body, resulting in a thickening of the mucoid. The effects of cystic fibrosis may be seen in many systems but primarily impacts the pancreas and lungs. Patients often present to the ED with gastrointestinal (GI) and/or respiratory issues stemming from obstructions caused by the thicker mucus their body produces. Isolation precautions should be initiated with these patients, as vulnerability to infection is an ever-present risk.[29]

In the GI system, the ability to digest food properly is impaired when the thick mucoid blocks needed digestive enzymes. Without these enzymes, food cannot be broken down into usable nutrients, so patients are often unable to utilize most fats which are then excreted in the stool. Typically, patients with cystic fibrosis are underweight and have pancreatic, bile duct, and liver obstructive issues as well.[11]

In the respiratory system, the same basic obstruction occurs from dehydrated mucus that is difficult to mobilize. Without consistent airway clearance therapy, patients with cystic fibrosis will present with an inability to ventilate due to bronchiole mucus obstructions as well as pneumonias, as the mucus retains and grows bacteria that easily get trapped in the pulmonary system. Over time, the lungs incur severe injury from the accumulation of these insults, and patients are unable to oxygenate and ventilate effectively.[15] Eventually, intubation may become inevitable, and death can occur shortly after.

Due to advances in care, life expectancy for patients with cystic fibrosis has improved over the last several decades and is now between 30 and 40 years of age.[15] In earlier times, cystic fibrosis was typically seen as a childhood disease because of the relatively short life expectancies for these patients. The medical world has adjusted to this increase in advances and life expectancy, and now adult specialty care has incorporated the adult patient with cystic fibrosis.[3]

Common reasons for ED visits by these patients include respiratory issues such as increased work of breathing, ineffective air exchange, and pneumonia, and/or GI issues such as abdominal pain, impaired pancreas or liver function, diabetic control due to pancreatic insufficiency, or renal impairment.[29]

Down Syndrome

Down syndrome is a genetic condition in which an extra chromosome appears in the patient's genetic profile. Also referred to as trisomy 21 (because the extra chromosome is found on chromosome 21), this syndrome can occur in a pregnancy at any age but has increased incidence in pregnancies of women older than 35 years of age.[14] Children with Down syndrome are at risk for some associated medical conditions that are commonly seen with this population, such as cardiac malformations. Septal defects are seen from birth, making cardiac surgery a common need in the first year of life.[14,23] Hypotonia, muscle weakness, and immune system dysfunction are other commonly seen issues in patients with Down syndrome. Respiratory infections are seen often due to these factors and are a major reason for ED visits. Death during the first year is more frequent for this population, mostly due to the cardiac issues, combined with respiratory challenges.[14]

A greater incidence of asymptomatic atlantoaxial instability is noted in patients with Down syndrome as well, with this condition affecting approximately 15% of this population.[14,23,43] Care should be taken with positioning and cervical spinal precautions implemented in certain cases, such as those involving trauma or intubation. Some care teams will opt to add a cervical collar when intubating a patient with Down syndrome even without a history of trauma, because of the extra stabilization it lends the patient. Also, patients with Down syndrome who present with neurologic symptoms such as incontinence, decreased sensation, neck pain, and others should be evaluated for cervical spine instability.[14]

Marfan Syndrome

Marfan syndrome, a connective tissue disorder, occurs in approximately 1 in 5,000–10,000 children.[10] This condition, which is caused by an autonomic dominant trait, is typically diagnosed by 3 years of age. Patients with Marfan syndrome can have issues with any system that contains connective tissue and will present to the ED for those issues that are acutely affecting their wellness status. Reasons for such presentations may include cardiac issues such as aortic dilation or aneurysms, mitral valve prolapses, and aortic regurgitation. Perfusion may be affected, and emergent care is typically required if this is the case.

Respiratory needs are also of concern for this population, as a spontaneous pneumothorax is a fairly common occurrence.[10] Ranging from a small simple pneumothorax that requires some level of intervention, to a larger one that severely affects ventilation efforts and needs a chest tube, these conditions require fast recognition, evaluation, and treatment efforts.

Marfan syndrome may also affect vision and skeletal systems and is typically recognized in the adolescent population by the physical markers of a long trunk and extended finger length. Atlantoaxial subluxation is a risk due to the laxity of the transverse ligament.[10,40]

Osteogenesis Imperfecta

Eight main categories of osteogenesis imperfecta exist, with several separate types falling into these categories, depending on which symptoms the patient has. An autosomal dominant condition, osteogenesis imperfecta occurs when the collagen produced by the body has a defect, affecting bone stability. Patients will have brittle bones that fracture easily and other symptoms such as blue sclera, weak musculature, dental issues, or short stature. Some patients also may have thinner skin and hearing loss in adolescence.[39]

In the emergency setting, these patients may present either with a known history of osteogenesis imperfecta and seeking treatment for fractures, or an unknown diagnosis that will present with fractures at an early age. This latter population may have the osteogenesis imperfecta diagnosis discovered while investigations for abuse are initiated due to the suspicious nature of the injuries. Psychosocial support for families is imperative when this is the case.[23]

RED FLAG

Handle patients with osteogenesis imperfecta with extreme care. Do not lift the patient's ankles to change a diaper or use the patient's extremities to roll for posterior exam. Lift infants using one hand under the buttocks/pelvis and one hand under the head/neck, not under the arms. Squeezing from a blood pressure cuff or tourniquet may cause injuries such as severe bruising and fractures.

Sickle Cell Disease

Sickle cell disease is an inherited blood disorder characterized by anemia and abnormally shaped red cells that diminish tissue perfusion. Patients with this disease are at risk for both acute and chronic medical complications that lead to shorter lifespans.[37] While the overall mortality rate has improved with the use of hydroxyurea, stem cell transplants, and prophylactic antibiotics, the burden of this disease remains high.[21]

Barriers to the rapid and aggressive pain management that is recommended for patients with sickle cell disease experiencing a vaso-occlusive episode include misconceptions about opioid addiction in this patient population, systemic racism, ED crowding, and frequent ED visits.[37] This example of unconscious (also known as implicit) bias's impact on patient care is further explored in the Emergency Nurses Association (ENA) topic brief *Management of Vaso-occlusive Episodes in Persons with Sickle Cell Disease in the Emergency Department.*[37] The American College of Emergency Physicians (ACEP) has an online guide, *Managing Sickle Cell Disease in the ED*, to help manage vaso-occlusive episodes in the ED.[5] **Figure 18-1** shows the ENA's *Caring for Children with Sickle Cell Disease in the ED* infographic.[20]

RED FLAG ⚠

Patients with sickle cell disease are triaged as being at high risk for significant illness. Life-threatening acute chest syndrome, anemia, sepsis, splenic sequestration, and stroke increase both morbidity and mortality in this population. Signs and symptoms of particular concern include the following[32]:

· Chest pain
· Fever
· Increasing pallor, lethargy, or jaundice
· Neurologic symptoms
· Newly palpable or enlarging spleen
· Right upper quadrant abdominal pain
· Shortness of breath

Data from Raphael, J. L., & Rogers, Z. R. (2022). Sickle cell disease in infancy and childhood: Routine health care maintenance and anticipatory guidance. *UpToDate*. Retrieved March 9, 2022, from https://www.uptodate.com/contents/sickle-cell-disease-in-infancy-and-childhood-routine-health-care-maintenance-and-anticipatory-guidance

Technology

Children with special healthcare needs are thriving more than ever before due to the many advanced technologies now available to aid in their care. Tracheostomies, long-term home ventilators, and the ability to support physical growth and nutrition with gastric tubes are just some examples of how technology has evolved to aid in supporting their needs. The following sections cover common healthcare technologies seen in the ED. Basic care of the pediatric patient with special needs requires baseline knowledge of these technologies.

Insulin Pumps

Children (typically age 8 and older) who have been diagnosed with type 1 or type 2 diabetes, and who are deemed good candidates, may opt for an insulin pump to manage

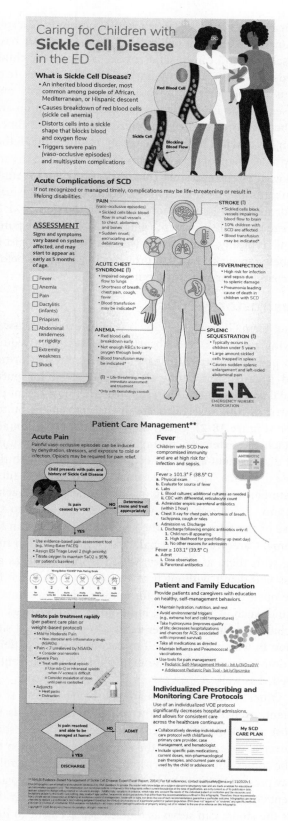

Figure 18-1 *Caring for children with sickle cell disease in the ED.*

Emergency Nurses Association. (2020). *Caring for children with sickle cell disease in the ED* [Infographic]. https://enau.ena.org/Users/LearningActivityAssetSingleViewer.aspx?LearningActivityAssetID=JmxUUrqcQq1z9mFJWTif%2bA%3d%3d

their insulin needs.[4,25] These external pumps have a sub-cutaneous access that delivers insulin on a regular basis (basal rate) and can be adjusted according to the child's needs based on activity, illness, or other events (e.g., bolus dosing for carbohydrate balance). Patients may present to the ED for issues concerning the pump and diabetes control, or they may present with another illness or injury and just happen to have an insulin pump. Either way, assessment of glucose is an essential first step in care, followed by the necessary treatment. If the pump's functioning is in question, remove this device and evaluate it for technical issues before restarting the pump. Make sure to monitor the patient's glucose level while the pump is off. Typically, consultation with an endocrinologist or diabetes specialty practice provider is warranted before discharge or for admission purposes.

Gastrostomy Tubes

Long-term GI challenges, such as failure to thrive, swallowing problems, and absorption issues, may require the pediatric patient to have a gastrotomy performed and a gastrostomy tube (G-tube) inserted for nutritional and pharmaceutical support. The most recent pediatric G-tube insertions are of the convenient button type (**Figure 18-2**). Given their minimal extrusion and detachable extension tubing, there is less opportunity for dislodgment and less need for securement with this style of device. The engineering design of these G-tubes is similar to an indwelling urinary catheter or a tracheostomy. A balloon filled with saline connected to the base of the tube gives it the stability to stay within the stoma. Caregivers will usually carry the extension tubing with them at all times, which is important, as access is difficult without it. An oral slip-tip syringe fits the open port and allows for adding small amounts of liquid, such as medicines, but boluses and feedings are a challenge without proper access. In an emergent situation in which nurses need to decompress the patient's abdomen, access with the extension tubing to vent is needed as well.

Other styles of G-tubes are still being used to some extent, even though the low-profile button type is the most prevalent. No matter which device is used, some universal caveats exist. If the stoma is fresher, when the tube comes out there is a risk for stoma closure. Families may present to the ED when this happens. If no replacement G-tube is present in the ED, a urinary catheter that fits the stoma can serve as a quick replacement to hold the stoma open until the correctly sized G-tube can be re-inserted. Dilation with incrementally larger urinary catheters may be needed to enable the original size G-tube to be secured,[13] and confirmation of placement through

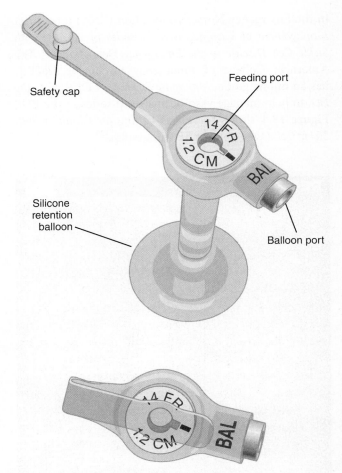

Figure 18-2 *Low-profile gastrostomy tube device (button).*
Courtesy of UC Regents.

gastric aspiration is acceptable if there is no history of trauma to the area.[41]

Ostomies

Ostomies are occasionally needed in pediatric patients for the treatment of disease, to repair injury, or for GI or urologic functional support. Although these patients commonly follow up on an outpatient basis with their surgeons and specialty providers, complications can occur that may bring these patients to the emergency setting. Obstruction, increased output, and stoma health are the major complaints on presentation. Evaluation and care of the ileostomy or colostomy in the pediatric population are similar to that in adult patients, including radiography studies to evaluate blockage, lab testing to determine the root causes of overproduction, and consults with system specialists and wound care experts to address the stoma itself. Some smaller patients are managed without stoma appliances if the output is minimal (such as infants with ileostomies) and use gauze and diapers for waste capture. Supplies such as colostomy appliances in pediatric sizes may be a challenge for some facilities, but can often be acquired through the family. An appropriate fit is imperative to maintaining skin integrity. If admission is not required for the patient with an ostomy, follow-up with their specialist is crucial to maintaining skin integrity and function.

Tracheostomies

Tracheostomies in children are necessary for a variety of reasons, including ventilator dependency, congenital anomalies of the airway, neuromuscular issues, and secretion management. These patients may present with complaints related to the tracheostomy tube and/or ventilator, or with something completely unrelated to these devices. Diligence when considering tracheostomy supplies and care is always warranted for the emergency nurse, as this can be a very difficult airway situation in a child. The danger is even greater with the infant, as the smaller the patient is, the more difficult the access to the stoma will be because of the shorter neck stature.[33]

Tracheostomies in pediatric patients are sized according to the internal diameter of the tube itself (and the tubes typically do not have an inner cannula, unlike the tubes used in adults) as well as based on length. The neonatal tracheostomy tube is a shorter version of the pediatric tracheostomy tube, which can cause confusion for the emergency nurse who is not familiar with this device. This factor also should be considered when preparing for care of the presenting patient, including having both the patient's size of tracheostomy tube and one smaller than that size available at the bedside. Obtaining a bag-mask device, tracheostomy spreaders, a functioning oxygen source, and suction with appropriately sized catheters will complete the recommended preparations. Typically, a standardized checklist for preparation of a patient with a tracheostomy should be readily available in anticipation of the need for tracheostomy change or emergency situation. Also, basic education classes for staff caring for patients with tracheostomies have helped to significantly decrease deaths in this population.[30]

Most often, patients with tracheostomy emergencies present with breathing issues (displaced or dislodged tube), respiratory infections, and/or difficulty managing secretions. If they are ventilator dependent, alarms will alert parents to an issue and either an ED visit or a call to emergency medical services is warranted. Multidisciplinary training for tracheostomy emergencies is recommended for healthcare staff who may come in contact with this population, as is a standardized plan for preparation and approach to evaluation and emergency care.[18]

Ventriculoperitoneal and Ventriculoatrial Shunts

The child with hydrocephalus (either congenital or acquired) experiences a buildup of pressure inside the cranium due to increased cerebrospinal fluid (CSF) or obstruction of flow of CSF. As the skull has little room for expansion in the infant, and none after the cranial sutures and fontanelles close, increased intercranial pressure (ICP) can occur. Increased ICP without treatment can lead to altered mental status, coma, and death. Shunt placement by neurosurgery can control the ICP by regulating CSF volume or flow.

Ventriculoperitoneal (VP) shunts are placed in a brain ventricle and guided to the patient's peritoneum. Ventriculoatrial (VA) shunts divert to the right atrium. Typically, both are placed with extra length on the tube to accommodate the child's growth. Some use magnet adjusters to open and close a valve noninvasively through the scalp, and can be measured and adjusted by the neurosurgical team right at the ED bed.

Increased ICP is of great concern for these patients. Neurologic assessments and vital signs should be constantly evaluated during their time in the ED, until the patient has been cleared or admitted by the neurosurgical team.

Baclofen Pumps

Intrathecal baclofen therapy is a very common treatment for patients with cerebral palsy who have varying levels of movement and function. Used to decrease spasticity, the oral version of this medication is associated with more side effects and less muscular relaxation compared to the intrathecal administration; thus, intrathecal pumps are a more popular option. These devices contain 5 to 6 weeks' worth of baclofen to help control spasticity and muscle tone, making movement smoother and less painful with active or passive motion.[22]

Occasionally, technological issues with the pump itself will cause it to stop working, thereby stopping the flow of helpful medicine. Caregivers will seek emergency care to evaluate signs of pain and discomfort associated with this malfunction, as baclofen withdrawal can be a medical emergency leading to anxiety, seizures, hyperthermia, disseminated intravascular coagulation, multi-organ system failure, and death, if severe enough and left untreated.[42] An emergency consult with the baclofen management team is warranted when these symptoms are present or to avoid reaching this point.

Emerging Trends

Ways that healthcare professionals can learn more about a patient in an emergency are being requested, developed, and utilized throughout the United States to facilitate care for CSHCN. For example, for the past 10 years southern Wisconsin has maintained a "Patient at Risk" service—an online database that is accessible to emergency medical services personnel to help them prepare for and provide care with a fuller understanding of the patient's history. Feeling it was underutilized, a study was conducted to examine emergency medical services staff's understanding and usage of this tool. Results determined that although the usage was less than anticipated, staff still wanted the resources available to them in case they were needed.[31]

Other means to provide history and information are available as well. A disaster "kit," for example, contains a copy of the patient's emergency information file (EIF), with the CSHCN basic medical information available when needed emergently and supplies that a family would need in any disaster until help arrives.[9]

Medical Homes

Recently, there has been a focus on ensuring CSHCN are associated with a "medical home" to help them maintain optimal health and well-being. Access to a medical home includes a usual source of care, a personal doctor or nurse, referral access, care coordination, and family-centered care.[24] Medical homes can adequately coordinate care for the child, both primary and subspecialty, as necessary. A recent study found that "providing access to a medical home for all children leads to improved preventive medical and dental care visits, reduced unmet medical and dental needs, reduced hospital emergency room visits, and improved child's physical and oral health."[2(p1504)]

Person-First Language

As mentioned in the preface of this text, the Emergency Nurses Association is committed to promoting diversity, equity, and inclusivity. One aspect of that commitment is use of person-first language, which is generally thought to be less stigmatizing and diminishes bias. Consider the difference between the terms "a schizophrenic" and "a patient with schizophrenia." Similarly, "homeless" is more stigmatizing than "a child experiencing homelessness." Using person-first language can diminish unconscious bias. However, some individuals prefer to embrace their condition as part of their personal identity. Examples may include patients with autism or hearing loss who prefer to be called autistic or Deaf, respectively.[16,19,44]

The American Psychological Association (APA) provides guidelines to help determine the best language to use in publications and acknowledges that language is evolving.[6,7,8] "Special needs," for example, is a euphemism that may be considered condescending or patronizing.[7] "CSHCN" is an example of person-first language that includes a specific definition associated with many healthcare and governmental services.

> **NOTE**
>
> **Empowering Language**
>
> Pay attention to and respect the words the child and the caregiver use to describe themselves. Consult the American Psychological Association guidelines:
>
> - American Psychological Association. (n.d.). *Bias-free language*. https://apastyle.apa.org/style-grammar-guidelines/bias-free-language
> - American Psychological Association. (2021, August). *Disability*. https://apastyle.apa.org/style-grammar-guidelines/bias-free-language/disability
> - American Psychological Association. (2021). *Inclusive language guidelines*. https://www.apa.org/about/apa/equity-diversity-inclusion/language-guidelines.pdf

Summary

Children with special healthcare needs require the nurse to have knowledge of a variety of issues and practices to help care for them. Conditions, risks, physical care techniques, communication techniques, and technology associated with the patient's baseline are just a few of the subjects in which emergency nurses need to be proficient. Parents are the source of truth when it comes to their children, or at least the best resource for information about their own child, as not every case involving a particular diagnosis is identical. Although differences are present between CSHCN and other patients seen in the emergency care setting, many similarities exist as well. Approaching CSHCN with a primary (ABCDE) and secondary assessment view, as would be done in any emergency case, is the best approach overall.

References

1. Ahmed, N. M., & Flynn, P. M. (2021). Fever in children with chemotherapy-induced neutropenia. *UpToDate*. Retrieved March 12, 2022, from https://www.uptodate.com/contents/fever-in-children-with-chemotherapy-induced-neutropenia

2. Akobirshoev, I., Parish, S., Mitra, M., & Dembo, R. (2019). Impact of medical home on health care of children with and without special health care needs: Update from the 2016 National Survey of Children's Health. *Maternal & Child Health Journal, 23*, 1500–1507. https://doi.org/10.1007/s10995-019-02774-9

3. Alishbayli, G. (2021). Evaluation of the health-related quality of life in Turkish cystic fibrosis patients. *Pediatrics International, 63*(8), 965–970. https://doi.org/10.1111/ped.14553

4. Al Shaikh, A., Al Zahrani, A. M., Qari, Y. H., AbuAlnasr, A. A., Alhawsawi, W. K., Alshehri, K. A., & Al Shaikh, S. A. (2020). Quality of life in children with diabetes treated with insulin pump compared with multiple daily injections in tertiary care center. *Clinical Medicine Insights: Endocrinology and Diabetes, 13,* Article 1179551420959077. https://doi.org/10.1177/1179551420959077

5. American College of Emergency Physicians. (2022). *Managing sickle cell disease in the ED.* https://www.acep.org/sickle-cell/

6. American Psychological Association. (n.d.). *Bias-free language.* https://apastyle.apa.org/style-grammar-guidelines/bias-free-language

7. American Psychological Association. (2021, August). *Disability.* https://apastyle.apa.org/style-grammar-guidelines/bias-free-language/disability

8. American Psychological Association. (2021). *Equity, diversity, and inclusion: Inclusive language guidelines.* https://www.apa.org/about/apa/equity-diversity-inclusion/language-guidelines.pdf

9. Bagwell, H. B., Liggin, R., Thompson, T., Lyle, K., Anthony, A., Baltz, M., Melguizo-Castro, M., Nick, T., & Kuo, D. Z. (2016). Disaster preparedness in families with children with special health care needs. *Clinical Pediatrics, 55*(11), 1036–1043. https://doi.org/10.1177/0009922816665087

10. Ball, J., Bindler, R., Cowen, K., & Shaw, M. (2017). Alterations in musculoskeletal function. *Principles of pediatric nursing: Caring for children* (7th ed., 821–860). Pearson.

11. Ball, J., Bindler, R., Cowen, K., & Shaw, M. (2017). Alterations in respiratory function. *Principles of pediatric nursing: Caring for children* (7th ed., 474–517). Pearson.

12. Barkoudah, E. (2021). Cerebral palsy: Clinical features and classification. *UpToDate.* Retrieved March 9, 2022, from https://www.uptodate.com/contents/cerebral-palsy-clinical-features-and-classification

13. Bhambani, S., Phan, T. H., Brown, L., & Thorp, A. W. (2017). Replacement of dislodged gastrostomy tubes after stoma dilation in the pediatric emergency department. *Western Journal of Emergency Medicine, 18*(4), 770–774. https://doi.org/10.5811/westjem.2017.3.31796

14. Bryant, R. (2022). Impact of cognitive or sensory impairment on the child and family. In M. J. Hockenberry, C. C. Rodgers, & D. Wilson (Eds.), *Wong's essentials of pediatric nursing* (11th ed., pp. 505–529). Elsevier.

15. Bryant, R. (2022). The child with respiratory dysfunction. In M. J. Hockenberry, C. C. Rodgers, & D. Wilson (Eds.), *Wong's essentials of pediatric nursing* (11th ed., pp. 619–677). Elsevier.

16. Carroll, S. M. (2019). Respecting and empowering vulnerable populations: Contemporary terminology. *Journal for Nurse Practitioners, 15*(3), 228–231. https://doi.org/10.1016/j.nurpra.2018.12.031

17. Dobrozsi, S., Trowbridge, A., Mack, J. W., & Rosenberg, A. R. (2019). Effective communication for newly diagnosed pediatric patient with cancer: Considerations for the patients, family members, providers, and multidisciplinary team. *American Society of Clinical Oncology Educational Book, 39,* 573–581. https://doi.org/10.1200/EDBK_238181

18. Doherty, C., Neal, R., English, C., Cooke, J., Atkinson, D., Bates, L., Moore, J., Monks, S., Bowler, M., Bruce, I. A., Bateman, N., Wyatt, M., Russell, J., Perkins, R., McGrath, B. A., & Paediatric Working Party of the National Tracheostomy Safety Project. (2018). Multidisciplinary guidelines for the management of paediatric tracheostomy emergencies. *Anaesthesia, 73*(11), 1400–1417. https://doi.org/10.1111/anae.14307

19. Dwyer, P. (2022). Stigma, incommensurability, or both? Pathology-first, person-first, and identity-first language and the challenges of discourse in divided autism communities. *Developmental and Behavioral Pediatrics, 43*(2), 111–113. https://doi.org/10.1097/DBP.0000000000001054

20. Emergency Nurses Association. (2020). *Caring for children with sickle cell disease in the ED* [Infographic]. https://enau.ena.org/Users/LearningActivityAssetSingleViewer.aspx?LearningActivityAssetID=JmxUUrqcQq1z9mFJWTlf%2bA%3d%3d

21. Field, J. J., & Vichinsky, E. P. (2022). Overview of the management and prognosis of sickle cell disease. *UpToDate.* Retrieved March 11, 2022, from https://www.uptodate.com/contents/overview-of-the-management-and-prognosis-of-sickle-cell-disease

22. Hockenberry, M. J. (2022). The child with neuromuscular or muscular dysfunction. In M. J. Hockenberry, C. C. Rodgers, & D. Wilson (Eds.), *Wong's essentials of pediatric nursing* (11th ed., pp. 1005–1046). Elsevier.

23. Kyle, T., & Carmen, S. (2021). Nursing care of the child with an alteration in mobility/neuromuscular or musculoskeletal disorder. *Essentials of Pediatric Nursing* (4th ed., pp. 743–804). Wolters Kluwer.

24. Lichtstein, J. C., Ghandour, R. M., & Mann, M. Y. (2018). Access to the medical home among children with and without special health care needs. *Pediatrics, 142*(6), e20181795. https://doi.org/10.1542/peds.2018-1795

25. Lyons, S. K., Ebekozien, O., Garrity, A., Buckingham, D., Odugbesan, O., Thomas, S., Rioles, N., Gallagher, K., Sonabend, R. Y., Lorincz, I., Alonso, G. T., Kamboj, M. K., & Lee, J. M. (2021). Increasing insulin pump use among 12- to 26-year-olds with type 1 diabetes: Results from the T1D Exchange Quality Improvement Collaborative. *Clinical Diabetes, 39*(3), 272–277. https://doi.org/10.2337/cd21-0027

26. McPherson, M., Arango, P., Fox, H. Lauver, C., McManus, M., Newacheck, P. W., Perrin, J. M., Shonkoff, J. P., & Strickland, B. (1998). A new definition of children with special health care needs. *Pediatrics, 102*(1), 137–139. https://doi.org/10.1542/peds.102.1.137

27. National Cancer Institute. (2019, May 10). *New drugs, new side effects: Complications of cancer immunotherapy.* https://www.cancer.gov/news-events/cancer-currents-blog/2019/cancer-immunotherapy-investigating-side-effects

28. National Cancer Institute. (2022, February 25). *Late effects of treatment for childhood cancer (PDQ®): Health professional version.* https://www.cancer.gov/types/childhood-cancers/late-effects-hp-pdq

29. Nelson, K. A., Hirsch, A. W., & Nagler, J. (2021). Pulmonary emergencies. In K. N. Shaw & R. G. Bachur (Eds.), *Fleisher & Ludwig's textbook of pediatric emergency medicine* (8th ed., pp. 946–949). Wolters Kluwer.

30. Ong, T., Liu, C. C., Elder, L., Hill, L., Abts, M., Dahl, J. P., Evans, K. N., Parikh, S. R., Soares, J. J., Striegl, A. M., Whitlock, K. B., & Johnson, K. E. (2020). The Trach Safe Initiative: A quality improvement initiative to reduce mortality among pediatric tracheostomy patients. *Otolaryngology—Head and Neck Surgery*, *163*(2), 221–231. https://doi.org/10.1177/0194599820911728

31. Piibe, Q., Kane, E., Melzer-Lange, M., & Beckmann, K. (2020). Patient at risk: Emergency medical service providers' opinions on improving an electronic emergency information form database for the medical care of children with special health care needs. *Disability and Health Journal*, *13*(2), Article 100852. https://doi.org/10.1016/j.dhjo.2019.100852

32. Raphael, J. L., & Rogers, Z. R. (2022). Sickle cell disease in infancy and childhood: Routine health care maintenance and anticipatory guidance. *UpToDate*. Retrieved March 9, 2022, from https://www.uptodate.com/contents/sickle-cell-disease-in-infancy-and-childhood-routine-health-care-maintenance-and-anticipatory-guidance

33. Ross, E., & Stephenson, K. (2019). Fifteen-minute consultation: Emergency management of tracheostomy problems in children. *Archives of Disease in Childhood: Education and Practice Edition*, *104*(4), 189–194. https://doi.org/10.1136/archdischild-2018-316099

34. Stephanos, K., & Dubbs, S. (2021). Pediatric hematologic and oncologic emergencies. *Emergency Medicine Clinics of North America*, *39*(3), 555–571. https://doi.org/10.1016/j.emc.2021.04.007

35. Stephanos, K., & Picard, L. (2018). Pediatric oncologic emergencies. *Emergency Medicine Clinics of North America, 36*(3), 527–535. https://doi.org/10.1016/j.emc.2018.04.007

36. Steuber, C. P. (2021). Overview of common presenting signs and symptoms of childhood cancer. *UpToDate*. Retrieved March 9, 2022, from https://www.uptodate.com/contents/overview-of-common-presenting-signs-and-symptoms-of-childhood-cancer

37. Tanabe, P., Alexander, A., & Frederick, E. (2021). *Management of vaso-occlusive episodes in persons with sickle cell disease in the emergency department* [Topic brief]. https://enau.ena.org/Users/LearningActivityInformation.aspx?LearningActivityID=0pmro02VpwQK%2b4luYF269A%3d%3d

38. The Royal Children's Hospital Melbourne. (2018, April). *Tracheostomy management*. https://www.rch.org.au/rchcpg/hospital_clinical_guideline_index/Tracheostomy_management/#Kit

39. Tillman, L. (2022). The child with musculoskeletal or articular dysfunction. In M. J. Hockenberry, C. C. Rodgers, & D. Wilson (Eds.), *Wong's essentials of pediatric nursing* (11th ed., pp. 969–1004). Elsevier.

40. Tzimenatos, L., Vance, C. W., & Kupperman, N. (2021). Neck stiffness. In K. N. Shaw & R. G. Bachur (Eds.), *Fleisher & Ludwig's textbook of pediatric medicine* (8th ed., pp. 324–332). Wolters Kluwer.

41. Weszelits, S. M., Ridosh, M. M., & O'Connor, A. (2021). Displaced gastrostomy tube in the pediatric emergency department: Implementing an evidence-based algorithm and quality improvement project. *Journal of Emergency Nursing*, *47*(1), 113–122. https://doi.org/10.1016/j.jen.2020.09.007

42. Winter, G., Beni-Adani, L., & Ben-Pazi, H. (2018). Intrathecal baclofen therapy: Practical approach: Clinical benefits and complication management. *Journal of Child Neurology*, *33*(11), 734–741. https://doi.org/10.1177/0883073818785074

43. Woodard, A., & Keilman, A.E. (2021). Neck trauma. In K. N. Shaw & R. G. Bachur (Eds.), *Fleisher & Ludwig's textbook of pediatric medicine* (8th ed., pp. 324–332). Wolters Kluwer.

44. Ziss, B. (2022). Does person-centered language focus on the person? *Journal of Developmental and Behavioral Pediatrics*, *43*(2), 114–115. https://doi.org/10.1097/DBP.0000000000001059

Pediatric Nursing Process

Skill Steps	Potential Interventions	Demonstrated?	
		Yes	No
Preparation and Triage (may occur after general impression if arriving without prenotification)			
1. Activate the team and assign roles.			
	"Is there any specific equipment that you would prepare?"		
2. Prepare the room.	May include but not limited to the following: › Length-based resuscitation tape › Pediatric equipment › Pediatric protocols and dosing guidelines		
3. Don personal protective equipment (PPE).	Consider potential safety threats to the team or need for decontamination		
	"The patient has just arrived."		
General Impression			
4. Assess the three components of the Pediatric Assessment Triangle (PAT) AND categorize the patient as "sick, sicker, or sickest": • Appearance • Work of breathing • Circulation to the skin	No alterations in the PAT = sick One alteration in the PAT = sicker Two or more alterations in the PAT = sickest		
5. Assess for obvious uncontrolled external hemorrhage or unresponsiveness/apnea and the need to reprioritize to C-ABC.	When alterations are identified, intervene as appropriate and reassess. May include but not limited to the following: › Assess for a pulse. › Control external hemorrhage. › Initiate chest compressions.		

(continues)

Skill Steps	Potential Interventions	Demonstrated?	
		Yes	**No**
Primary Survey			
Alertness and Airway with Simultaneous Cervical Spine Stabilization			
6. Assess level of consciousness using AVPU.	*Note:* If unresponsiveness was identified in Step 5, credit is also given here.	**	
7. Open the airway.	May include but not limited to the following: › If cervical spinal injury is suspected, provide manual cervical spinal stabilization AND demonstrate manual opening of the airway using the jaw-thrust maneuver. › When no trauma is suspected, open the airway with a head tilt–chin lift or jaw-thrust maneuver. › When the patient is alert and can cooperate, it is acceptable to ask the patient to open their mouth to assess the airway.	**	
8. Assess the patency and protection of the airway (identifies at least FOUR): · Bony deformity · Edema · Fluids (blood, vomit, or secretions) · Foreign objects · Loose or missing teeth · Sounds (snoring, gurgling, or stridor) · Tongue obstruction · Vocalization	When alterations are identified, intervene as appropriate and reassess. May include but not limited to the following: › Anticipate the need for intubation. › Insert an oral or nasopharyngeal airway. › Place padding under shoulders/torso. › Position patient to optimize airway. › Remove any loose teeth or foreign objects. › Suction the airway.	**	
Breathing and Ventilation			

9. Assess breathing effectiveness (identifies at least FOUR):
· Breath sounds
· Depth, pattern, and general rate of respirations
· Increased work of breathing
  · Abnormal positioning
  · Grunting
  · Head bobbing
  · Nasal flaring
	When alterations are identified, intervene as appropriate and reassess.
	May include but not limited to the following:
	› Anticipate need for a chest tube.
	› Anticipate need for drug-assisted intubation.
	› Anticipate need for medications.
	› Anticipate need for needle decompression.
	› Apply oxygen.
	› Provide bag-mask ventilations.
		**	

Skill Steps	Potential Interventions	Demonstrated?	
		Yes	**No**
• Retractions/accessory muscle use • Tachypnea • Open wounds or deformities • Skin color • Spontaneous breathing • Subcutaneous emphysema • Symmetrical chest rise		**	
10. If intubated, assess endotracheal tube (ETT) placement (must identify ALL THREE): i. Attach a CO_2 detector device; after 5 to 6 breaths, assess for evidence of exhaled CO_2. ii. Simultaneously observe for rise and fall of the chest with assisted ventilations. iii. Auscultate over the epigastrium for gurgling AND lungs for bilateral breath sounds.	*Note:* If the learner chooses a capnography sensor instead of the one-time-use detection device, credit is given in Step 23.	**	
11. If intubated, assess ETT position by noting the number at the teeth or gums AND secure the ETT.			
12. If intubated, begin mechanical ventilation or continue assisted ventilation.			
Circulation and Control of Hemorrhage			
13. Assess circulation (must identify ALL THREE): • Assess capillary refill. • Inspect AND palpate the skin for color, temperature, and moisture. • Palpate a pulse.	When alterations are identified, intervene as appropriate and reassess. May include but not limited to the following: › Anticipate goal-directed therapy for shock. › Apply a cardiac monitor—credit given in Step 21. › Apply a pelvic binder. › Assess patency of prehospital IV line. › Compare central and peripheral pulses.	**	

(continues)

Skill Steps	Potential Interventions	Demonstrated?	
		Yes	No
Primary Survey (*continued*)			
	› Consider sources of internal hemorrhage.		
	› Control external hemorrhage.		
	› Draw labs—credit given in Step 20.		
	› Facilitate FAST and/or radiographs to identify source of internal hemorrhage.		
	› Initiate chest compressions and advanced life support.		
	› Obtain intravenous (IV) or intraosseous (IO) access:		
	· Two sites may be needed.		
	· To administer a fluid bolus, determine weight in kilograms.		
	· Use the push–pull, rapid infuser, or other method as appropriate for patient weight and IV access.		
	· 20 mL/kg for infant/child.		
	· 10–20 mL/kg for blood depending on component (packed cells or whole).		
	· 10 mL/kg with frequent reassessments for neonates, cardiogenic shock, or other risk of volume overload.		
	› Palpate central pulse if peripheral pulse is absent.		
	Disability (Neurologic Status)		

14. Assess neurologic status using the Glasgow Coma Scale (GCS):
  · Best eye opening
  · Best verbal response
  · Best motor response
	When alterations are identified, intervene as appropriate and reassess.
	
	May include but not limited to the following:
	› Assess bedside glucose.
	› Anticipate the need for drug-assisted intubation.
	› Anticipate the need for head computed tomography (CT).
	
	Note: The GCS score is documented as non-testable if a factor, such as sedation or paralytics, is interfering with communication. Determine the score prior to administering medication for intubation if possible.
		**	

15. Assess pupils.			

		Demonstrated?	
Skill Steps	**Potential Interventions**	**Yes**	**No**
Exposure and Environmental Control			
16. Remove all clothing AND inspect for obvious abnormalities or injuries.	When newly identified life-threatening alterations are identified, intervene as appropriate and reassess. If a transport device is in place, it is removed. If there are no contraindications, the patient may be turned to quickly assess the posterior. This can be deferred until after the head-to-toe and imaging if needed to evaluate spinal and pelvic stability.	**	
17. Provide warmth (identifies at least ONE): · Blankets · Increase room temperature · Warmed fluids · Warming lights			

Note: During testing, if the learner did not intervene to correct life-threatening findings in the primary survey and/or did not complete all double-starred criteria, the instructor will review the primary survey and notify the course director.

Full Set of Vital Signs and Family Presence			
18. Obtain a full set of vital signs and weight in kilograms (if not determined earlier).	› Blood pressure (BP): mm Hg › Heart rate (HR): beats/minute › Respiratory rate (RR): breaths/minute › Temperature: °F (°C) › Oxygen saturation (SpO_2): % › Weight: kg		
19. Facilitate family presence.			
Get Adjuncts and Give Comfort (LMNOP)			
20. **L:** Consider the need for laboratory analysis.	May include but not limited to the following: › Blood gases › Blood glucose › Blood cross/type and screen › Coagulation studies › Complete blood count › Cultures › Lactate › Metabolic panel › Pregnancy › Toxicology screen		

(continues)

Skill Steps	Potential Interventions	Demonstrated?	
		Yes	**No**
Primary Survey (*continued*)			
21. **M:** Attach patient to a cardiac monitor.	Set monitor to record frequent blood pressures. Consider need for 12-lead electrocardiogram (ECG)—credit given in Step 45.		
22. **N:** Consider the need for insertion of nasogastric or orogastric tube.	Consider venting preexisting feeding tubes when the patient is intubated or if the abdomen is distended.		
23. **O:** Assess oxygenation and continuous end-tidal capnography (if available).	May include but not limited to the following: › Increase or decrease rate of assisted ventilation. › Wean oxygen (consider parameters other than oximetry due to hypothermia, vasoconstriction, and skin color's impact on pulse oximetry measurements). *Note:* Capnography is highly recommended for all patients and is vital for sedated or ventilated patients.		
24. **P:** Assess pain using an appropriate pain scale.		*	
25. Give appropriate nonpharmacologic comfort measures (identifies at least ONE): · Distraction · Family presence · Placing padding over bony prominences · Repositioning · Splinting · Verbal reassurance · Other, as appropriate	*Note:* Applying ice to swollen areas may be appropriate but consider hypothermia risk for major trauma and very small patients. Warmth may also be appropriate, but consider burn risk.		
26. Consider obtaining order for analgesic medication.			
Consideration of Need for Definitive Care			

"Is there a need to consider transfer to a pediatric-capable facility, surgery, or critical care?"

Skill Steps	Potential Interventions	Demonstrated?	
		Yes	No
Secondary Survey			
History and Head-to-Toe Assessment			
27. Obtain pertinent history (identifies at least ONE): · Medical records/documents · Prehospital report · SAMPLE			

Note: The learner describes and demonstrates the head-to-toe assessment by describing the appropriate inspection techniques and demonstrating the appropriate auscultation and palpation techniques.

28. Inspect and palpate head for abnormalities.			
29. Inspect and palpate face for abnormalities.			
30. Inspect and palpate neck for abnormalities.	Demonstrate removal AND reapplication of cervical collar for assessment (if indicated).		
31. Inspect and palpate chest for abnormalities.			
32. Auscultate breath sounds.			
33. Auscultate heart sounds.			
34. Inspect the abdomen for abnormalities.			
35. Auscultate bowel sounds.			
36. Palpate all four quadrants of the abdomen for abnormalities.			
37. Inspect and palpate the flanks for abnormalities.			
38. Inspect the pelvis for abnormalities.			
39. Apply gentle pressure over iliac crests downward and medially.			
40. Apply gentle pressure on the symphysis pubis (if iliac crests are stable).			
41. Inspect the perineum for abnormalities.			

(continues)

		Demonstrated?	
Skill Steps	**Potential Interventions**	**Yes**	**No**
Secondary Survey (*continued*)			
42. Consider how to measure urinary output.	› Assess for contraindications for an indwelling urinary catheter. › External catheter. › Weighing diapers.		
43. Inspect and palpate all four extremities for neurovascular status and abnormalities.			
Inspect Posterior Surfaces			
Note: If the patient has a suspected spinal or pelvic injury, obtain imaging PRIOR to turning the patient. The log roll maneuver may cause secondary injuries including spinal injury or hemorrhage. Instructor prompt: "*Imaging has been performed, so it is safe to turn the patient*" or "*It is not safe to turn the patient.*"			
44. Inspect and palpate posterior surfaces.	Not required if suspected spinal or pelvic injury.	*	
Note: Summarize abnormalities identified, listed below, throughout the scenario. If the learner has not already identified them all, the instructor will ask for any additional noted.			
"What interventions or diagnostics can you anticipate for this patient?"			
45. Identify at least THREE interventions or diagnostics.	May include but not limited to the following: › Antibiotics › Consults › Head CT for any alterations in mental status › Imaging (other radiographs, CT, ultrasonography [US], interventional radiology as indicated) › Law enforcement › Mandatory reporting › Psychosocial support › Social services › Splinting › Tetanus immunization › Wound care		

Skill Steps	Potential Interventions	Demonstrated?	
		Yes	No
Just Keep Reevaluating			
"What findings will you continue to reevaluate while the patient is in your care?"			
46. Reevaluate vital signs.			
47. Reevaluate all identified abnormalities and effectiveness of interventions.			
48. Reevaluate primary survey.			
49. Reevaluate pain.			

Definitive Care or Transport

"What is the definitive care for this patient?"			
50. Consider the need for transfer to a pediatric-capable facility or admission.			
"Is there anything you would like to add?"			

Double-starred (**) criteria to be done in order—assessments and interventions must be completed prior to moving to the next step:

** Alertness and airway

** Breathing

** Circulation

** Disability

** Exposure

Single-starred (*) criteria to be done, though the sequence not critical:

* Reassessment of primary survey interventions

* Blood glucose if any mental status alterations identified

* Pain assessment using an appropriate scale

* Inspection of posterior surfaces (unless contraindicated by suspected spine or pelvic injury)

Skills Performance Results

Evaluation Form

Evaluator: _____

Learner: _____

❑ Station successfully completed.

- All ** critical steps demonstrated in order

- All * demonstrated

- Demonstrated at least _____ of _____ points (70%)

❑ Incomplete. Needs minimal instruction before reevaluation.

❑ Incomplete. Needs considerable instruction before reevaluation.

Potential instructor (must achieve 90%)   ❑ Yes   ❑ No

Demonstrated points   Number   Percentage

Total possible   =   _____ / 100%

Learner demonstrated   =   _____ / _____

Index

Note: Page numbers followed by *b*, *f*, *t* denote boxes, figures and tables, respectively.